MOSES WASN'T FAT

TOM CIOLA

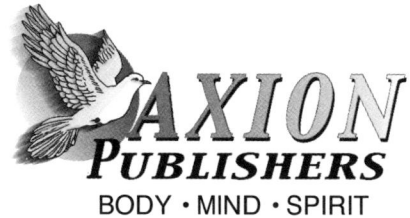

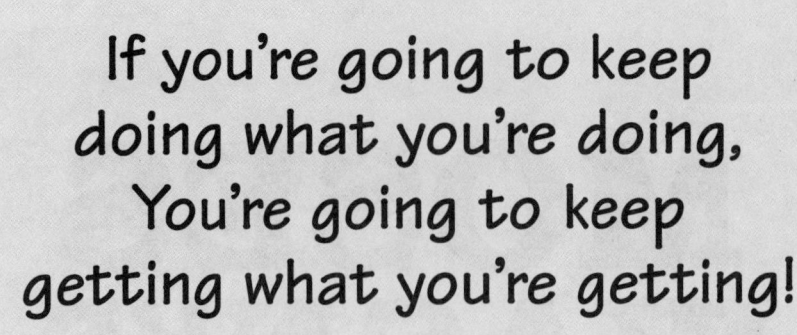

All scripture quotations used in this book are from the *New King James* version of the Bible. In addition to the name *Jesus*, I have also chosen to use the name *Yahshua*, the Hebrew version of His Holy Name.

Library of Congress Control Number 00-135837

ISBN: 0-9706607-0-7

Copyright © 2001 by Thomas Ciola
All rights reserved. No part of this book may be reproduced, distributed, or transmitted in any form or by any means, electronic or mechanical, including photocopying, recording, or by any information storage or retrieval system, without written permission from the publisher.

Address all correspondences to:
 Axion Publishers,
 731 Kirkman Road,
 Orlando, FL 32811
 1-407-472-0120
 www.moseswasntfat.com

Printed in the United States of America

TABLE OF CONTENTS

The 10 Commandments Of Health i
Dedication iii
Forward v
Preface vii
Chapter 1. Our Journey Begins 1
Chapter 2. Out Of Babylon: Freedom From Diet Confusion 7
Chapter 3. Developing A Winner's Attitude 15
Chapter 4. Goals, Plans, Action 21
Chapter 5. What To Do When You Get Discouraged 27
Chapter 6. Health & Fitness Through Faith & Prayer 33
Chapter 7. Eat Of Eden 39
Chapter 8. Behold How The LORD Has Made Our Food 45
Chapter 9. Edifying Enzymes 55
Chapter 10. Losing Weight And Getting Healthy With Biblical Nutrition 61
Chapter 11. To Eat Meat Or Not To Eat Meat – That Is The Question 67
Chapter 12. Some Healthful Foods From The Holy Book 77
Chapter 13. Food… Lies… And The World Of Big Business 87
Chapter 14. How To Regulate Metabolism For Faster Weight Loss 101
Chapter 15. Does The Bible Hold The Secret To Appetite Regulation 107
Chapter 16. Fasting For Physical And Spiritual Blessings 111
Chapter 17. To Stay Healthy & Fit, You Have To Exercise 117
Chapter 18. Do Good And Forget It – Do Bad And Regret It 131
Chapter 19. I Pray The Lord My Soul To Keep 135
Chapter 20. Self Control Through Behavior Modification 139
Chapter 21. Without Accountability You're Doomed To Fail 145
Chapter 22. Putting It All Together 153
Epilogue 163
Appendix 165
    Appendix A: Questions
    Appendix B: Dieter's Profile
    Appendix C: Charts
    Appendix D: Additional Prayers
    Appendix E: On Choices
    Appendix F: Menus
    Appendix G: Blends, Recipes, Shakes
    Appendix H: Web Sites

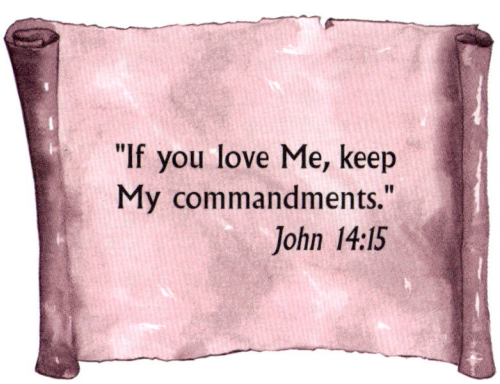

"If you love Me, keep My commandments."
John 14:15

THE TEN COMMANDMENTS OF HEALTH

I. Thou shalt take into thy body each day, pure oxygenated air, the Breath of Life. Thou shalt breath of it deeply, so that it may bathe each and every part of thy body. For God breathed into Adam and he became a living soul.

II. Each day, thou shalt bathe the outside of thy body in pure, clean, Living Waters and each day thou shalt bathe the inside of thy body by drinking an abundance of pure, clean, Living Waters.

III. Thou shalt eat each day from the earth's table of abundance of natural, unprocessed, whole foods which the LORD thy God has provided for thee. Remember to eat thy foods slowly, tranquilly, and never to excess.

IV. Know ye not that thy body is the Temple of the Holy Spirit and that thou must abstain from all that would pollute God's Holy Temple? Therefore, do not defile thy body with drugs, alcohol, tobacco, artificial foods, chemical food additives, refined foods and all foods stripped of their nutritional value.

V. Thou shalt not allow a day to pass without some form of physical exercise, for life is movement and exercise is movement.

VI. Thou shalt entrust the dark hours of thy day to calm, restful sleep, for God called the light Day, and the darkness He called Night.

VII. Remember the Sabbath Day to keep it holy. Six days shalt thou labor, and do all thy work; but the Seventh Day is the Sabbath of the Lord thy God. In it thou shalt not do any work, thou, nor thy son, nor thy daughter, thy manservant, nor thy maidservant, nor thy cattle, nor thy stranger that is within thy gates. For in six days the LORD made heaven and earth, the sea, and all that is in them, and rested the Seventh Day; wherefore the LORD blessed the Sabbath Day, and hallowed it.

VIII. Thou shalt permit no day to pass without allowing the Light of the Sun to touch upon thy skin.

IX. Thou must set aside one day a month to abstain from the consumption of all foods. This shall be a day of prayer and meditation to the LORD thy God.

X. Thou shalt let no day pass without performing at least one good deed for thy neighbor.

Dedication

While most people think of their lives as a steady-flowing continuum from the cradle to the grave, this isn't really how it works. Instead, life is a series of defining moments – mountain peaks of memorable significance which, in retrospect, always stand high as we walk through the many fields of every day living. Graduation, a move to a new home or city, a new job, birth of a child, death of a parent, meeting a new friend, accepting the Lord Jesus Christ as Savior. In fact, the true calendar of our lives is highlighted around such events. In some way, I'm hoping that your reading this book may be such a defining moment in your life.

As I prepared to write this book, I recalled one of these very significant times in my life. It was in 1970, shortly after I had opened my first combination health club and health food store in Central New York. Something about Dan Mansberger exuded power as he first walked through the front door. Young, solidly muscular, boyish good looks. He asked to see the health club and as I began the tour, little did I know that he was about to change my life forever. I asked him about the flecks of wood chips that were all over his clothing and scattered in his hair. He told me that he cut down trees for a living. I guess that explained his powerful built. Our conversation flowed easily as we walked the gym floor and an instant friendship developed between us. Dan joined my club that day.

Over the ensuing months, I was amazed by the natural strength of this young tree cutter. For someone who had never lifted weights, he took to the iron incredibly fast. In all of my years in the health and fitness business, I have never met anyone with the natural, God-given strength of Dan Mansberger. In just a matter of months, I had him competing in his first powerlifting competition wherein he managed a respectable second place among a field of seasoned competitors. He was hooked and I was proud.

But there was another equally strong side to Dan in those days and that was his burning love for the Lord. I'm not sure how he and I got on the topic of religion, but once we did, we never stopped. I was a wishy-washy Christian back then, with a belief system that had just been diluted by four years of a very liberal college education. Dan was a strong believer in the Bible who had met and accepted Yahshua (Jesus) as his Savior. An ideological collision was inevitable. Evolution was the trigger.

"Don't tell me you don't believe in evolution," I remember smugly taunting Dan one day with all of my best bred college learning to back me up?

"Tom, God created everything right from the beginning just as the Bible says," Dan retorted. "I'll bring you in some books to prove it."

I agreed I would read what he gave me but I asked him to also keep an open mind and read what I would give him. He agreed also. Sure enough, the next day Dan handed me two little books that posited that "in the beginning God created the heavens and the earth." I told Dan I would have my books for him to read the next day, certain that my college science books would end this matter once and for all.

I took Dan's books home with me that evening and began to read. . . and read. . . and read. . . I couldn't believe what I was reading and how it opened my eyes. Truth is often like that. I felt truly ashamed for my erroneous beliefs and began to wonder what else in my life was built upon sand. This was a defining moment!

"Got the books for me?" Dan inquired the next day as he came in for his workout.

"Dan, you were right. I read your books last night and I have to admit I was totally wrong. Evolution is not only false – it's a satanic lie! I can't believe I fell for it. Buddy, thank you so much for making me see the truth." And with that admission on my part came two years of intensive Bible study with my good friend Dan Mansberger, who led me to one truth after another. This book could never have been written without him.

I wish I could say that Dan and I remained friends right up to today but such was not meant to be. I remember perfectly that night in 1972 when I came home from work and my wife told me that there had been a terrible tragedy. Two men were cutting down a tree when their boom truck severed an electrical power line. The man in the truck was killed instantly. His partner, my strong and good friend Dan, jumped onto the truck in a valiant effort to save his co-worker. He too was electrocuted, cut down in the prime of his life, leaving behind a beautiful wife and a newborn baby. My loss and my grief I carry with me to this day.

I think what hurts the most is that I never had a chance to say thank you to Dan for getting me started in my love and appreciation of the Bible. Little do we know how wonderfully God works through us. If it hadn't been for one strapping young man with a burning love for God and the courage to defend his beliefs, **Moses Wasn't Fat** might never have been written. My hope is that this book will be for you what Dan Mansberger was for me.

Dan, some day in the Kingdom of God, we will pick up our friendship where we left off. And then, I want to be able to give you a proper thank you. Rest in peace my dear friend.

Tom Ciola
October, 2000

Foreword

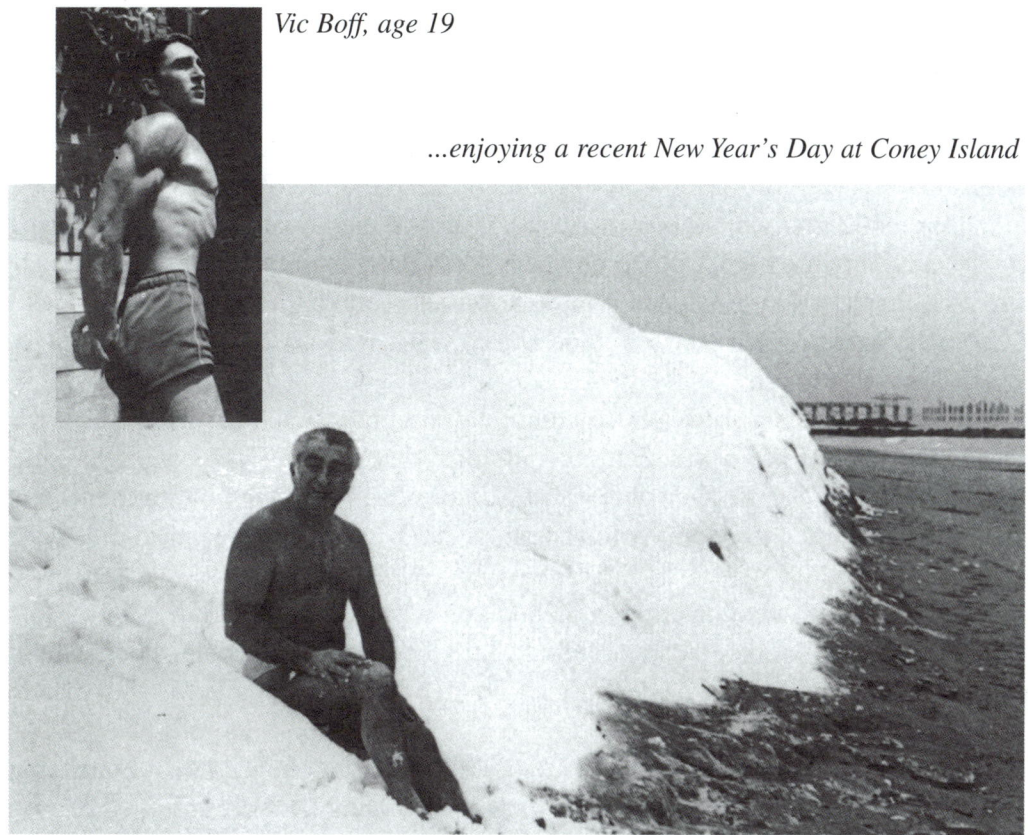

Vic Boff, age 19

...enjoying a recent New Year's Day at Coney Island

Photo: Aldo L 'Orefice

By Vic Boff

Health and fitness have always been the most important part of my life. From my earliest memories even as a boy, strong, well-built men have impressed me. I too wanted to have a physique and strength like my boyhood heroes. And with this goal in mind, I began a wholehearted lifetime pursuit into the study and practice of what we used to call physical culture back in the old days. My journey took me down a variety of paths, and over the course of many decades I have had the good fortune to meet and become friends with some of the best known names in the health and physical culture field.

One thing I learned early on is that the state of our health is truly under our own control. Nature has laid down several rules to good health and long life. Follow them and you will be rewarded. Break them and you will pay a severe price. Fortunately, the road to good health has been marked out for us by what I like to call *The Four Great Physicians of Life* – fresh air, restful sleep, pure water, and wholesome, natural foods. When you respect your body, work in harmony with nature, and let these four great physicians direct you, then you will reap a blessing of health that all the money in the world could never buy.

Unfortunately, too many people have never been exposed to the universal and timeless truths of health and fitness. This is readily apparent by the ever-diminishing state of people's health, not only in our nation, but also throughout the world. What we need to stop this tragic decline and win people back over to the "physical culture lifestyle" is a massive re-education program. Granted, there are more books and magazines on health and fitness out now than ever before. But sadly, too many of them contain inaccurate and sometimes even harmful information. That's why it gives me such great pleasure to recommend to you Tom Ciola's great book *Moses Wasn't Fat*.

Through the years, Tom and I have had many long and interesting discussions on health and fitness. To his credit, he has always been a cordial and willing listener to some of my long discourses on this subject. That's why I was equally as willing to listen to him when he first started to talk to me about the Bible and health. While our religious backgrounds are different, I had already reached some of the same conclusions that he was now bringing to my attention. My study of nature and her magnificent design of life left no doubt in my mind that there had to be a higher creative force beyond man directing our lives and providing order to the universe. Additionally, it has always been readily apparent to me that there is also a negative or dark force that is seeking to rob us of our health. I view it somewhat abstractly as a struggle between good and evil, whereas Tom sees it as a literal battle between God and the devil.

I must admit I was intrigued as he began to point out to me how much the Bible has to say on health, fitness and nutrition. I had never really thought of it that way and in listening to Tom, I began to find a whole new appreciation for the Bible. So much of what he pointed out to me fit precisely with what I had already learned through my long years of study. But then again, truth is truth no matter where you first meet it.

When Tom told me of his intentions to write a book on what the Bible has to say on health and fitness, I strongly encouraged him to do so. After all, I too had written a "Bible" book called *Vic Boff's Body Builder's Bible For Men And Women*. Granted it had nothing to do with the Holy Scriptures.

Thankfully, Tom did write the book and you are holding it in your hands now. I must admit I chuckled when he told me the title, but Tom has a knack for coming up with unforgettable names. Nevertheless, this is truly a book that will change your life. Tom has done a fantastic job of presenting a total approach to health and fitness based on the ancient wisdom of the Bible. I can honestly say, based on all of my years of experience, that if you follow this book's advice, your life and your health are going to change for the better. I am very thankful to Tom for writing this long-needed book and I am also glad to call him my friend.

Vic Boff,
Founder and President of The Association of Old Time Barbell and Strongmen

Preface

I have been a student of the Bible for approximately 30 years now and coincidentally, I have also been a student of health and fitness for about the same amount of time. Over those many years, I have read literally hundreds of books on diet, health, nutrition, exercise, religion, theology and the Bible. While I have enjoyed both pursuits immensely, it has only been over the past few years that I have come to see the powerful relationship between the Bible and health. What surprised me is that it took me so long to make the connection between the two. Also, when I finally did see the link, I had no idea where this pursuit was going to lead me. What truly amazed me, however, is just how quickly things opened up for me once I made this connection. It was all there right before my eyes, yet I was too blind to see. But now I do see and it's time to share what I have found with as many people as possible.

The Bible – God's written word – is the most popular, most respected, most widely read, most quoted book in the history of the world. Through it, He wants to give you all of your answers if you will only let Him. Its wisdom and guidance is timeless and its words have brought spiritual direction and hope to countless millions of people. But there's another side to the Good Book that often gets overlooked amidst its spiritual theme and that's the message of health that it also offers. Many people are surprised to learn that the Bible can also be used as a guide to physical health and well being.

Even though *Moses Wasn't Fat* was written to help people lose weight, it is much more than a diet book. It is a book about developing a healthy, God-glorifying lifestyle. Most diet books focus only on the <u>process of losing weight</u> and therein lies their high failure rate. For any diet program to be effective, it must <u>embrace a total health plan for living</u>. That is precisely what the book *Moses Wasn't Fat* is all about.

You will meet a theme over and over again in the book – namely that God's natural Bible foods and herbs are your best "medicine." You are never going to find good health in a prescription pill or at the doctor's office. Therein, at best, you will only find a way to treat your illness *symptoms*. True, lasting, God-given health can only be achieved when you live your life according to God's TEN COMMANDMENTS OF HEALTH. Like Job, you too must learn to develop faith, trust and understanding of God's wisdom. Hopefully, this book will help show you the way. It is far different from any other diet book you may have read. The *Moses Diet & Health Program* begins exactly where God would want it to – with a strong belief in Him.

> "Yahshua (Jesus) said to him, 'If you can believe, all things are possible to him who believes.'" **(Mark 9:23)**

Trying to follow any health building plan that does not include God is ultimately doomed to failure. *Moses Wasn't Fat* is going to lead you on a journey out of the bondage of physical travail into the promised land of radiant good health. Much of the information it contains has never been discussed before. Some of it may even cause a certain degree of discomfort to those people who erroneously believe that the condition of their bodies has nothing to do with their salvation. Perhaps this book will help them change their minds.

While the title may seem cute, the subject matter is deadly serious. Deadly because Satan – knowing that a strong, healthy body is a glorious temple for the Holy Spirit – will do all in his power to destroy you both *physically* as well as *spiritually*. If he could do it, he would stop you from reading this book right now. He knows that the truth contained herein can liberate you from his physical oppression – an oppression he inflicted on the human race all the way back since the Garden of Eden.

Undeniably, nutrition and physical health are linked to the first sin of Adam and Eve in the Garden. For proof of this, just recall how Satan's very first attack against mankind dealt with eating improperly *("but of the tree of knowledge of good and evil you shall not eat,"* **(Genesis 2:17)** as well as his desire to destroy our physical bodies *("for in the day that you eat of it you shall surely die."* **(Genesis 2:17)**

Now ask yourself something. Do you honestly believe Satan would discard a plan of attack that worked so well for him in the Garden? Hardly! He is cunningly intelligent and he is every bit as much engaged today in physical warfare against us as he is in a spiritual war. Whereas God is the author of life, health, peace, and harmony, Satan is the author of sickness, disease, poor health, and ultimately even death itself. You better believe he's out to destroy you physically because if you don't think so, then you give him an open invitation to wreak havoc upon your body. You must learn how to repel him so that your physical temple is worthy of the indwelling of the Holy Spirit. Yet, even though we are still under the curse of Eden, God wants us to enjoy a healthy and long life.

> *"So all the days of Noah were <u>nine hundred and fifty years</u>; and he died."* **(Genesis 9:29)**

> *"Honor your father and your mother, <u>that your days may be long</u> upon the land which the LORD your God is giving you."* **(Exodus 20:12)**

> *"Moses was <u>one hundred and twenty years old when he died</u>. His eyes were not dim nor his natural vigor diminished."* **(Deuteronomy 9:7)**

> *"With <u>long life</u> shall I satisfy him, and show him my salvation."* **(Psalm 91:16)**

> *"<u>Old men and old women</u> shall again sit in the streets of Jerusalem, each one with his staff in his hand <u>because of great age</u>.* **(Zechariah 8:4)**

For too long now, many Christians have erroneously looked upon their physical bodies almost as an impediment to their eternal salvation when in fact our bodies are the actual contact point with God's Spirit.

> *"Do you not know that <u>you are the temple of God</u> and that <u>the Spirit of God dwells in you</u>? If anyone defiles the temple of God, God will destroy him. For the temple of God is holy, <u>which temple you are</u>."* **(1 Corinthians 3:16-17)**

> *"And what agreement has the temple of God with idols? <u>For you are the temple of the living God</u>. As God has said: '<u>I will dwell in them</u> and walk among them. I will be their God and they shall be My people.'"* **(2 Corinthians 6:16)**

To me, these scriptures are very clear. Even in our imperfect, fallen state, the Holy Spirit seeks to dwell within us, foreshadowing a time when we will be given perfected, glorified bodies and the indwelling will be forever. Is it not true that God designed Adam and Eve to live forever in physical bodies in the Garden of Eden? Had they not sinned, they would be in glorified physical bodies just the same as we will be given one day. Therefore, it is wrong for us to overlook or underplay the importance of our bodies and the kind of care we take of them.

When God created Adam's body from the soil of the earth and then breathed into it His Holy Spirit, He intended from that point on for man's body to be a bridge, a connection point between heaven and earth. This heaven-earth union through our bodies is precisely what will take place in the New World when we are given glorified bodies. This is the deeper meaning of what Yahshua (Jesus) meant when he said: *"whatever you bind on earth will be bound in heaven, and whatever you loose on earth will be loosed in heaven."* **(Matthew 16:19)** Indeed our bodies are very important, and although they may be imperfect now, we have an obligation to God to keep them physically fit and spiritually holy.

Now take a good, honest look at yourself. Is the condition of your physical body worthy of the indwelling of the Holy Spirit or has Satan convinced you that it really doesn't matter? Just remember one thing, however, he's the master deceiver. After all, he argues, if you have accepted Yahshua (Jesus) as your Savior, then you already have eternal salvation so the condition of your body isn't really all that important. Is he right?

Well just ask yourself further what it takes to get the body out of shape: overeating, over drinking, lack of regular exercise, misuse of drugs, faulty nutrition. Do any of these things sound like they are of God? Of course not! So if the things that destroy our body temples aren't from God, how is it then that we rationalize our poor physical condition by saying that it has nothing to do with our relationship to God? This is faulty logic and it accounts for much of the poor health and physical condition of so many Christians today.

If any of this makes sense to you, then it is my sincere hope that this book will serve as a construction guide to the rebuilding of your temple so that it truly may become worthy of the indwelling of the Holy Spirit. Trying to put into practice a health-for-life plan that doesn't include God is doomed to failure. That's why *Moses Wasn't Fat* places such an important emphasis on belief and trust in God. That's also why so many readers of this book have been successful in turning the state of their health around.

I know that many of you purchased this book seeking to lose weight. The good news is that when you follow the program contained herein, you *will* lose weight. But always keep in mind that this book is about so much more than dieting. It's about a whole biblically based lifestyle. It is designed to give you an integrated approach to health. To be successful, you must put all of the steps together. Only then will you experience the dramatic transformational effect this program is going to have on both your physical and spiritual well being. *Moses Wasn't Fat* will outline a system for living which will not only help bring your bodyweight to its proper level, but will take you into new areas of good health and well being that are your God-given heritage.

Maybe you aren't even aware of it but Satan has launched a two-fold attack against you. He seeks to destroy you both *physically* and *spiritually*. This book will show you how to defeat Satan's *physical* attack so that you will have the strength and inner fortitude to defeat his *spiritual* attack.

I have made every effort to keep it as non-technical and easy to understand as possible so that you can put this information into practice immediately. I have written this book with the full understanding that I will have to account for it to the Lord some day. Therefore, I have undertaken this project with all of the seriousness and dedication it deserves. My wish is that you will read it with the same commitment. May God bless you and give you good health and long life. Now let's begin our journey to the Promised Land.

SHALOM-SHALOM

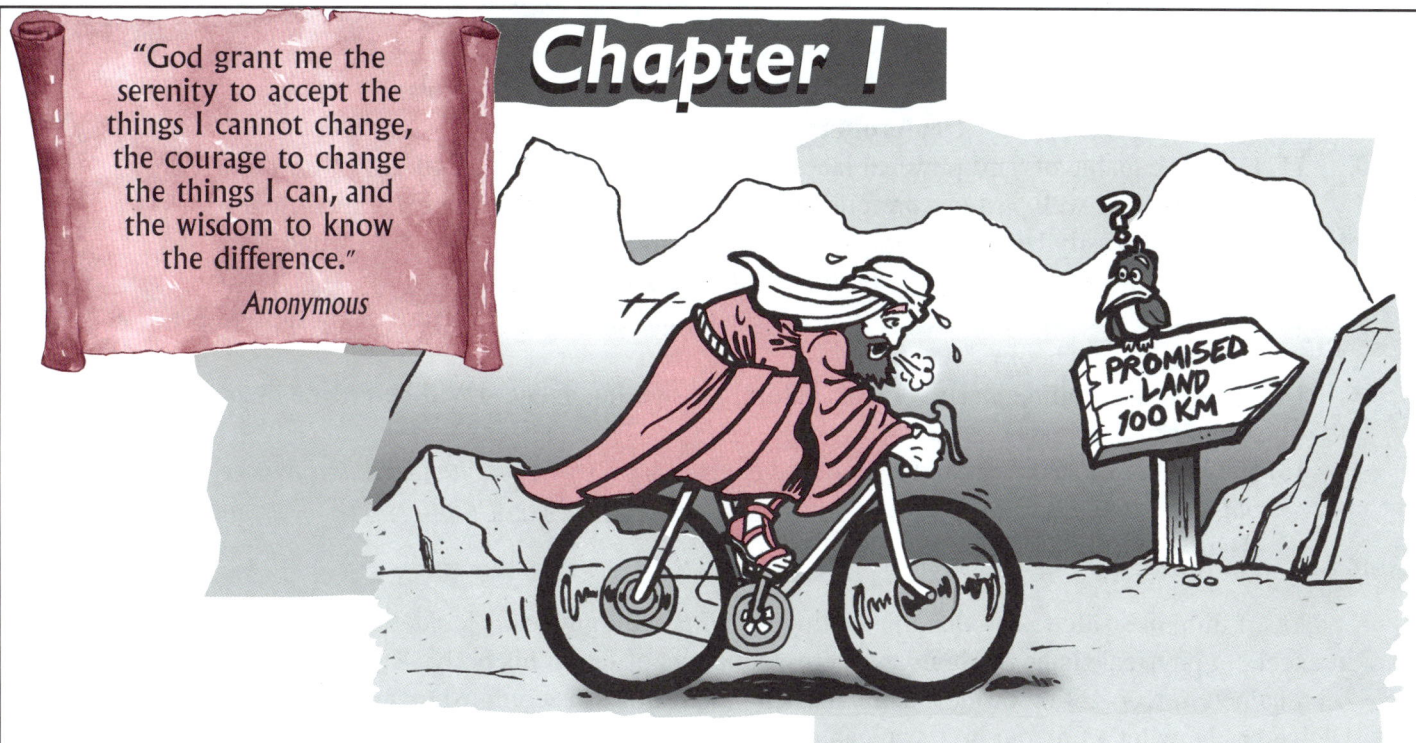

> "God grant me the serenity to accept the things I cannot change, the courage to change the things I can, and the wisdom to know the difference."
> Anonymous

Chapter 1

Our Journey Begins.

You Have The Creative Power Of God Within You. Therefore, You Have The Ability To Create Your Own Reality And Be The Master Of Your Own Destiny.

So Moses wasn't fat? Who says so? Is it in the Bible? Well... sort of. Let's examine the evidence for such a bold and unusual claim. Here is what we do know about Moses:

1. He started out as a baby on a proper diet of natural mother's milk rather than bottled baby formula. **(Exodus 2:9)**
2. He was apparently athletic, possessed physical fighting skills, and was well capable of defending himself. **(Exodus 2:17-19)**
3. As a shepherd and the deliverer of Israel, he was an ardent walker. **(Exodus 3:1; 4:20; Deuteronomy 2:7)**
4. He had the agility and the strength to climb high mountains. **(Exodus 3:1-4; Exodus 19:14;20)**
5. He cut an impressive and powerful image not only among his own people but even among the Egyptians. **(Exodus 11:3)**
6. He was disease free at least for the last third of his life. **(Exodus 15:26)**
7. Every day, of the last 40 years of his life, he was able to eat the most nutritious and perfect food ever created. A food made directly by God Himself. **(Exodus 16:4; 16:35)**
8. He had the opportunity to drink the purest spring water on earth. **(Exodus 17:6)**
9. He had excellent aerobic conditioning and impressive muscular coordination that enabled him to carry the two stone tablets of the Law down from the heights of Mt. Sinai. **(Exodus 32:15)**

10. He was known to fast for 40 days and 40 nights on several occasions. **(Exodus 24:18; 34:28; Deuteronomy 9:9)**
11. He was capable of hard physical labor, even in his 80's. **(Exodus 40:18) (Numbers 7:1)**
12. When he was well past our present day age of retirement, this biblical senior citizen was capable of easily bending over and lying face down outstretched on the ground. No evidence of a fat, out-of-shape body here. **(Numbers 20:6)**
13. He ate a diet of wholesome, unprocessed, natural foods. (Will be proven by subsequent chapters of this book)
14. He used olive oil regularly – God's natural fat-fighting agent. (Will be proven in a later chapter of this book)
15. He lived to be 120 years old in perfect health. "Moses was one hundred and twenty years old when he died. <u>His eyes were not dim nor his natural vigor diminished</u>." **(Deuteronomy 34:7)**

Yes, I think it's safe to say that this distinguished Bible figure, this hand picked agent of God, was in excellent physical shape, without any excess amounts of fat on his body. Therefore, this book has been named in recognition of the exemplary health and fitness accomplishments of Moses – God's Deliverer. Now let's find out how you can do the same thing.

WHAT IS THIS THING CALLED HEALTH?

Is good health something that every one of us can attain or does God want us to pass through this life suffering from weight problems, arthritis, indigestion, tooth decay, hypertension, headaches, allergies, acne, constipation, diarrhea, colitis, ulcers, colds, sinus problems, backaches, osteoporosis or perhaps even worse – heart disease, cancer, diabetes, Alzheimer's disease, strokes? Unfortunately, many people believe that such ailments are an unavoidable part of life and they look upon them as some sort of test from God. Some will even cite the Book of Job as proof of their belief. What they fail to realize are two very important points.

First of all, even though God permitted these things to happen to Job, it was actually Satan who brought about the plagues. This should be proof that sickness and disease are not part of God's world, but rather Satan's. Secondly, rather than go to his grave condemned with his physical disease, Job is not only ultimately cleansed by God of his ailments, but is actually rewarded *double*. Therefore, the real question we should be asking ourselves is what was it that Job did to allow God to heal him. The answer is an important one.

For one thing, Job never loses his faith and trust in God, which leads him to tell the LORD,

> "I know that you can do everything, and that no purpose of Yours can be withheld from You." **(Job 42:1)**

It is this proclamation of faith in the last chapter of the book that seems to finally put Job's healing process in motion.

But that's not all. In addition to this, Job also comes to realize that God's intellect is far superior to that of man and that the starting point of all understanding (and healing) is to acknowledge this. This Job does.

> "Therefore I have uttered what I did not understand, things too wonderful for me which I did not know." **(Job 42:3)**

In other words, Job and his well-meaning friends were looking at his problems through faulty human understanding. Yet, only by admitting that God is above all, did Job finally get healed. God was simply demonstrating that we must learn to do things His way rather than our own way.

Now here's an interesting observation. The two things that eventually effect Job's cure – namely trust and understanding – are the very same things cited in Proverbs 3.

> *"Trust in the LORD with all your heart and lean not on your own understanding; in all your ways acknowledge Him and He shall direct your paths."* **(Proverbs 3:5-6)**

Isn't this amazing? It actually seems that God has linked the Book of Job to this Proverb. Want further proof of the connection? Let's keep reading the Proverb.

> *"Do not be wise in your own eyes; fear the LORD and depart from evil. It will be <u>health to your flesh and strength to your bones.</u>"* **(Proverbs 3: 7-8)**

When you trust in God and make Him your health building partner, then He will begin to change your life. But when you have doubts, or try to do it your own way, then you surround yourself with a negative energy field that repels God's Holy Spirit and makes His help very difficult. There is an invisible chain that links your heart to the heart of God. This means that God feels what you feel. When you hurt, He hurts and when you rejoice, He rejoices with you. And most importantly, when you succeed, He succeeds.

On The Meaning Of Shalom

If the importance of Bible words were ever to be determined by the number of times they appear in the text, then we would have to accord the word "peace" with near the top honors. This interesting word appears over 400 times in the Bible where we are exhorted time and time again to be at peace, receive peace, or give peace.

Yahshua (Jesus) said, *"<u>Peace</u> I leave with you; my <u>peace</u> I give you."* **(John 14:27)**

"The LORD will bless His people with <u>peace</u>." **(Psalm 29:11)**

"Depart from evil and do good. Seek <u>peace</u> and pursue it." **(Psalm 34:14)**

"Then He said to the woman, 'Your faith has saved you. Go in <u>peace</u>.'" **(Luke 7:50)**

"Grace to you and <u>peace</u> be multiplied." **(1Peter 1:2)**

Let's take a closer look at this very interesting word peace. It is a translation of the Hebrew word ***shalom*** (number 7965 in the Strong's Concordance). According to Strong's, the word shalom means *safe, well, happy, friendly, health, perfect, prosperity, peace, <u>good health</u>, whole*. Please notice that **peace** and **health** and **well being** are all linked to the meaning of the word shalom. Thus, when the Bible exhorts you to be at peace, it is also saying that you should be in good health. In other words, health gives you peace and peace gives you health.

Therefore, here is even further evidence that shalom-peace-health is part of our God-given birthright and that disease is contrary to His will for us.

And did you know that the reason Jerusalem is called the City of Peace is because the ending of its name – ***salem*** – is just another variation of the word shalom. Therefore, the coming New Jerusalem is a worldwide system of complete peace and wholeness where there will be no sickness, disease or death.

One more important point. The Bible uses an interesting technique when it wants to really emphasize a point. It repeats a word or a thought *twice* – that's right, *twice* – for extra emphasis and importance. We meet an interesting example of this principle with the use of the word shalom in the book of Isaiah – *twice*.

> *"You will keep him in <u>perfect peace</u>, whose mind is stayed on You, because he trusts in You."* **(Isaiah 26:3)**

> *"'<u>Peace, peace</u> to him who is far off and to him who is near,' says the LORD."* **(Isaiah 57:19)**

The underlined words in both scripture examples are the word shalom. Based on the meaning of shalom as noted above from Strong's Concordance, another very acceptable translation of this doublet phrase would be ***perfect health***. I'd like to think that translation is more in keeping with the philosophy of this book.

And so, I wish you – ***Shalom-Shalom!***

His will is that people will see His grace & glory through each of us & come to

And that's why God does not want us to suffer. His greatest joy is for us to be blessed and for His will to be completed in our lives. Therefore, He wants to bless us with a healthy, long life. Don't forget our friend Moses. He made it to 120 in perfect health (see point 15 above). The only curse passed on to all of us as a result of Adam and Eve's fall in the Garden is death. (Yes, even Moses died.) Other than that, as a child of God, you are deserving of a strong, healthy body and don't you ever let anyone tell you otherwise.

→ We deserve nothing

But what about instantaneous healing miracles? Doesn't God often simply heal people of their physical ailments? Let's take a closer look at that issue. Many if not all of the physical ailments we suffer are brought about ultimately by our breaking God's laws of health.(see TEN COMMANDMENTS OF HEALTH) *Period – not just re: health* In other words, we bring about our own sickness; and then without any attempt at changing our ways, we expect God to heal us. In order for God to do this, He would have to break His own laws – and He will not do that. Instead, He wants us to acknowledge Him, just as Job did, in both the truth and understanding of His ways. Only then can He begin to work a "miracle" in our lives. How many times have you heard the expression *"God helps those who help themselves?"* Granted, it may not be in the Bible, but this oft-repeated saying is definitely true. Just remember this important point. Miracles often come in a ***can***: yes I can – yes I can – yes I can.

SATAN IS DESTROYING THE HEALTH OF OUR NATION

Sadly, many people in America have forsaken God's TEN COMMANDMENTS OF HEALTH and then they wonder why they get sick. Consequently, our nation is now in the worst physical condition it has ever been in. According to a study reported in the October 2000 issue of the *American Journal of Clinical Nutrition*, Americans have been gorging themselves on junk foods for many years now. Empty calorie snack foods – typically high in fats, oils, sugars and food additives – continue to be a large part of our diets accounting for nearly 30 percent of daily caloric intake. The report went on to state that those people who are following this type of diet are much less likely to be getting proper amounts of vitamins, minerals and other nutrients important for good health.

It should come as no surprise that Satan is behind this attack. In his clever treachery, he has us eating just about anything while believing that we can escape any consequences. But not to worry! If we do get sick, he has all of his medicines waiting to "help" us. In a cunning twist, he has led us to believe that pharmaceutical drugs as well as some of the most questionable medical therapies hold the answer to our "health."

As he often does, he has even gotten us to reverse the meaning of words. For instance, we speak of "*health*" when we really mean "*illness.*" We go to the doctor and to the hospital for *health care* when we really mean *sickness care*. Insurance companies sell us *health insurance* when they really mean *sickness insurance*. We call doctors and nurses *health practitioners* when we really mean *sickness practitioners*.

Furthermore, most cities have nearly as many medical clinics as McDonalds restaurants and our hospitals are literally bursting at the seams, always adding a new wing. This is rather strange when you consider that by some estimates, doctors actually cause between 230,000 to 284,000 deaths per year in the U.S.

Just about everyone over 40 is on one type of medicine or another. In fact, we get downright upset if, after a visit to the doctor, he (or she) doesn't write us a prescription. After all, doesn't he have a magic pill in his panoply of medicines for just about everything that ails us? Are you aware of the fact that our English word "pharmaceutical" comes from the Greek word **pharmakeia** which means *sorcery, magic, witchcraft?* Don't you find that a bit strange?

But what does the Bible have to say about the use of substances that can heal and strengthen us? The answer is found in the Book of Revelation. *"The leaves of the tree (of Life) were for the healing of the nations.* **(Revelation 22:2)** Of course, these leaves represent God's natural healing herbs just as He outlined all the way back in the book of Genesis.

> *"And God said, 'See, I have given you every herb that yields seed which is on the face of all the earth, and every tree whose fruit yields seed; to you it shall be for food.'"* **(Genesis 1:29)**

God's natural foods and herbs are our true "medicine." Not witchcraft and sorcery.

> *"He causes the grass to grow for the cattle, and the <u>vegetation (herbs)</u> for the service of man."* **(Psalms 104:14)**

> *"For the earth which drinks in the rain that often comes upon it, and bears <u>herbs useful for those by whom it was cultivated</u>, receives blessing from God."* **(Hebrews 6:7)**

Another one of Satan's clever deceptions is that aging always equates to ailments, sickness, suffering and a general physical breakdown. Consequently, many of us enter into our middle age believing that physical breakdown is inevitable. Is this the truth? Just look at Moses once again. He made it to 120 years in excellent physical condition.

GOD WANTS YOU TO BE HEALTHY

Let me say it one more time. God does not want us to suffer. He wants so very much to help us but we must be willing to meet Him half way. Thankfully, He has the answer to every problem of life and the thing that really matters is that He cares about us. He wants us to enjoy good health 365 days a year, every year of our lives. Each day of your life should be filled with unbounded energy, a zest for living, a bounce in your walk, a sparkle in your eyes, an inner vibrancy and an outer vitality that states loudly and clearly to everyone you meet that you are a child of the Living God. Yes, He wants to be there for you. So call on His name and He will assist you. He can work this "miracle" in your life when you surrender your will to His will. And then through your faith and prayers, as well as by following His TEN COMMANDMENTS OF HEALTH, He will be able to give you the good health that is your birthright. Just turn your faith loose, trust in God and then go for the victory.

You now hold in your hands a book that can totally change your life. What you do with it is entirely up to you. But I do want to make this important promise to you. If you follow the advice contained in it, you are going to have a fuller, healthier, holier life as you discover and put into practice the ancient health wisdom of the Bible.

Whether your problem is simply that you are overweight or if you suffer from any of the other ailments listed above, the Bible has answers for you right now. But let me advise you once again that ***Moses Wasn't Fat*** is not about curing anything. It is not a quick fix diet manual. Instead, it is a lifestyle book based on solid biblical wisdom which, when followed, will help bring you to the state of health God wants for you and all of His children.

Be cautioned that Satan is doing all in his power to keep these truths hidden from you. Thus, you have been deceived, told half-truths and out-and-out lies in his efforts to deny you good health and ultimately destroy you. Furthermore, when you do discover the truth, he will use every means possible to dissuade you from implementing it in your life. Be watchful, therefore, for at the core of your quest for healthful, Godly living, there rages an even higher battle between good and evil.

In closing this chapter then, I would like to leave you with the words of Yahshua (Jesus) who summarized the goal of this book best when he said,

> *"And you shall know the truth, and the truth shall set you free."* **(John 8:32)**

5

What Does It Mean If Good Health Doesn't Come?

What if you follow all of the advice in this book and still are plagued with health problems? What does this mean? Has God forsaken His promises? Have you somehow proven to be unworthy of good health? Was the information contained in this book spurious? While the answer to all three questions is definitely no, the overriding question really is why would this happen at all?

First of all, we must accept the fact that while God created a once perfect world and He has plans to do so again in the future, we are currently living under a curse. Even when we live our lives according to God's health laws, much of what happens to us, much of what impacts our well being, is beyond our immediate control. For instance, weak genetics and tendencies towards certain illnesses may very well be the consequence of parents who violated one or more of God's TEN COMMANDMENTS OF HEALTH. Indeed, God warned us in the Book of Deuteronomy that both blessings and *curses* could be passed on generationally.

> *"But it shall come to pass, if you do not obey the voice of the LORD your God, to observe carefully all His commandments and His statutes which I command you today, that all these curses will come upon you and overtake you: Cursed shall you be in the city, and cursed shall you be in the country. Cursed shall be your basket and your kneading bowl. Cursed shall be the fruit of your body and the produce of your land."* **(Deuteronomy 28: 15-18)**

Secondly, while we may be able to control all of the health factors within our own lives, we still are obliged to live in a world where others may not share our Godly views and beliefs. Thus the world grows more polluted almost by the day, with many potentially harmful elements being dumped into our air, food and water. In the highly controversial case of genetically modified foods, for example, we may not even know that we are eating them. Remember what I said earlier? God always wants to heal us, but He cannot break His own laws to do so.

While God speaks to us as individuals, He also speaks to us collectively as nations. Ideally, He wants everyone in a nation to abide by His law for then He is able to pour forth His blessings upon the whole land. But because so many people in our country have strayed from God's law, then societal disease is now spreading like a cancer through our nation, just as cancer spreads in the bodies of individuals.

Does this mean then that it is a waste of time to follow a system like the *Moses Diet & Health Program*? Absolutely not! The facts prove just the opposite. I can promise you that everyone who follows this program is going to have a better quality spiritual life as well as experiencing at least some higher level of physical health. And while you may not reach the level of Moses' achievement, you are still going to be greatly rewarded for your efforts.

Now one last point. Must we have good health in order to be saved? The answer to that question is decidedly **NO** for I am sure that the Kingdom of God will be filled with many people who walked this earth in less than perfect health. The good news is that all those who have accepted the atoning blood of Yahshua (Jesus), be they healthy or be they sick, are heirs to the Kingdom of God.

> *In that day the deaf shall hear the words of the book, and the eyes of the blind shall see out of obscurity and out of darkness. The humble also shall increase their joy in the LORD, and the poor among men shall rejoice in the Holy One of Israel. For the terrible one is brought to nothing."* **(Isaiah 29: 18-20)**

Chapter 2

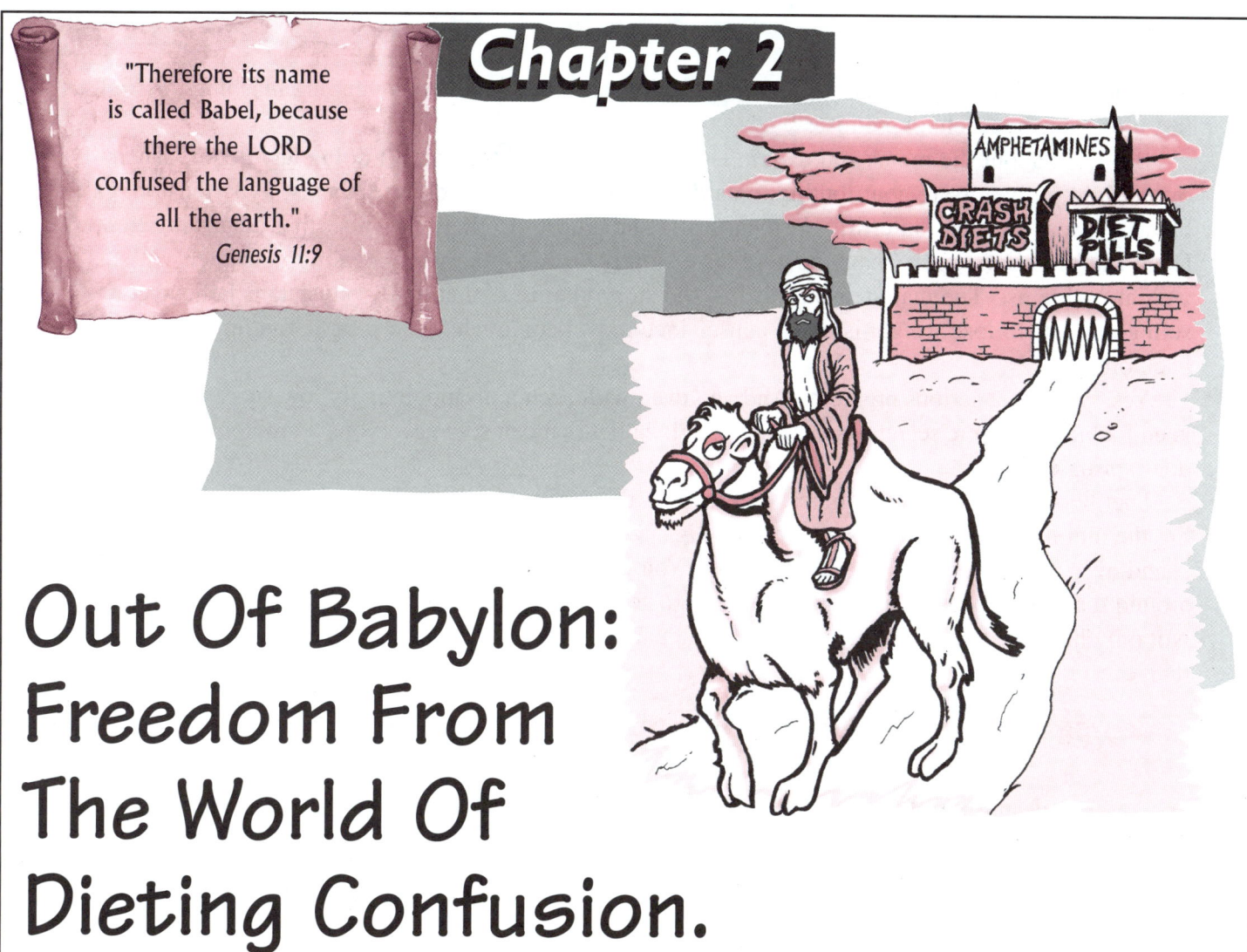

"Therefore its name is called Babel, because there the LORD confused the language of all the earth."
Genesis 11:9

Out Of Babylon: Freedom From The World Of Dieting Confusion.

It's Much More Difficult To Unlearn A Lie Than It Is To Accept A New Truth.

There's an epidemic spreading throughout our country today and it is not a respecter of race, age, gender, income or education. Some people fight it all their lives, while with others, it sneaks up a little bit at a time. In either case, once it claims its victim, it is an extremely stubborn and difficult adversary to beat. Of course, I'm talking about **FAT** – undesirable weight gain.

Back in the 1960s, it was estimated that about 25 percent of Americans were overweight. Today, some government sources place that number at nearly 40 percent. If they're correct, then over 100 million people in this country are now overweight. Wow! Pretty startling isn't it?

According to a recent article in *Newsweek* magazine, some six million American children alone are now fat enough to endanger their health with an additional five million on the threshold. "The children we see today are 30 percent heavier than the ones who were referred to us in the 1990s," says pediatric endocrinologist, Dr. Naomi Neufeld. According to Dr. Theresa A. Nicklas, Professor of Pediatrics at the Baylor College of Medicine, obesity in America has now reached epidemic proportions and it is the most prevalent disease among children and young adults.

Newsweek goes on to report that a study of preschool children at New York City Head Start Centers found overweight children three and four years old with signs of elevated blood pressure and cholesterol. Is it any wonder, now that many schools allow soda and junk snack vending machines, as well as fast food outlets on school premises?

But what about the moms and dads? The sad news is that they aren't doing any better. Their overweight problems are contributing to cardiovascular disease, strokes, diabetes, hypertension, gall bladder disease, cancer, infertility, osteoarthritis and a host of other ailments. In a disturbing Reuters Health Information report, many doctors have simply decided to give up dealing with their patients' weight problems. The main reason for this, the story claims, is that many physicians believe counseling patients to lose weight is a lost cause since most people who lose weight end up putting it all back on.

Yes, we have a serious problem. And yet, even with such a disappointingly low success rate, we keep looking for some secret answer – the magic bullet that can solve everyone's problem. I guess hope does spring eternal.

Diet books, diet pills, diet clinics, diet foods – they're everywhere. Do you have any idea just how big the diet industry is? Here's a clue. It's big – very **B-I-G**! Would you believe Americans alone spend over $30 billion a year to lose weight? You might guess with that kind of money being thrown around that we'd have finally figured out how to solve this ubiquitous problem. Well guess again! Not only have we not solved the problem, it actually keeps getting worse. Americans are now fatter than ever.

WEIGHT LOSS MARKETERS ARE LYING THROUGH THEIR TEETH

And yet, despite all of this dismal failure, the diet industry keeps on rolling along, pushing one weight loss hoax after another on an ever-gullible public. If deep down, you've always had a sneaking suspicion that the diet industry is a big racket – you're right! Here's just a brief sampling of some recent advertising lies you may have seen.

- **Lose weight fast without dieting or counting calories.**
- **Now you can lose inches without strenuous exercise.**
- **Great new diet pill melts fat right out of your body.**
- **New diet formula helps you lose up to two pounds per day.**
- **New patented product finally conquers weight problems.**
- **Amazing new pill traps fat and drives it from your body.**
- **A new diet that's guaranteed to slash your body fat.**
- **Doctor discovers powerful, new fat loss ingredient.**
- **Lose up to 10 lbs. this weekend with new Hollywood diet.**
- **Burn off fat while you sleep.**
- **New pill blocks body chemical that causes weight gain.**
- **Physician accidentally stumbles on secret to weight loss.**
- **New capsule guaranteed to soak up fat FAST!**
- **Eat everything you want and still lose weight.**
- **Miracle diet aid clinically proven to burn a pound of fat daily.**
- **Lose 60 pounds in 6 weeks or your money back.**
- **Fantastic new diet pill works like a drug without side effects.**

And on and on it goes. It would actually be laughable if it weren't so sad. This isn't just about lying. It's about treachery and stealing too – a clever way to extract millions of dollars from desperate

Dieter's Euphoria

Many people put off starting a diet because they believe it is going to be an unpleasant experience. This is not necessarily true. While there is some discipline and self denial involved, dieting can actually be an uplifting experience. New studies have shown that the shedding of excess fat can actually be a mood booster.

In the past, it was believed that dieting was a downer and that dieters often become depressed, anxious and suffer negative mood swings. Some counselors even went so far as to discourage people from dieting so as not to make them miserable. These erroneous conclusions were based on psychological studies conducted in hospitals with patients on near-starvation diet programs. This research simply has no bearing on the average person who follows a sensible lifestyle changing diet program.

More recent and reliable studies have found that mood actually improves as pounds are shed. Even more exciting is the fact that dieters who start out with a negative mood show the greatest improvement in temperament and that this improvement is noticeable after losing the first ten pounds.

people. I'm willing to bet that many of you have already been victimized by these blatant hucksters. But you need not feel ashamed. These con artists know how to prey upon your discouragement, vulnerability and despair. What they fail to tell you is that there is no quick fix, no magic formula, no super pill that will solve your weight problems. None of them would dare tell you the truth – namely that losing weight is only 20 percent of the battle but keeping it off is 80 percent of the battle. And the only way to lose weight and keep it off permanently is to make healthy dietary and lifestyle changes.

Just use some logic for a minute. If any one of these products really worked, don't you think the word would spread like wildfire – especially with upwards of 100 million people desperately overweight? Wouldn't that product be the talk of the nation? The story would be all over the media. They wouldn't be able to manufacture this wonder pill fast enough.

Now ask yourself. Have you ever heard of any of these products doing that? Hardly! In fact, sooner or later, every one of them disappears, making room for the next round of hoaxes – often from the same companies.

I can't urge you enough to stop sending your hard-earned money to these con artists. Please trust me. There is no pill, no powder, no drink, no magic potion that is going to effortlessly make you lose weight, let alone keep it off forever. There is no quick fix, no shortcut to a lean, fit body. It can only be done through changing your lifestyle.

BEWARE OF CRASH DIETING

If there's anything worse than falling for the diet pill hucksters, it's crash dieting. At least with most diet pills, other than throwing away your money, chances are you are not doing any damage to your body. Not so with crash dieting. Extremely low calorie diets that promise rapid weight loss can cause severe damage to your health. (Maybe that's why they're called "crash diets.") For example, crash diet programs under 1000 calories may increase the risk of cholesterol saturation in the bile, subsequently leading to the formation of gallstones.

Also, sooner or later, crash dieting leads to relentless food cravings which leads to bingeing, which leads to weight loss failure. But that's not all. Once you go off them, crash diets *always* lead to a rapid regaining of the lost weight plus some additional fat pounds on top of that. Crash diets are the classic cause of the so-called dieting "yo-yo syndrome" not to mention that they will ultimately play havoc with your metabolism. (This whole metabolism issue is discussed in detail in Chapter 14.) My warning to you on crash dieting is this. **DON'T DO IT!** Remember this very important principle. The faster you lose weight, the worse the diet is for you and the faster you will put all of the weight back on.

SO WHAT'S THE ANSWER?

While dieters continue to search frantically for a solution to their weight problems, the answer has been staring us all in the face for thousands of years. That answer is in the Bible. Granted, a diet and health program based on the Bible may not be as flashy and exciting as the latest diet fad. Nevertheless, it does work – and fabulously well, at that! The reason for this is because it offers a complete package – a total approach to effective and lasting weight control based on the ageless wisdom of the Bible.

When To Start A Diet

Picking the proper time to start a diet is very important since it can have a great bearing on your success.

START A DIET
- When you are highly motivated and committed. *this may never happen*
- When you have a definite plan to follow.
- When you have all of the knowledge and tools you need.
- When you are in total control of your environment. *this is never!*

DON'T START A DIET
- If you have just given up smoking or drinking.
- If you are pregnant.
- If you are sick.
- If you are battling depression. ** could actually be therapeutic*
- If you have an overriding medical problem.
- If you are going away on vacation or business.
- Between Thanksgiving and Christmas.

By the way, when I speak of weight control I don't necessarily mean just fat loss since much of our overall bodyweight involves muscles, bone and water as well as fat. That's why the **Moses Diet & Health Program** discussed in this book deals with so much more than just fat loss. It is a lifestyle plan designed to help you build your body into a suitable temple for the Holy Spirit. Unbiased diet research has demonstrated over and over again that permanent weight loss can only be sustained through positive changes in lifestyle. Anything else is doomed to failure.

In order to break free of the diet yo-yo syndrome, you will need to put your trust in God. There isn't a weight problem in the world that cannot be conquered by prayer and faith in the LORD. No bad habit, no weakness, no health problem is too hard for Him to correct. Just let His guiding words in the Bible show you the way. And once you zero in on your destination, God the Father, through the intercession of His Son Yahshua (Jesus), is going to give you the determination you need to sustain you all the way there.

If you have been searching for a way to finally get control of your weight problems, you need look no further. You are about to discover a new power in the Bible. The **Moses Diet & Health Program** integrates an ten-point lifestyle plan that is going to change your life forever. I promise you that if you follow this program faithfully you will conquer your weight problems once and for all.

MOSES' TEN TOOLS FOR BUILDING A NEW TEMPLE:

1. Faith
2. Prayer
3. Goal Setting Techniques
4. Cleansing/Purifying
5. Organization
6. Proper Eating
7. Supplementation
8. Exercise
9. Behavior Modification
10. Accountability

There's absolutely no doubt about it. The *Moses Diet & Health Program* is going to exponentially boost your odds for success. I know you can do it. God knows you can do it. Now all that remains is for you to know you can do it. Regardless of whatever else you have tried in the past, regardless of your previous failures, this is a new beginning. This is your Genesis!

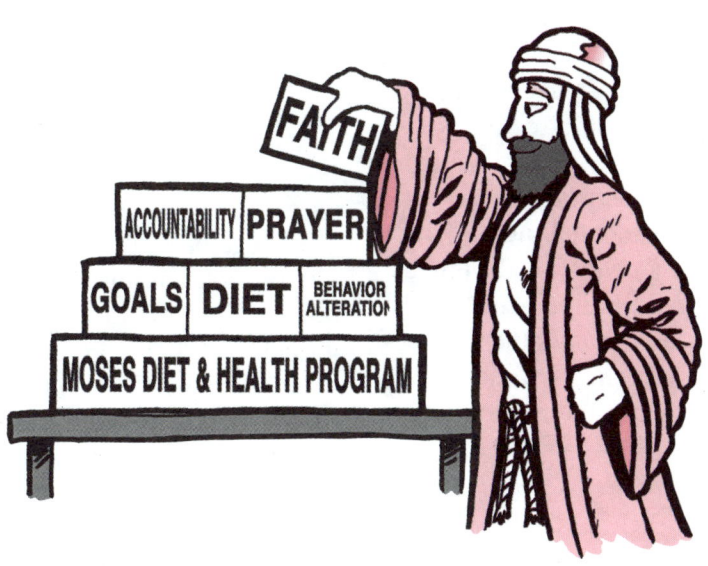

A Brief Review Of The Diet Industry

There are so many books, pills, exercise programs, courses, etc. for dieting and weight control that it is virtually impossible to critique them all here. However, here is a brief review of some of the current and popular ones.

DIET PILLS (PRESCRIPTION)

(**Amphetamines**) Prescription diet pills have been around for over 50 years. The first type to become popular were amphetamines when it was discovered that amphetamine-type medications (so-called uppers) also had the ability to suppress the appetite. Very addictive with lots of unpleasant side effects including hyperactivity, nervousness, headaches, irritability, sweating, constipation and dry mouth. Definitely not a biblically based strategy. Should NEVER be used for weight control. Some common types and brand names include: **Benzedrine, Dexadrine, Ionamin, Phentermine, Adipex-P, Tenuate Dospan Fastin, Gradumet (Desoxyn), Didrex, Duromine, Teronac, Sanorex, Mazindol.**

(**Non-Amphetamines**) Pharmaceutical companies continue to search for effective weight control drugs. Relatively new medications include Sibutramine, (*Meridia*® and *Reductil*®) designed to create a feeling of fullness and Orlistat (*Xenical*®) which is designed to block fat absorption. All have numerous side effects. Neither these, nor any other prescription drugs represent a biblically based strategy for weight control and should not be used.

DIET PILLS (NON-PRESCRIPTION)

(**Herbal/Nutritional**) There are many different types of herbal/nutritional diet pills and they are reputed to work in a variety of ways. (Increase metabolism, block carbohydrate and fat absorption, burn fat, stimulate the thyroid, reduce water, etc.) Common ingredients used include: ephedra/mahuang, guarana, kola nut, garcina cambogia (HCA), ginseng, yerba mate, white willow bark, spirulina, chromium, carnitine, amino acids, kelp, lecithin, cider vinegar, grapefruit powder). There are many different brands on the market and some products are named to sound similar to prescription diet pills. While the majority of these products are harmless and may, in some small way, temporarily contribute to weight loss, they are not designed to treat the long range causes of weight problems. This can only be achieved through lifestyle changes.

(**Others**) There are several non-herbal/nutritional chemical substances that are being used for weight control. One of the most popular is *phenylpropanolamine*. It is an FDA approved appetite suppressant. It is found in numerous over-the-counter medications such as cough syrups, cold and allergy medicines. It is the main ingredient in two very popular non-prescription diet products: *Dexatrim*® and *Acutrim*®. Phenylpropanolamine can have mild side effects and definitely has no place in a biblically based diet and health program.

MEAL REPLACERS
(SHAKES, POWDERS)

These products are usually high protein, low fat preparations that also contain a variety of vitamins and minerals. They come in numerous flavors, in both pre-blended liquid form and powders and are designed to be low calorie meal substitutes. When used in conjunction with a well-rounded weight loss program, they definitely can be helpful. Some common brands include: *Slim Fast*®, *METrx*®, *Success*®.

DIET BOOKS & PROGRAMS

Every season brings a new crop of diet books and programs. Here is a review of some of the currently popular ones.

(Dr. Atkins' Diet Revolution) This highly controversial diet continues to be one of the most popular weight loss programs in the country. Based on the premise that carbohydrates make us fat, the Atkins program seeks to drastically reduce carbohydrate intake. Instead, dieters are urged to eat high protein, high fat meals. "Cut out carbohydrates and fat will automatically become the number one fuel," claims diet creator Dr. Robert Atkins. While this diet program definitely promotes weight loss, it is extremely unhealthy and unbiblical since it virtually eliminates carbohydrates – a nutrient found in large quantities in nearly all of God's Eden-type foods.

(The Zone Diet) Popularized by the book *Enter The Zone* by Barry Sears PhD., this diet is based on the premise that elevated insulin levels lead to excess fat. It attempts to regulate insulin levels by maintaining a balance at each meal of 40 percent carbohydrate, 30 percent protein and 30 percent fat. The Zone Diet permits three meals a day and two snacks. The suggested nutrient balances are acceptable and allow for a good variety of biblically based foods. This diet program with some modifications may be used in conjunction with a biblically based lifestyle.

(The Carbohydrate Addict's Diet) As with the Atkins program, once again carbohydrates come under attack. The book's main premise is that many people suffer from a form of carbohydrate addiction which, when indulged, leads to weight gain. Besides the usual low carbohydrate meals, this program does offer an unusual twist. Dieters are encouraged to eat one "reward" meal daily of anything they want. Once again this diet would not be biblically sound since it greatly alters the natural balance of protein, fat and carbohydrate as found in God's Eden-type foods.

(Eat Great, Lose Weight) Here's Suzanne Somers latest contribution to the world of dieting confusion. Her program purports to restructure your metabolism so that you will burn fat and have more energy. The method? A food-combining strategy that prohibits eating proteins and fats at the same meal. There is no supportable scientific evidence for this approach and it is certainly unbiblical since most of God's Eden foods contain protein, fat and carbohydrate all in one. Not recommended.

(Sugar Busters) While most nutritionists would agree that we are definitely consuming too much refined sugar, this book goes one step further and incriminates sugar (and insulin) in weight gain. Therefore, the diet attempts to promote weight loss by eliminating food combinations that boost insulin. So far – so good. But the program becomes unbiblical when it starts prohibiting natural, God-made foods such as carrots, corn, beets, potatoes, and recommending that fruits be eaten by themselves. It also tends to be high in animal products. Not recommended.

(The Weigh Down Diet) This scripture-guided diet program by registered dietician Gwen Shamblin has become very popular of late among Christians. Shamblin maintains that dieting actually is counter-productive leading only to ongoing weight problems. Instead, she encourages participants to submit to God and to trust the inherent monitors of hunger and fullness that He has built into the human body. Her main mantra is to eat only when you are prompted by hunger since eating for other reasons may actually border on being sinful. While I am sure that Shamblin's intentions are good, her diet program is not. She not only condones the consumption of junk foods such as chocolate brownies, over-processed snacks and diet sodas, she implies that God finds the eating of these foods in moderation to be quite acceptable. *"God is the genius chef behind lasagna and chocolate cheesecake. He did not put bagels and cream cheese on earth to torture us."* (page 46) Furthermore, she underplays the importance of exercise. *"exercise will not help you to lose weight faster."* (page 32) Not recommended.

(**Richard Simmons**) Every year brings a new Richard Simmons TV diet infomercial – which is usually a variant on the same four themes: meal planning, exercise, accountability and a high dosage of motivation from Richard himself. Simmons has helped thousands of very obese people change their lives and for this he needs to be congratulated, (although of late some questions have been raised regarding the legitimacy of his endorsers). His diet and nutritional programs tend to be sound and effective. His multi-faceted approach to weight control is a proven strategy and is similar to some of the principles in the *Moses Diet & Health Program*.

SURGICAL ALTERNATIVES

(**Stomach Stapling**) A radical surgical procedure whereby the volume capacity of the stomach is reduced by actually being stapled smaller. Cautiously recommended as a last resort only for the very obese who are facing a life-threatening situation. Can cause nutritional deficiencies and acute diarrhea.

(**Tummy Tuck**) Cosmetic surgical procedure designed to remove excess loose skin resulting from rapid weight loss.

(**Suction Lipectomy**) A relatively new surgical technique whereby body fat is literally sucked out of problem areas of the body by the insertion of a long, thin vacuuming instrument. Can be painful. May leave scaring or unnatural appearance to the treated area. Extremely contrary to the philosophy of this book and the TEN COMMANDMENTS OF HEALTH. Definitely not recommended.

(**Jaw Wiring**) Procedure whereby the jaw is wired shut for an extended period of time to prevent the consumption of solid foods. The patient must rely on liquid nourishment for the duration. This is a foolish procedure and a poor excuse for not getting healthy God's way. Definitely not recommended.

MISCELLANEOUS

(**Fasting**) While fasting certainly has an important place in a health-building program and is definitely biblical, it is never recommended as a procedure for weight loss.

(**Liquid Protein Diets**) Once very popular but now fallen from grace, LPDs still have an occasional resurgence. The dieter consumes only liquid protein and vitamin supplements for an extended period of time in a form of controlled fasting. Unmonitored LPDs can be harmful and even life threatening. Never recommended.

(**Mono-Dieting**) This very unhealthy diet technique is based on eating only one food product until the desired weight is lost. Cottage cheese, brown rice, grapefruits and potatoes are examples of foods that have been used in mono-dieting. Extremely boring and unhealthy. Never recommended.

(**Rubber Suits & Body Wraps**) Two techniques based on the idea that fat can be either sweat out or squeezed out of the body. Unscientific, unproven. Not recommended.

(**Passive "Exercise" Machines**) Rollers, massagers, electric vibrators, electric muscle stimulators. Don't work.
Save your money.

Chapter 3

"With God – all things are possible."
Matthew 19:26

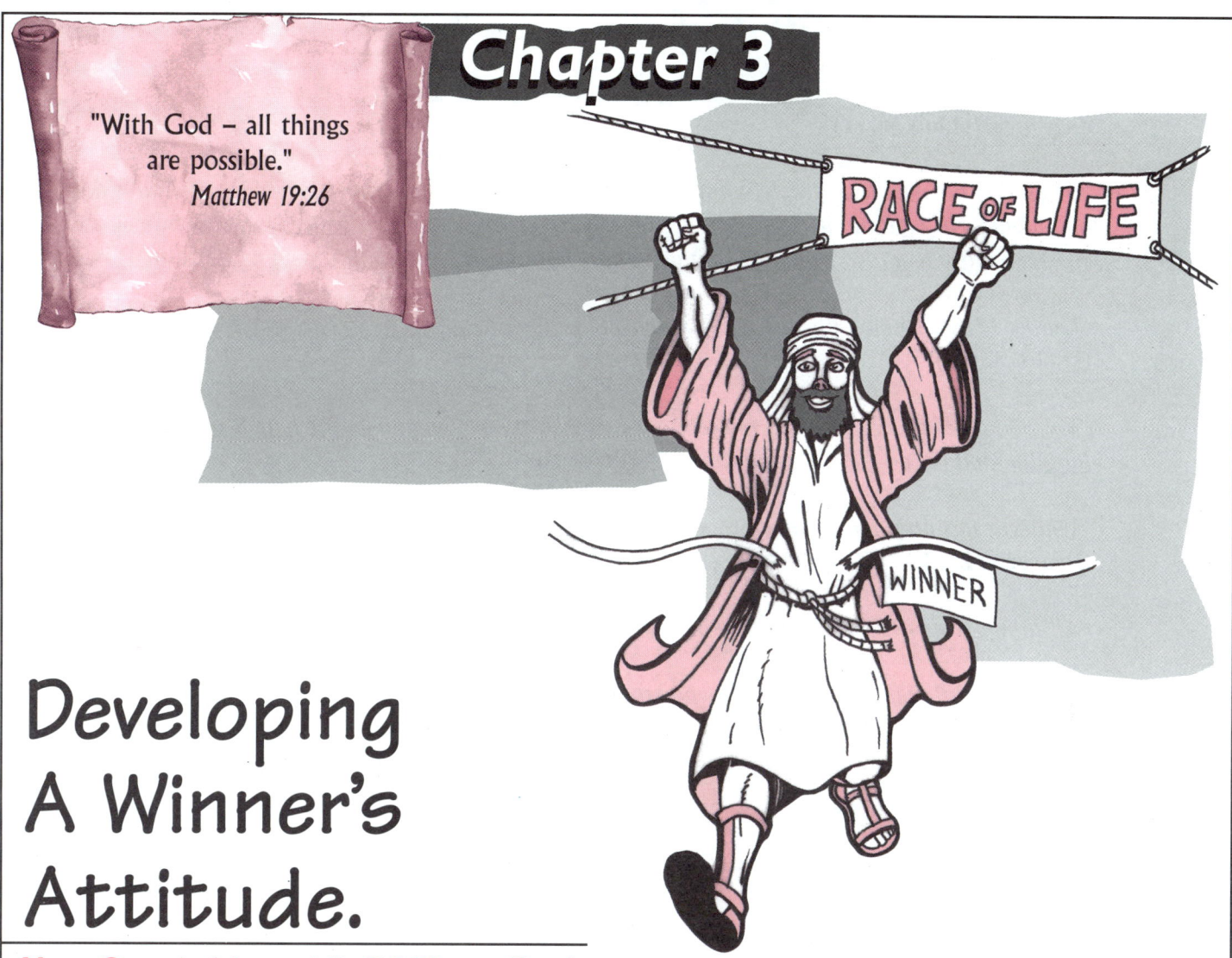

Developing A Winner's Attitude.

You Can Achieve All Of Your Goals Through Faith In God And Faith In Yourself!

Right now, as you sit reading this book, there are over 6,000,000,000 people in the world. Having some trouble reading that large number? It's six B-I-L-L-I-O-N!! Now add to that, the thousands more born daily and pretty soon you're talking about a whole lot of people.

So how many of these six billion are leading successful, healthy, productive, God-filled lives? How many are achieving their physical, financial, vocational, and spiritual goals? How many even have any goals? How many are truly happy? How many are living by what Robert Schuller likes to call "Possibility Thinking?"

Unfortunately, only a very small number. This is very sad since God truly wants all six billion of His children to be successful, productive, holy, healthy and happy when we live according to His word. Here are just a few Scripture verses that illustrate God's rewards for those who do His will.

> "This Book of the Law shall not depart from your mouth, but you shall meditate on it day and night, that you may observe to do according to all that is written in it. For then you will make your way <u>prosperous</u>, and then you will have <u>good success</u>." **(Joshua 1:8)**

"If they obey and serve Him, they shall spend their days in prosperity, and their years in pleasures." **(Job 36:11)**

"Blessed is the man (whose) delight is in the law of the LORD, and in His law he meditates day and night. He shall be like a tree planted by the rivers of water, that brings forth its fruit in its season, whose leaf also shall not whither; and whatever he does shall prosper." **(Psalm 1:1-3)**

"Let the LORD be magnified, who has pleasure in the prosperity of His servant." **(Psalm 35:27)**

"My son, do not forget my law, but let your heart keep my commands; for length of days and long life and peace they will add to you." **(Proverbs 3:1-2)**

"Whoever has no rule over his own spirit is like a city broken down, without walls." **(Proverbs 25:28)**

"All things are possible to him who believes." **(Mark 9:23)**

"I can do all things through Christ who strengthens me." **(Philippians 4:13)**

"For God has not given us a spirit of fear, but of power and love and of a sound mind." **(2 Timothy 1:7)**

"Beloved, I pray that you may prosper in all things and be in health, just as your soul prospers." **(3 John: 2)**

SATAN WANTS TO HOLD YOU BACK

There's no doubt about it. God would like for all of His children to be successful, holy, healthy, and happy. Winners! So why, then, are so few people on this earth enjoying the fulfilling and productive lives that God desires for them? Why are so many people barely managing to get by – living lives, shall we say, of quiet desperation?

Perhaps it's because there is also an evil force on this planet that would like nothing better than to see each and every one of us totally destroyed. That's right. Satan knows that there is virtually unlimited potential for greatness in all of us once we bond with our Creator. Therefore, he does all in his power to keep us from reaching our God-given potential. He does this in many subtle ways.

For one thing, he has most people convinced that they will never achieve anything noteworthy in their lives. Success is something reserved only for a special few lucky ones. The rest of us are doomed to mediocrity – or so he would have us believe. Hence, very few people even begin to tap into the vast reservoir of skills and talents which our Heavenly Father has freely gifted to all of us. Yahshua (Jesus) discusses this very point in the parable of the talents in **Matthew 25:14**. In this story, a wealthy nobleman is called away on business. Before leaving, he calls in three of his servants and entrusts them with varying amounts of his money (interestingly enough called talents in the King James Version). Upon his return, he calls the three in for an accounting. Two of the three have used their ingenuity to double his money, which greatly pleases the master. *"Well done good and faithful servant,"* he tells both of them. But not so for the third servant. In fear of losing his master's money, this servant buries it and hands it back to the master upon his return. This infuriates the nobleman who instructs his aids to take the talent from this man and give it to the first servant. He then further instructs them to cast this poor wretch into the outer darkness. This parable should leave no doubt in your mind as to how Yahshua (Jesus) feels about the wasting of talents. It is a very serious sin that will need to be accounted for some day. Satan knows this too and thus, he feeds us a steady diet of lies day after day, trying to convince us of our mediocrity. Unfortunately, he has been very successful with this ploy and as a result, most people go to their graves with their music still in them. Don't assign your life to the bin of mediocrity. Never settle for halfway performance. Strive to live every day to your fullest potential. God wants it no other way.

TO CONQUER YOUR FEARS RUN TO THEM

Still another way that Satan blocks you from becoming a winner and reaching your full potential is through fear – fear of the unknown, fear of failure, fear of humiliation, fear of change. While fear is a normal and common human emotion, fear needs to be conquered in order to become a winner. *"Do not fear for I am with you."* (**Genesis 26:24**) Therefore, the surest way to conquer all of your fears is not to run away from them but to run towards them. Seek out that which you fear, face it head on, challenge it and then find a way to neutralize it. Sometimes the very act of *doing* is all you will need to overcome fear.

Have you ever hesitated to do something out of fear and then, once you got your courage up and did the thing, you found out that your fears were unwarranted? And can you recall that feeling of satisfaction you had once you vanquished your fear? With such a good feeling attached to overcoming your fears, why would you want to walk around day after day filled with all of the negative emotions that fears impart?

Here are a few words of wisdom to help you conquer your fears.

- No fear is ever conquered by flight.
- To complete a difficult task, your desire for success must exceed your fear of failure.
- Believe in God, then believe in yourself and you are ready to conquer the world.
- If you allow fears to dominate your thoughts, they will eventually drive everything else out and become your belief system.
- You're only as brave as the fear that stops you.
- Nothing will cause more stress, tension and anxiety than a recurrent fear from which you keep running.
- Courage is not the absence of fear but the ability to go forward even with fear.
- A coward dies a thousand times but a brave man dies but once.
- Sometimes a touch of fear enables us to give our best performance.
- If you'd like to experience one of life's most exhilarating highs, find that thing which you fear the most and then go out and overcome it.
- When you can accept the pain – you've conquered the fear.
- *"Yea, though I walk through the valley of the shadow of death, I will fear no evil."* **(Psalm 23:4)**
- *"In God I have put my trust; I will not fear, what can flesh do to me?"* **(Psalm 56:4)**
- *"For God has not given us a spirit of fear, but of power and love and of a sound mind."* **(2 Timothy 1:7)**

IF YOU WANT TO ACHIEVE – YOU'VE GOT TO BELIEVE!

Once you are truly committed to getting fit and healthy, never let anything get in your way or distract you. You are worthy of your dreams because they are blessed by God. Your Heavenly Father has given you the power to recreate yourself – to become a new person both physically and spiritually. When you walk together with God, there is no end to the progress you will make. Today is only the beginning of what you will be tomorrow as the little achievements you make each day will soon add up to a new life and a new you.

Words are the very power of creation. They bring into reality that which never existed before. God has given you the powerful gift of speech. Use it wisely. State what it is you want to achieve and you will automatically put the creative force in motion. Then once you have stated it, go out and do it to the very best of your ability. Remember that from the moment you were conceived, God put His Holy Spirit in you. Therefore, for as long as you live, you have the ability to change your destiny. Only death takes away another chance.

Far too few people ever achieve their true potential. Few grasp that they can expand their limitations almost endlessly since most limitations are self-imposed. In actuality, there is virtually no limit to the human spirit and there is proof of this all around us. What was thought impossible yesterday becomes possible today and commonplace tomorrow.

Most people tiptoe through life trying to make it safely to their death. Don't you fall for this satanic ploy. Instead, strive to lead a full, productive, healthy, God-centered life and send Satan reeling back to hell where he belongs. All of us have what it takes to become winners because a winner is simply a dreamer who has never given up. To be a winner you must stop living your life by accident and start living it on purpose. Don't just drift into the future – create it! Write your own play. Become your own director. And just remember that the big victories only come about through a series of small wins. That's why the big changes you are seeking to make in your life will be the consequences of the little things you do day in and day out, every week, every month and every year.

As you now make your preparations to change your life for the better, I want you to begin as a winner. I want you to start with the certainty that your victory is already assured through the life, death and resurrection of Yahshua the Messiah (Jesus Christ).

> *"Therefore, if anyone is in Christ, he is a new creature; old things have passed away; behold, all things have become new."* **(2 Corinthians 5:17)**

It's going to be easy to succeed on this program because all you're going to need is the faith of a mustard seed.

> *"If you have faith as a mustard seed. . . nothing will be impossible for you."* **(Matthew 17:20)**

Power Affirmations

Have you ever heard about *Power Affirmations?* They're short, key phrases that you memorize and then recite to yourself when you feel that you are wavering from a goal. Here are a few Power Affirmations for you to use on the *Moses Diet & Health Program.* Feel free to memorize them, adapt them or add to the list with some Power Affirmations of your own.

- I can do all things through Christ who strengthens me.
- With God on my side, how can I lose?
- I am a child of God and God doesn't make inferior products.
- I will put all of my trust in God and lean not on my own understanding.
- Thank you God for giving me this chance to demonstrate that I have self-discipline.
- If not now – when?
- When in doubt – don't!
- Lord, accept this act of self-denial as a demonstration of my love for You.
- Every day, in every way, I am getting a little bit better.
- Carpe Diem.
- If it's to be, it's up to me.
- I can be anything I choose to be.
- Lord, may I never have enough common sense to stop.
- No pain – no gain!
- I believe in myself because God believes in me.
- By His stripes I am healed.
- The future begins today.
- Each day is a brand new beginning.
- Never surrender.
- Success is a process.
- The only way out is through.
- Only death takes away another chance.
- Everything is changeable through prayer
- I refuse to dwell on my previous mistakes.
- SHOW TIME!!

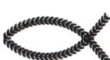

Chapter 4

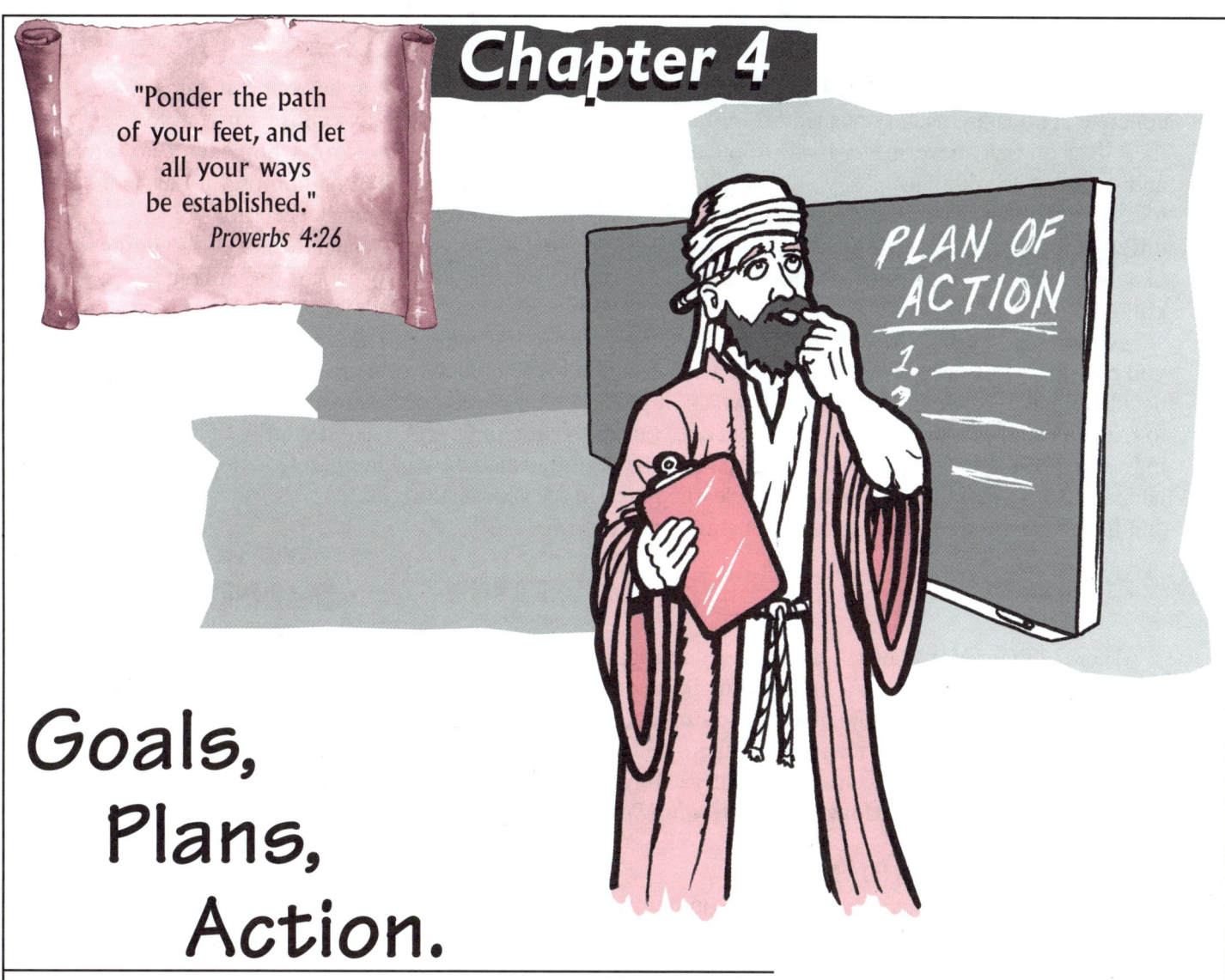

"Ponder the path of your feet, and let all your ways be established."
Proverbs 4:26

Goals, Plans, Action.

If You Fail To Plan – You Better Plan On Failing.

In the previous chapter you learned that all great achievements, all positive changes, all successes, first begin in the mind with a winner's attitude before they can ever be converted into tangible results in the real world.

"For as he thinks in his heart, so is he." (**Proverbs 23:7**)

In this chapter I am going to show you the important role that planning plays in achieving your goals. Without a good plan of attack, you will never turn your diet and health goals into reality.

"Through wisdom a house is built, and by understanding it is established." (**Proverbs 24:3**)

Can you imagine a construction company erecting a skyscraper without blueprints? Can you imagine a general leading his troops into battle without a strategy? Can you imagine God creating the world without a plan? (See **Job 37** & **38**) Yet, this is exactly how most people live their lives – ricocheting off of each new day without any sense of order, direction or planning. One week simply rolls into the next without any real attempt to impart a structure or purpose to their lives. Sure, they have some kind of hazy outline in their heads of what it is they would like to accomplish, but any concrete actions are usually pushed off into the future – indefinitely! They've chosen instead to live their lives on that "never-never land" tropical island called the *Isle of Some Day*. "Someday I'll do this and someday I'll do that." They are living their lives by accident rather than on purpose. It has been wisely stated that insanity is doing the same thing the same way every day and expecting different results. Have you fallen into this mindset? Have you convinced yourself that you're doing okay – moving forward with your life while you're really standing still – or worse yet – maybe even going backwards?

As you read through *Moses Wasn't Fat*, you are going to be faced with an important choice. Either you can finish this book, place it away on a shelf and go back to your world, or you can consciously decide to make a change right now. So what's it going to be? Action or procrastination? Are you ready to make a change? Are you ready to clean out your physical temple and make it worthy of the indwelling of the Holy Spirit? Nothing can ever be accomplished by wishing. Only action makes things happen. So if you're ready, it's time you learned how to set your health and fitness goals and follow an action plan to achieve them.

A SIX-STEP PLAN FOR SETTING YOUR GOALS

There are numerous books and audio tape programs available on goal achievement. (I think my library contains nearly every one.) But no matter how many different sources I've studied, there seems to be a recurring consistency of advice in all of them. Here now, is a six-step goal-setting strategy that I want you to study carefully and refer back to often as you follow the *Moses Diet & Health Program*.

(1) SET SPECIFIC GOALS

You can't accomplish anything if you don't really know what it is you want to do. Therefore, you need to get a pen and paper right now and make a list of all of your health and fitness goals. No one has to ever see your list so don't hold back. Put down everything you can think of no matter how far fetched it might seem to you right now. You can always edit down your list later.

But please try to be very specific rather than general. For instance, don't simply say: "I want to lose weight." Instead, say something like this: "I want to lose 15 pounds in the next six weeks." The more specific you make your goals, the easier it is to reach them. And don't forget to give yourself a target date for accomplishment wherever it's pertinent. Try to come up with a minimum of ten goals. Here are some more examples to help you compile your list:

> **a.** I will exercise a minimum of 30 minutes for four days every week.
> **b.** I will read at least one book a month on health and fitness.
> **c.** I will read the Bible for 15 minutes every evening before bed.
> **d.** I will no longer keep non-nutritious foods like diet soda, cookies, candy, cakes, fattening snacks in my home.
> **e.** I will keep my refrigerator well stocked with plenty of raw fruits and vegetables and I will eat some every single day.
> **f.** Before I consume anything, I will always ask myself this question – "Does this food help build my body temple or does it pollute it?"
> **g.** I will enroll in a natural foods cooking class within two months or less.

How To Establish Good Habits:

1. Make a big deal out of starting a new habit.
2. Once you begin, try to make no exceptions.
3. Strive to acquire good habits quickly.
4. The more times you perform a good habit, the more engrained it becomes.
5. Each time you say no to a bad habit, the stronger you become.

(2) CONSTANTLY REFER TO YOUR GOALS

Goals that are written down once and never looked at again are a total waste of time. If you are to achieve your goals, then you must constantly refer back to them. Therefore, you must write them down (by hand and not type written) and read them at least once each and every day (aloud, if possible). Don't underestimate the power of this suggestion. It works amazingly well.

Some people write their goals on 3x5 index cards and carry them with them and refer to them throughout the day. I like to write mine out on bright fluorescent index cards (available at any office supply store), keep them stacked on my desk and every hour put the bottom one on top.

If you do nothing else, I want you to promise me that you will read your list of goals every night before you go to bed.

(3) BELIEVE YOUR GOALS ARE WORTHWHILE

To keep yourself motivated and moving forward, you must believe with all your heart that the goals you have listed are worthy goals to achieve. This should be easy for you since everything about the *Moses Diet & Health Program* is geared to making your body temple worthy of God's Spirit.

"Delight yourself also in the LORD, and He shall give you the desires of your heart." **(Psalm 37:4)**

(4) BELIEVE YOUR GOALS ARE TRULY ACHIEVABLE

While goals may often be difficult to accomplish, nevertheless, they should always be realistically achievable.

"All things are possible to him who believes." **(Mark 9:23)**

If the goals you wrote down in step one are too unrealistic, then you are simply setting yourself up for frustration and failure. If you've listed something simply because it sounds nice or you think it's the kind of goal you're supposed to have, then that's not really a goal. For instance, a goal to exercise two hours every day or to read the whole Bible in a month would be unrealistic.

(5) HAVE FAITH THAT GOD WILL PROVIDE WHATEVER THINGS ARE NECESSARY TO ACHIEVE YOUR GOAL

Once you make a commitment to reach a worthwhile goal, you put supernatural forces in motion to help you achieve it. Be constantly on the lookout for new ideas, inspirations and unanticipated circumstances that seem to appear almost miraculously to help push you towards your goal.

"Commit your way to the LORD, trust also in Him, and He shall bring it to pass." **(Psalm 37:5)**

(6) STRIVE FOR PERFECTION BUT BE HAPPY WITH ON-GOING IMPROVEMENTS

As you strive to achieve your new health and fitness goals, keep the thought in mind of the perfect person God wants you to be.

"Therefore you shall be perfect, just as your Father in heaven is perfect." **(Matthew 5:48)**

Nevertheless, be aware that true perfection is something that is reserved for those who make it into the coming Kingdom of God. Therefore, since perfection is hopefully awaiting you at a future date, keep striving for constant improvement now – it's the next best thing. And what ever you do, never fall victim to the all-or-nothing mentality that believes if you can't be perfect, why bother at all. Instead stay focused on your steady improvements. They're all that really matter.

NEXT YOU NEED A PLAN FOR REACHING YOUR GOALS

Now you've got some goals to strive for. So far – so good! That already puts you among a very select group of people on this earth. What you need next is a plan – a step-by-step process to follow that will turn your goals into reality. But don't be dismayed. It's easier than you think.

(1) BREAK EACH GOAL DOWN INTO A SERIES OF MINI-STEPS

There's an old saying that says even an elephant can be eaten one fork at a time. And so it is with your goals. When you only look at the end goals alone, then they may often seem overwhelming. The trick is to break them down into a series of smaller steps. Then, rather than focusing on the bigger challenge, you can now proceed one mini-step at a time. Keep knocking off the mini-steps and guess what? You eventually reach your goal. It almost sounds too easy, doesn't it? Well let's look at an example.

Suppose one of your goals is to run a mile in 10 minutes or less within three months (12 weeks). And suppose further that you haven't run in several years. You accept the goal as believable, worthwhile and achievable. Now what? Mini-steps. You want to list as many mini-steps as you can because the more you list the more it enables you to continue your forward progress. Your mini-step list might look something like this:

1. buy a good pair of running shoes
2. buy a good pair of running shorts and top
3. buy a stop watch
4. find a local track to run around
5. decide what time of day to run and then stick to it
6. buy running magazines and cut out photos for inspiration
7. set up a notebook for keeping time and distance
8. write the main goal and all of the mini-step goals down on 3x5 index cards
9. carry the goal cards every day and read once every hour
10. WEEK ONE: walk one mile (four laps) every other day. Target time 25 minutes or less
11. WEEK TWO: walk one mile every day for six days. Rest on seventh day. Target time 25 minutes or less
12. WEEK THREE: run one lap, walk one lap. Repeat this sequence four times. No time goal set. (6 days, rest 1)
13. WEEK FOUR: run two laps in 7 minutes or less then walk one lap. Repeat sequence. (6 days, rest 1)
14. WEEK FIVE: run three laps in 12 minutes or less then walk one lap. Repeat sequence. (6 days, rest 1)
15. WEEK SIX: run four laps in 15 minutes or less then walk one lap. Repeat sequence. (6 days, rest 1)
16. WEEK SEVEN: run five laps in 18 minutes or less then walk one lap. Run two more laps in 6.5 minutes or less and walk one lap. (run 2 – rest 1; run 2 – rest 2)
17. WEEK EIGHT: run six laps in 20 minutes or less then walk one lap. Run two more laps in 7 minutes or less and walk one lap. (run 2 – rest 1; run 2 – rest 2)
18. WEEK NINE: run eight laps in 25 minutes or less and walk one lap. (Every other day, rest seventh day)
19. WEEK TEN: run eight laps in 23 minutes or less on first day and run four laps in 12 minutes or less on next day. Repeat this cycle three times this week.

> *The secret to accomplishment is to get started and the secret to getting started is to break a complex or overwhelming task into small, manageable tasks and then start on the first one.*

20. WEEK ELEVEN: run eight laps in 21.5 minutes or less on first day and run four laps in 11 minutes or less on next day. Repeat this cycle three times this week.
21. WEEK TWELVE: run eight laps in 20.5 minutes or less on first day and run four laps in 10 minutes or less on next day.
*** GOAL ACHIEVED! ***

Do you see how easy and logical that is? Rather than fret over the bigger goal, you simply have to meet each week's smaller goals and then let the big picture take care of itself. And by the way, if you fail to meet a mini-step goal on time, simply move everything back. Even with this delay, you will still reach your bigger goal sooner or later. Start using this mini-step technique and I guarantee you that you will reach every one of your goals. Remember – by the yard it's hard; but inch by inch it's a cinch.

(2) SET UP A RECORDING SYSTEM AND MONITOR YOUR PROGRESS

In order to get the most out of your goal quests and the mini-step program, you are going to need some way of recording your progress. I have found that a three-ring notebook with separate column or graph paper for each goal works best.

And here's another great tip. Rather than writing down each mini-step as you complete it, list each of them ahead of time. Now every time you complete a mini-step, run a yellow highlight marker through the listing. Something about seeing the yellow lines adding up and progressing towards the bigger goal serves as a great motivator.

Don't forget to review each separate goal sheet in your progress book every day whether there has been movement or not. This will force you to account to yourself for your actions or non-actions. Never skip a day and don't rely on your memory. You must be able to see the steady progress you are making daily. Without this type of feedback and accountability you will have neither the incentive to keep progressing nor any way to know how you are really doing. Remember – something committed to writing is more apt to be completed.

(3) RE-EVALUATE AS OFTEN AS NECESSARY

No matter how diligently you think your goals through and organize your plans, you are still going to have to constantly evaluate where you are at, how you are doing, should you add new goals, rewrite or discard current ones. Don't ever feel guilty or ashamed about making changes to your goals. This is just a normal part of all accomplishment. Did you know that airplane pilots must make hundreds of flight corrections during the course of a flight in order to reach their destination? They don't simply point the plane in the desired direction and hang on. And it's the same way when you're driving a car. Notice it next time. You will make constant adjustments to the steering wheel in order to stay on the road. Reaching your goals is just like that. You will always be making adjustments, corrections and changes on the way to your destination. This is the way anyone who has ever succeeded has done it.

(4) BE DOGGEDLY PERSISTENT

Once you have established worthwhile goals, don't let anything stand in your way. Commit all of your energy and resolve to making them come true. Learn to fight discouragement and overcome all setbacks. Trust in the LORD with all your heart and trust in your own abilities and greatness to succeed.

"Come unto Me, all you that labor and are heavy laden, and I will give you rest."
(Matthew 11:28)

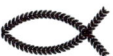

Chapter 5

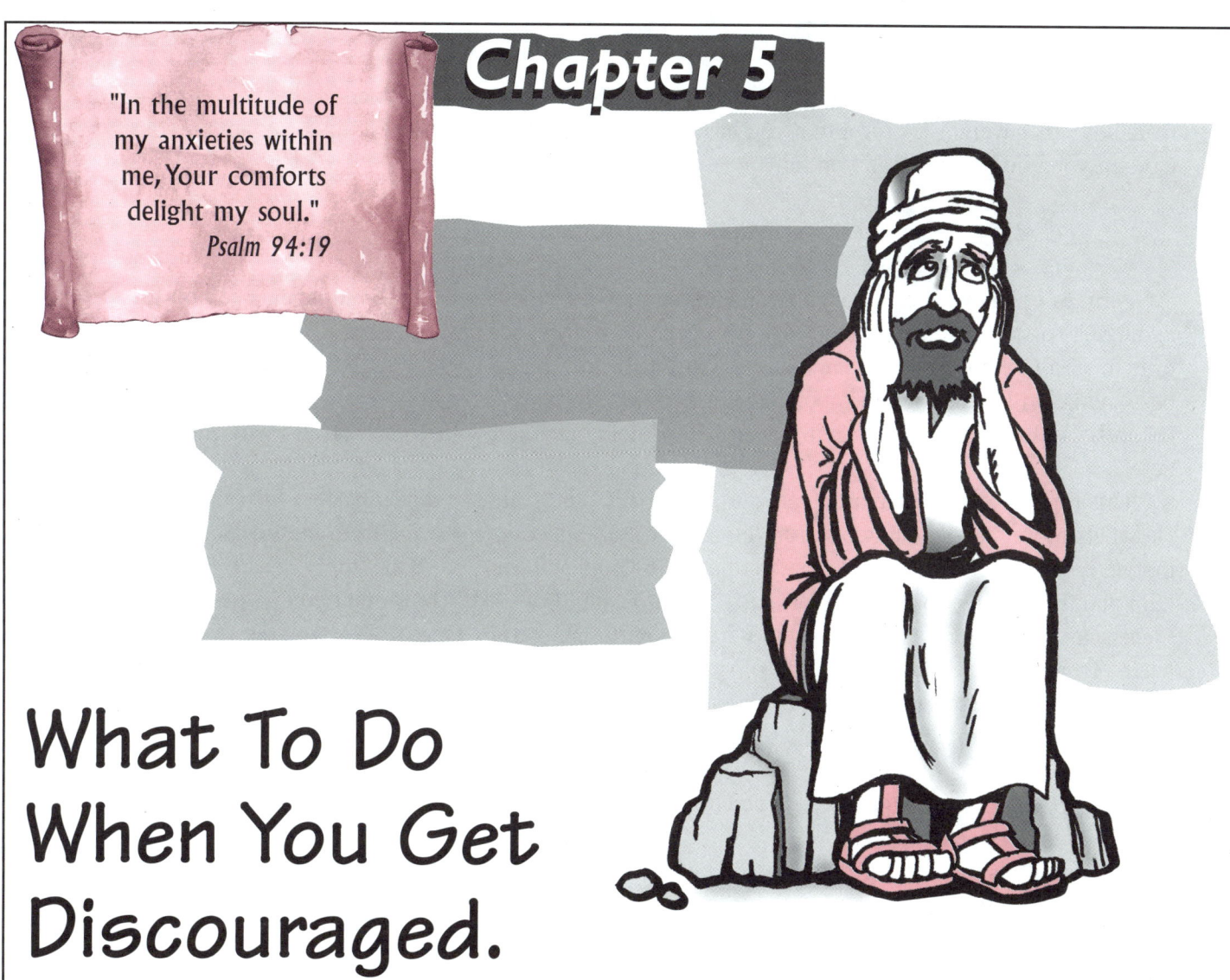

"In the multitude of my anxieties within me, Your comforts delight my soul."
Psalm 94:19

What To Do When You Get Discouraged.

You Never Fail Until You Stop Trying!

There are two things you absolutely must have in order to succeed on this program – *enthusiasm* and *motivation*. I cannot stress enough to you how much enthusiasm and motivation will be the two key elements for making your success strategy work. Granted just about everyone starts a new diet program with plenty of enthusiasm and motivation. (Think about all those New Year's resolutions.) The trick, however, is to stay enthusiastic and motivated in order to continue progressing towards your goals. It is sustained enthusiasm and sustained motivation that separate achievers from dreamers, winners from losers.

Yet, no matter how motivated and enthusiastic you are, no matter how diligently you plan, no matter how determined you are to succeed, no matter how many promises you make to yourself and to God, there are going to be times when you will get discouraged. There are going to be times when you will experience setbacks. This is just an unavoidable part of all successful achievement programs. Winners know this, anticipate it, and make plans to work around it. If you believe the ***Moses Diet & Health Program's*** road to success will be smooth sailing with no bumps along the way, then you have already set yourself up for a crash. Life is a series of ups and downs. Once you understand this, you can be ready for the downs when they come and you will already have a plan in place to work through them. This is wisdom.

First of all, keep in mind that the ***Moses Diet & Health Program*** outlined in this book is different from any other weight loss program you have ever seen. Significantly, with this program you have God on your side so how can you fail?

"If God is for us, who can be against us?" **(Romans 8:31)**

Perhaps you have tried other programs in the past with the greatest intentions, only to quit in agonizing frustration. Forget the past. It's over! Don't let your past attempts discourage you. It's time to stop looking backward and start looking forward. Satan wants you to be obsessed with your past and he will forever try to sabotage your current efforts by constantly reminding you of your failures. As long as you keep trying, then God is not concerned with your past. So why should you be?

This time you will be breaking new ground. This time you have a new partner in your corner and He wants more than anything else for you to succeed. Success will come from the supernatural power that enters your life when you accept God as your "personal trainer." You simply need to have faith in Him and the courage to ask Him for help. You are a child of God. He formed you in the womb. **(Jeremiah 1:5)** He is waiting for you to call on Him. He will be there to give you the strength you need. Trust in Him. The Bible is full of stories of ordinary people who put their trust in God and went on to accomplish extraordinary achievements. Have faith in Him for that faith will let you face all of your discouragement and all of your setbacks and still be victorious.

"All things work together for good to those who love God." **(Romans 8:28)**

While faith is the starting point, it's going to take a special, *proactive* faith to reach your goals. Your faith must go beyond a passive trust in God. Your faith must be more than just believing. You need to turn your belief into action.

"Faith without works is dead." **(James 2:20)**

Do you recall the story of the woman with the blood issue in the New Testament? **(Mark 5:25)** She had faith that Yahshua (Jesus) could heal her but it was only when she took action and reached out and touched his garment that she was healed. Now it's time for you to reach out and touch His garment. Once you begin the ***Moses Diet & Health Program***, a miracle work will be underway in your body. Never let doubt or discouragement defeat you. These negatives come from Satan. He hates it when God's children begin a temple cleansing process. He is so confident that he can beat you that he is expecting you to quit after just a few setbacks. What he doesn't know is that this time you are going to use God's help to outlast him. **This time he loses**.

"When you pass through the waters, I will be with you; and through the rivers, they shall not overflow you. When you walk through the fire, you shall not be burned. Nor shall the flame scorch you. For I am the LORD your God, the Holy One of Israel, your Savior." **(Isaiah 43:2-3)**

WHAT IS THIS THING CALLED FAILURE?

First of all, I want you to forget everything you have ever learned about failure because there is really no such thing. It is totally an invention of the devil. I want you to erase the word "failure" from your vocabulary. I don't ever want you to use it again. Instead, from this moment on, I want you to use the word "setback." And please don't ever confuse a setback with a failure. You learn from setbacks. You quit with a failure. A setback can only become a failure if you let it. Thus, you are never really a failure as long as you keep on trying. Yes, you are going to have setbacks; but you must learn to see them as minor glitches that help get you to your goal. And yes, you will make some mistakes along the way; but understand that some of our greatest learning comes from the mistakes we make. Try to focus on and celebrate your progress, no matter how gradual it might be, rather than beating yourself up over temporary setbacks. And most importantly, you must never allow yourself to fail.

A 12 POINT PLAN FOR DEALING WITH SETBACKS

(1) When you suffer a setback or a make a mistake, let it go as quickly as possible. Just say to yourself: "It's OVER!" and then move on.
(2) Setbacks dwelled upon quickly become failures. Therefore, never dwell on your past mistakes or setbacks. The past is over the second that you cut it loose.
(3) See conquered setbacks as something that actually makes you stronger.
(4) See a setback as a chance to start again with a fresh new resolve and renewed vigor.
(5) Your chance of success is going to be in direct proportion to the number of times you have a set back and keep on trying.
(6) If you dwell on your previous setbacks, you are destined to repeat them. Instead, dwell on God's grace, your plan, and your goal.
(7) Strive to re-ignite your original desire as quickly as possible after a setback.
(8) Remember that regardless of how many setbacks you encounter, the future is always a clean slate.
(9) Never have enough "common sense" to stop.
(10) Accept God as your partner and "personal trainer" and then place your trust in Him during periods of setback.
(11) Write down your goals and read them daily, and let nothing ever deter you from reaching them.
(12) Always remember how the Success Shuffle works. "Three steps forward and one step back." You're never going to change it. That's just the way things work. So you might as well learn to live with it.

MISCELLANEOUS THOUGHTS ON FAILURE, SETBACKS AND SUCCESS

- Mistakes are only mistakes when they are repeated.
- It is far better to temporarily fail in a cause that will succeed than to temporarily succeed in a cause that will fail.
- Beware of the temptation to quit too early.
- Death is the only thing that takes away another chance.
- Persistence is that little voice you hear at the end of the day that says, "I'll try again tomorrow."
- Before you can get it perfect, you will make several imperfect starts.
- You may be disappointed if you fail – but you're doomed if you don't try.
- For some people, their fear of failure is stronger than their desire to succeed.
- God did not create us to fail.
- Stagnation is worse than failure.
- It's not how hard you fall but how far you bounce back.
- All growth comes with setbacks.

- No matter where you have been, no matter what you have done, you can always start over.
- Regardless of the past, your future is always a clean slate.
- What to do when you make a mistake:
    (1) admit it
    (2) learn from it
    (3) don't repeat it
- There really are no mistakes. Only lessons.
- Failure is never an option.
- <u>The Law of Persistence</u>: you may try and you may fail but the more you try, the more you increase your chances of success.
- A winner is just a dreamer who has never given up.
- You can always spot people who have given up. They're the ones who tell you what could have been or what was.
- Even failure is noteworthy in a great attempt.

> **"Failure is only an opportunity to more intelligently begin again."**
>
> *-Henry Ford*

IMPORTANCE OF POSITIVE, SUPPORTIVE PEOPLE

Whereas God is the author of individuality, Satan is the author of collectivism – the herd mentality. His philosophy is flawed. "You've got to go along to get along, don't rock the boat, everybody else does it this way." You can always spot those underachievers who have bought into his logic. They want to look like, act like, dress like, live like and be like everyone else. Hence, the world is in no short supply of collective thinking naysayers – negative people who will try to sabotage your health plans by telling you that you will never succeed.

Therefore, you must learn to classify the people in your life into two groups: those who encourage and support you to make progress and reach your goals, and those who discourage and distract you from accomplishing your goals. It goes without saying that you need to avoid as much as possible those negative, "toxic" people who would hinder your progress. Those who do not build you up will inevitably pull you down. Words have the power to encourage you or discourage you. A few negative words from a family member or friend may be all it takes to derail your well-intentioned efforts. Instead, try to get your family members behind you. Tell them how much this program means to you. Ask for their help and encouragement. A simple word of reassurance from a loved one may be just enough to keep you going.

The worth of any relationship should be measured by the contribution it makes to helping you attain the goals you have established for your life. Remember – ultimately it's not what others believe that matters – it's what you believe.

"All things are possible to him who believes." **(Mark 9:23)**

Hence, if the ***Moses Diet & Health Program*** is to succeed for you, then the way you feel should never be influenced by the thoughts in someone else's head. You may not be able to change those people who upset you, but you can surely change how you react to them. Just be careful that you don't blame others for your own shortcomings.

And perhaps by persevering and reaching your goals, your success and newfound level of health and fitness may be just the spark needed to motivate your detractors to change their lives. God does work in strange ways. He may actually use your achievements as the instrument to touch their hearts.

IMPORTANT NOTE: This chapter may very well be the most important one in the whole book because if you allow any setback to become a failure, then you run the risk of quitting the whole program. Therefore, it is imperative that you re-read it every time you have a setback. This is not a suggestion. It is an order! Always remember that hope springs eternal. There is a light behind every shadow. There can be no shadow unless a light is shining somewhere. Always have the perseverance to ride out each and every setback. God created you with the strength to handle every obstacle you will ever encounter. Ask Him for His guidance and then trust in your abilities to listen to Him. God has a better tomorrow waiting for you. Don't quit! Don't get discouraged! Give God and this program the time they both need to work a miracle in your life. I know that with God's help, you will find the courage to overcome all setbacks. With God on your side, you cannot fail. Just look to the rainbow He put in the sky and know that His word and His promises are eternal.

The Road To Success

You failed many times in your life although you may not remember some of them.

- The first time you tried to walk, you fell down.
- The first time you tried to talk, you could hardly make a sound.
- The first time you dressed yourself, you may have looked like a clown.
  BUT YOU DIDN'T GIVE UP!
- Did you hit the ball the first time you swung a bat?
- Did you make a cartwheel the first time you tried that?
- Did you jerk the car the first time you drove stick shift?

Sometimes the greatest in their field also suffer the most setbacks.

- Albert Einstein was four years old before he could speak.
- Isaac Newton was a poor student and called "unpromising."
- Beethoven's music teacher once called him hopeless as a composer.
- While working in a dry goods store at 21, F.W. Woolworth was not permitted to wait on customers because he was told he "didn't have enough sense to close a sale."
- Professional basketball stars Bob Cousy and Michael Jordan were both cut from their high school basketball teams.
- Walt Disney was once fired by a newspaper editor who claimed he "lacked imagination and had no good ideas."
- Winston Churchill failed sixth grade.
- Babe Ruth struck out 1,330 times, but he also hit 714 home runs.
- R. H. Macy failed seven times before his store in New York became successful.
- Abraham Lincoln ran for public office several times unsuccessfully before being elected President of the United States.
- Thomas Edison experimented with hundreds of substances to place inside the light bulb before coming upon tungsten.

All successful people will suffer setbacks on their journey. That's just part of life. Don't despair over your setbacks. Instead, think about all of the chances for achievement you miss if you don't even try.

Don't Quit

When things go wrong as they sometimes will,
When the road you're trudging seems all up hill,
When the funds are low and the debts are high,
And you want to smile but you have to sigh,
When care is pressing you down a bit,
Rest if you must, but don't you quit.

Life is queer with its twists and turns,
As everyone of us sometimes learns,
And many a failure turns about,
When we might have won had we stuck it out;
Don't give up though the pace seems slow,
You may succeed with another blow.

Success is failure turned inside out,
The silver tint of the clouds of doubt.
And you never can tell how close you are,
It may be near when it seems so far;
So stick to the fight when you're hardest hit,
It's when things seem their worst that you must not quit.

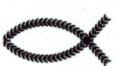

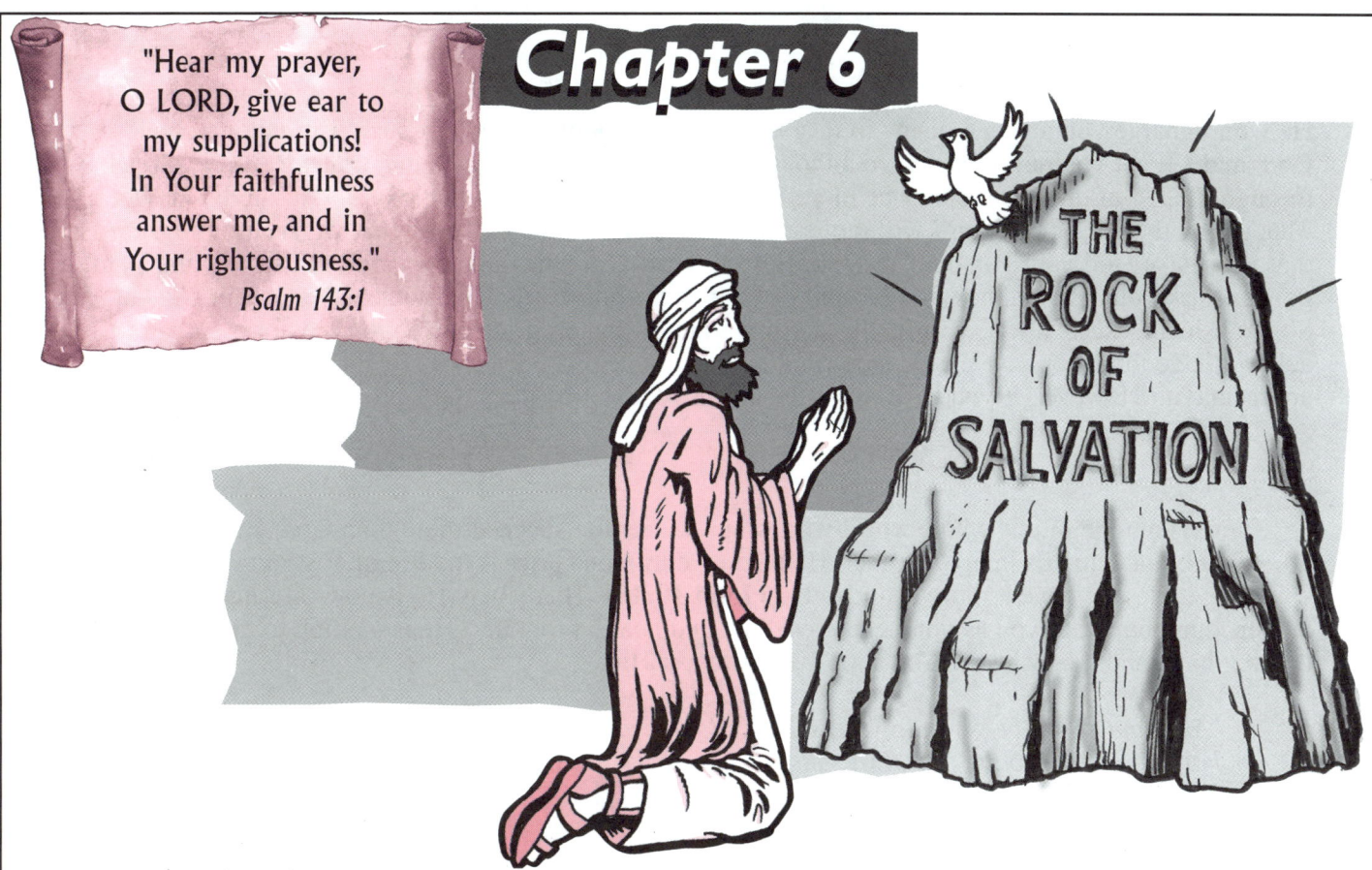

"Hear my prayer, O LORD, give ear to my supplications! In Your faithfulness answer me, and in Your righteousness."
Psalm 143:1

Health & Fitness Through Faith & Prayer.

The LORD Is Waiting For You To Call Upon Him. He Will Lead You To Success When You Make Him Your "Personal Trainer."

Have you noticed how fashionable it is these days to have a personal trainer? Hollywood stars, professional athletes, politicians – everyone's got their own personal trainer. And if you've ever heard any of these people talk about their personal trainers, you will immediately notice how much they credit their progress and success to their trainer.

So what makes a good personal trainer? If you were out shopping around today for your own personal trainer, just what qualifications would you be looking for? Your list might look something like this.

1. extensive knowledge
2. motivational
3. easy to talk to
4. understanding
5. reliable
6. trustworthy
7. patient
8. forgiving
9. accessible
10. supportive
11. practice what they teach

Wouldn't you agree that if you found a personal trainer with all of these attributes, that person could play an important role in your health and fitness program? Would you not be tempted to immediately hire that person?

Well, the good news is that there indeed is such a personal trainer available to you right now and He won't charge you a single penny to take you on as a "client." Yes, of course I'm talking about God, and I'll bet you never even gave a thought to making Him your personal trainer? But just read through the list of qualifications once more. Does He not meet every single one? Assuredly He does. That's why the very first thing I will request of you in following the **Moses Diet & Health Program** is that you make God your Personal Trainer. Before we take another step forward in this program, I am going to ask you here and now to place all of your faith and trust in God your Father and in His faithful Son Yahshua (Jesus Christ). This is the starting point of this program and if you are not prepared to acknowledge this, then you should stop right now and give this book away to someone who would appreciate it. However, if you have made this acknowledgement, then let's proceed.

GOD WANTS YOU TO SUCCEED

There is no one in this whole world who wants to see you succeed more than God, Himself. After all, you are made in His image. In fact, He paid an enormous price – the life of His Son – so that you could have life and have it more abundantly. **(John 10:10)** That's why He is now offering His support and encouragement to you as you begin your diet and health program. He is waiting to give you a helping hand and a new heart. You simply have to ask Him.

> *"Ask, and it will be given to you; seek, and you will find; knock, and it will be opened to you. For everyone who asks receives, and he who seeks finds, and to him who knocks, it will be opened."* **(Matthew 7:7-8)**

When God becomes involved in your life, your victory is assured.

> *"Thanks be to God, who gives us the victory through our Lord Jesus Christ."*
> **(1 Corinthians 15:57)**

The important point is that the victory comes through Him when you learn to trust Him and allow Him to give you the strength you need to succeed. Yes, you can do all things through Christ who strengthens you. **(Philippians 4:13)** And as you learn to trust in God, He will lead you from strength to strength rather than from weakness to weakness.

> *"Yet in all these things we are more than conquerors through Him who loved us."*
> **(Romans 8:37)**

As you begin to entrust your life to your Personal Trainer, He is going to help you do what you cannot do alone. There is no obstacle too big to stop Him and there is no problem He cannot solve. You need to open your heart and your mind to His instructions and He will come and teach you.

> *"The LORD is near to all who call upon Him, to all who call upon Him in truth."*
> **(Psalm 145:18)**

God knows the heartache you have experienced trying to do it on your own. If you have tried other diet and health programs and failed, just let it go. This time it's going to be different. This time you have a new Trainer in your corner. This time you cannot fail.

> *"With God all things are possible."* **(Matthew 19:26)**

This time you are going to let God become totally involved in what you are doing. And when He comes to your aid, He brings all of the power of heaven along with Him. How can you possibly fail with this kind of support?

LORD, TEACH US TO PRAY

Now that I've hopefully convinced you to bring God aboard as your Personal Trainer, the question is, how do you ask Him and how do you access His help? There is only one way and that is through prayer. It will be through your prayers that you will open up the entry point for God's instructions and guidance into your life.

But before we get into the specifics of praying I want to take a minute to share with you just how powerful prayer can be especially when it comes to your health and well being. There have been many studies conducted recently that have demonstrated that people who pray regularly not only recover faster from illnesses, but also tend to be healthier. According to Dr. Larry Dossey, author of the book **Healing Words: The Power of Prayer**, (Harper) and the former chief of staff at Medical City Hospital in Dallas, "prayer is not just a matter of illusion or belief. It really works." Dr. Dossey has spent the last 15 years of his life collecting literature and research on prayer. "Prayer has been studied in the lab and experiments show results aren't due to coincidence or chance. There are things the mind can do that the brain and body can't," he states.

Supporting Dr. Dossey's research is Dr. Herbert Benson, a professor at Harvard Medical School who reports that through prayer you can actually change the way your body works, triggering a specific set of physiological changes. "If prayer were a drug we wouldn't be able to make it fast enough," Benson further notes.

One recent study found that consistent praying actually has the power to lower the heart rate, slow respiration and brain wave activity, reduce blood pressure, relieve anxiety and in some cases even help patients avoid surgery.

Another study in Maryland of 100,000 regular churchgoers found that they had fifty percent fewer deaths from coronary artery disease as well as fifty-six percent fewer emphysema deaths.

A recent Gallup poll measuring the degree of people's happiness found that more than half the people surveyed who read the Bible daily or weekly and attended church regularly said they were very happy.

And you can also add a longer life span to the list of benefits for those who pray and attend church services regularly. That's the finding of two decades worth of research conducted by the National Institute for Health Care Research (NIHR) which tested for a correlation between religious activity and longevity. "People who actively participate in religious activities like going to church regularly, tend to live longer," said Dr. David B. Larson, president of NIHR. "It's about 30 percent more for men and 60 percent for women," he added. Interestingly, it didn't seem to matter to which denomination the subjects went.

A study of the success rate of drug treatment centers in Texas showed that 45 percent of patients in religious drug treatment centers were able to successfully break their drug habit, compared to a meager five percent success rate in secular, state run centers.

There is no doubt that there is great power in prayer. Yahshua (Jesus) knew this when He said:

> *"Have faith in God for assuredly I say to you, whoever says to this mountain, 'Be removed and be cast into the sea,' and does not doubt in his heart, but believes those things he says will be done, he will have whatever he says. Therefore I say to you, whatever things you ask when you pray, believe that you receive them, and you will have them."* **(Mark 11: 22-24)**

I am sure that many of you reading this book already have a strong prayer life and this is good. For you, I will shortly address the issue of how to properly pray to the LORD for help and guidance in your diet and health program. But first I want to speak to those of you who are unaccustomed to praying and perhaps feel a bit uneasy about this whole subject. As I stated earlier, prayer is going to be a big part of this program. You must learn to integrate daily prayer into your life in order to stay with a lifelong health program. Remember this – prayerless people are powerless people.

First of all, you do not have to feel awkward or self-conscious when you pray since you will be doing it in complete privacy. Your prayers are going to be a private and personal matter between you and God. In fact, Yahshua (Jesus) told us to pray in exactly that manner:

> *"But you, when you pray, go into your room, and when you have shut your door, pray to your Father who is in the secret place; and your Father who sees in secret will reward you openly."* **(Matthew 6:6)**

If you have not been praying because you really aren't sure how to go about it, rest assured that it is nowhere near as difficult as you may be imagining. In just a minute I will show you how easy it really is. But before we go there, let me explain what prayer is all about.

There are two main types of prayer – *ritualistic prayer* and *personal prayer*. Unfortunately, many people are familiar only with the first type. Ritualistic prayer is what people usually do in church. It is formalized, methodic and often formulaic. It is most often accompanied by kneeling, clasped hands and bowed heads. While ritualistic prayer has its place, it is not the type of prayer you will be doing with this program. Instead, on this program you are going to have, one-on-one, personal, intimate discussions with the LORD. I want you to tell Him about your hopes, your dreams, your worries, your fears and your anxieties. Remember – He is your Personal Trainer. He can't help you if you aren't honest with Him. Think of it more as a conversation rather than "prayer." Talk to God as you would to your very best friend for He is precisely that. Pour out your heart to Him and don't be afraid to tell Him how you are doing. Yes, He already knows but the very act of your telling Him enables Him to come into your life and assist you. Tell Him what's on your mind. If you have slipped, simply ask Him to give you strength and courage to continue. Don't try to ignore your shortcomings. And most importantly of all, when you slip up or have a bad day don't feel too ashamed to pray. That's the time you will need God the most. He has a lot invested in you. After all, what personal trainer wants their student to fail? You must never be afraid to talk to the LORD. Open your heart and your soul to His wisdom and understanding and He will find a way to reach you. Believe this with your whole heart for it is the truth. Everything is changeable through prayer.

By all means tell Him your hopes and dreams and desires. But your prayers to God must not be about wishing, fantasizing, hoping, or dreaming that God will do all of the work for you. You can't ask Him to perform a "miracle" without any effort on your part. This is the wrong way to pray. No personal trainer can wave a magic wand and instantly get you into shape. You need to follow his program. Well it's the same with God. You must ask God to give you the strength to reach your goals but then you have to do your part.

WHEN AND HOW TO PRAY

Of course, you can and should pray to God as often as you think of Him but the two times you absolutely must pray in order for this program to be effective are first thing in the morning and the last thing at night. Every morning in prayer you will renew your commitment to God to live according to His laws – both spiritual and physical. You must ask Him to give you the strength and determination to stay focused on your goals. And you must tell Him that you trust in Him to help you through your day.

Every evening, just before retiring, you must review your day with Him and thank Him for being with you. Acknowledge where you succeeded and where you slipped. Recommit yourself to your goals and ask Him to let a good night's sleep prepare you for your next day's challenges.

Here now are two sample prayers that you can either use as they are or feel free to alter to fit your personal needs.

A Morning Prayer

Heavenly Father – Author of Life – I give You all honor and glory as this majestic day begins, for it was Your wisdom and divine intellect which brought forth the very first day. And it was You Father, who formed Adam from the dust of the earth and shaped him into your image and likeness. And it was You who breathed into Adam and made him a living soul. And it was You who provided everything that he needed to be healthy and strong:

- **+ nutritious, whole food,**
- **+ crystal clear Living Water,**
- **+ clean, fresh air,**
- **+ and radiant, invigorating sunshine.**

So now I come before You, O great Creator, through the body and blood of my Lord and Savior Yahshua (Jesus Christ), and ask that You allow these same elements of food, water, air and sunshine to enter my body and make me grow in both health and strength so that I may become a worthy Temple for Your Holy Spirit.

Guide my actions today so that I do nothing injurious to this body that You have entrusted to me. Help me to make the right choices in the quantity and types of food that I consume. Let nothing pass into or out of my mouth that does not magnify and glorify Your Temple.

Let me drink freely of Your clean, life-sustaining water and as I do so, let it remind me of the day when I will drink of the Everlasting Waters that come from the throne of Heaven.

Forgive me for any wrongs I may have committed in the past against my body and give me the strength and motivation to always keep it worthy of Your indwelling. I pray also that You keep me from sickness, disease, and bodily weakness and deliver me from the evil temptations of the son of darkness.

For the Heavens are Yours, and the Earth is Yours, and my body is Yours, as it was in the beginning, is now and ever shall be, into the coming age of Shalom.
Amen

An Evening Prayer

Heavenly Father and Most High Lord, as this day now draws to a close, I want to say Thank You for all of the blessings You have given me today. Thank You also Father for watching over me and protecting me from harm. Thank You for giving me the courage and determination to pursue all of my goals – both those that strengthen me spiritually and those that strengthen me physically.

Thank You also for dwelling with me today for without You in me I am as the grass that blows aimlessly in the wind or the clouds that float purposelessly in the sky.

But because You love me Father, You have allowed the blood of Your Son, Yahshua (Jesus Christ), to redeem me from sin and death. Therefore, may I always prove worthy of such a great gift.

Father, You know my heart before I even speak, so You already know how much I want my body to be a worthy dwelling place for Your Holy Spirit. Thank You for guiding my actions and leading me to make the difficult but right choices. I know that with Your divine guidance, even though I may stumble, I will ultimately succeed in purifying my body temple and make it worthy of Your indwelling.

Let the ending of this day remind me that all things must pass – including me. Yet even now I reach for everlasting life as I recall the words of Your Son, my King Yahshua (Jesus), who said that Heaven and Earth would pass away but His words would never pass away. And His words were the words of eternal life.

Therefore, even though my days on this Earth are numbered, I will still do all in my power to keep both my body and my soul holy and pure until I breathe my last breath.

My Father, I praise Your sweet and Holy Name and pledge my complete love to You for as long as there is life within my body.
Amen

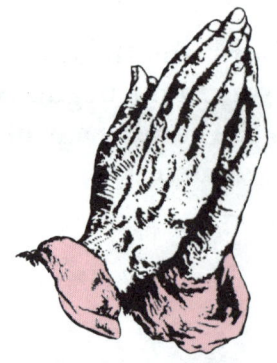

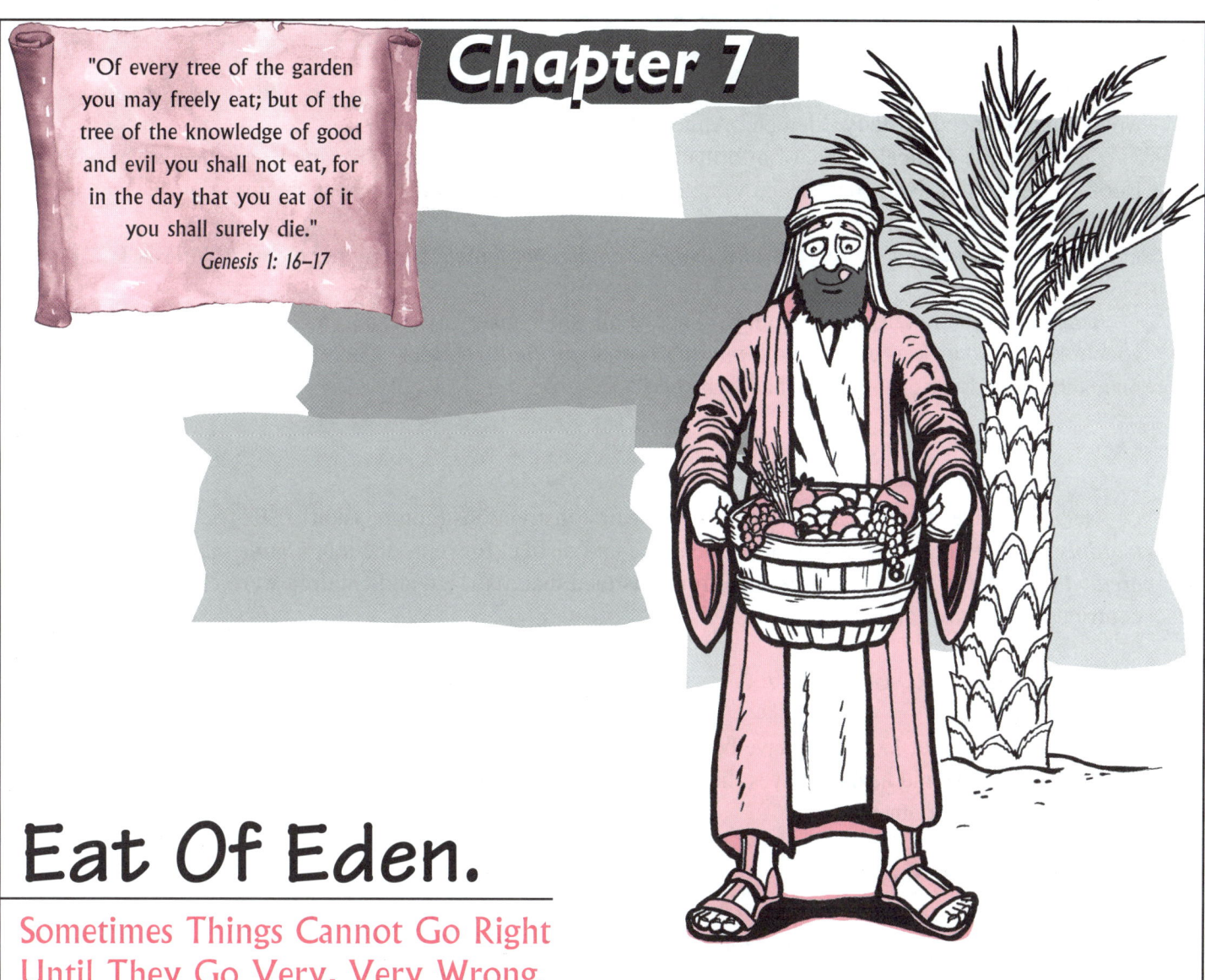

> "Of every tree of the garden you may freely eat; but of the tree of the knowledge of good and evil you shall not eat, for in the day that you eat of it you shall surely die."
> Genesis 1: 16-17

Chapter 7

Eat Of Eden.

Sometimes Things Cannot Go Right Until They Go Very, Very Wrong.

Have you ever wondered why God designed our bodies so that we must eat to stay alive? Have you ever really thought about the act of eating? I mean really sat there and pondered why it is that two or three times per day, for each and every day of your life, you must take external material called food, place it through a slit in the front of your head and then swallow it down inside your body? It sounds kind of strange when you look at it like that, doesn't it? Yet that is exactly what each and every one of us must do to stay alive. But why? Couldn't God have designed us in a different way? The answers to these questions are very important to the conclusions drawn in *Moses Wasn't Fat*.

EDEN WAS PERFECTION

Before answering them, I am going to first state a premise that is consistently maintained throughout this book. ***Everything physiological about Adam and Eve in the Garden of Eden before they sinned was exactly the way God ideally intended it to be for all of us and it is the way we shall be once again in the Kingdom of God. Eden was not some temporary abode for the man and the woman, a brief holdover tank from which they would later be removed. Eden was to be their home forever and <u>everything about their bodies was perfectly designed in order for them to continue</u>***

dwelling there. Therefore, if we want to know what is absolutely best for our health, physiology and well being, we need to study Eden before the fall.

Our principle biblical source of information for this study is found in the first three chapters of the Book of Genesis. It is in chapter one verse 27 that we first meet God's highest creation.

> *"So God created man in His own image. . . male and female He created them."* **(Genesis 1:27)**

This immediately tells us two things. First of all, since man was created in God's image, we can conclude that Adam was created both *physically* and *spiritually* perfect. Therefore, everything about man and his body prior to the fall had to be perfect.

HEALTH AND THE FAMILY

Next God gives the man and the woman their first instructions (commission). *"Be fruitful and multiply."* Since their bodies were made separate and distinct for reproduction, (*"male and female He created them"*), we can properly assume from this then that marriage and children were also meant to contribute to our overall health.

> *"And the LORD God said, 'It is not good that man should be alone.'"* **(Genesis 2:18)**

And as a matter of fact, there have been numerous studies which have shown that happily married couples live longer and healthier lives than single people and that a harmonious, God-centered family is a very healthy environment.

> *"You shall be happy and it shall be well with you. Your wife shall be like a fruitful vine in the very heart of your house, your children like olive plants all around the table. Behold, thus shall the man be blessed who fears the LORD."* **(Psalm 128: 2-4)**

HEALTH AND ANIMALS

God continues in Genesis, *"fill the earth and <u>subdue</u> it; have dominion over the fish of the sea, over the birds of the air, and over every living thing that moves on the earth."* This word "subdue" is a very interesting word in Hebrew. It's **kabash** and it means *conquer, subjugate, bring into subjection, dominate.* But it is also closely related to two other Hebrew words – **kebel** and **kabar** which both carry the meaning intertwine or link together. What God was telling the man then was to bring a harmony upon the earth and intertwine all living things with him. From this it's obvious to me that Adam, and all human beings, were meant to have an intimate, loving and harmonious relationship with all of the animals. As further proof of this, God brings all the animals to Adam and has him name them (**Genesis 2:19**). Please note that the act of naming in the Bible is a very intimate and bonding event. Certainly then, meat eating had no part in the original Eden diet.

I would even go a step further and postulate that there was some form of symbiotic relationship between Adam and the animals. In other words, some sort of biological, physical, and perhaps chemical event took place between Adam and the animals when they were in contact with each other. Perhaps it was some form of electro-magnetic frequency that bonded them to each other. If so, then Adam needed to communicate with the animals for his health and perfection, and they needed to communicate with him for their health and perfection.

If I am correct in this assumption, might we also conclude that having pets today is a healthy thing to do? Not surprisingly, there actually have been some very interesting studies done which found that people who have a loving relationship with a pet are healthier and better balanced. Dog owners, for instance, live longer and suffer fewer physical and mental ailments than other people, according to Dr. Larry Dossey, author of the book *Reinventing Medicine*.

Eden's Foods

To Achieve Normal Bodyweight And Good Health, Eat Regularly From God's Eden Menu.

- Fruits
- Vegetables
- Legumes
- Beans
- Grain/Cereal
- Spices
- Seeds
- Sprouts
- Herbs
- Nuts

HEALTH AND FOOD

Immediately after God discusses the animals in Genesis, the very next topic discussed is *food*.

> *"And God said, ' See, I have given you every herb that yields seed which is on the face of all the earth, and every <u>tree</u> whose fruit yields seed; <u>to you it shall be for food</u>."*
> **(Genesis 1:29)**

Bingo!! We have now uncovered exactly what it was that perfect man was to eat before the fall in the Garden. And therefore, if we are to seek after our original Adamic perfection – and we should – (*"Therefore you shall be perfect, just as your Father in heaven is perfect."* **Matthew 5:48**), then it behooves us to find out exactly what this perfect Eden diet was. Let's find out.

Re-read Genesis 1:29 above. Notice first of all that God identifies two basic *plant* sources of nourishment for man – herbs and trees. The Hebrew word for herb is ***eseb*** which means *green, grass, tender shoot* or *herb*. Falling under this broad definition then would be a wide variety of foods including cereals (wheat, barley, rice, etc.), vegetables, beans, legumes, berry plants, herbs and spices.

Furthermore, the seed producing trees would also give us a huge variety of fruits and nuts, including two important Bible foods – grapes and olives. Not to be overlooked is the fact that God more than likely intended for us to eat even the seeds themselves since modern science is now uncovering a host of health-building factors in seeds and pits. Noticeably absent from this Eden menu, however, is any form of animal products (meat, fish, milk, dairy, eggs). Also absent are food additives, artificial preservatives, colorants, fungicides, mold inhibitors, extenders, artificial flavorings – you know – the usual stuff we eat every single day of our lives.

One other key point here. The Bible mentions nothing about the use of fire, ovens, or microwaves in Eden. Might we assume then that perfect foods for perfect humans were meant to be eaten raw? More than likely yes!

DOES IT REALLY MATTER?

So now we have created a template of the perfect foods that God ordained for perfect man's original Eden diet. The question is this. Is there merit to still eating this way or doesn't it really matter anymore? Many Bible scholars will present strong arguments that it really doesn't matter anymore. We have been saved by the blood of Yahshua (Jesus), they reason, so worrying about the foods we eat or don't eat smacks of "legalism" and only distracts us from the free gift of salvation that God has graciously bestowed on us.

Can they be right? Do they really mean to say that what we eat doesn't matter anymore? Does a high fat diet of over processed and over chemicalized junk foods really not matter anymore? Just bless it all in the name of Yahshua (Jesus)! Is it true that God doesn't care what we eat as long as we accept Yahshua (Jesus) as our Savior? This whole line of reasoning is absurd and has accounted for many of the health problems now confronting Christians!

Of course it matters what we eat since we now know conclusively that certain types of eating patterns can cause all kinds of illnesses and ultimately death. This being the case, then why would we not opt for the most perfect diet God ever created for man – the Eden diet? While in Eden, Adam and Eve ate freely from all of the trees including the Tree of Life (**Genesis 2:16**). In the Book of Revelation we are told that we are once again eating freely from the Tree of Life (**Revelation 22:2**). Why would we choose to eat any differently in this fallen, cursed time in between? The answer is because of our own selfishness. We have put our likes and wants and tastes and appetites ahead of what God wants. Rather than force us to live by His rules – which God never does – He is allowing us to temporarily do it our way.

WHAT ABOUT MEAT?

But didn't God tell Noah after the great flood that he and his family could now eat animal flesh?

> *"Every moving thing that lives shall be food for you. I have given you all things even as the green herbs."* (**Genesis 9:3**)

But notice what else God said after the flood.

> *"And the fear of you and the dread of you shall be on every beast of the earth, on every bird of the air, of all that move on the earth and on all the fish of the sea."* (**Genesis 9:2**)

Can you see what's happened here? Did you notice how contradictory this all is to the peace and harmony I mentioned earlier that originally existed in Eden between Adam and all of the animals? Something quite seriously wrong has now obviously taken place. This is not the world as God intended. It is a changed, fallen world. You can almost hear God saying to man, "You wanted it, now you've got it." (Some Bible scholars believe that the eating of animal flesh was one of the contributing factors to the violence that was upon the world before the flood.)

We encounter another strange phenomenon at the time of the flood when men become meat eaters. Man's life span is shortened from multiple centuries to 120 years.

> *"And the LORD said, 'My spirit shall not strive with man forever, for he is indeed flesh; yet his days shall be one hundred and twenty years.'"* (**Genesis 6:3**)

Some scholars (and nutritionists) have made the connection between eating meat and a shorter life span. I happen to agree. So what is really happening then is that both the earth and man are going through a process of *devolution* not *evolution*. Things keep getting worse not better. In fact, by the time the Psalms are written, man's life span is even shorter.

> *"The days of our lives are seventy years; and if by reason of strength they are eighty years."* (**Psalm 90:10**)

But how could it be any other way since, as we noted above, man was to be God's instrument of harmony on the earth? As man goes, so goes the earth.

YES - IT'S WORTH IT

So just ask yourself this. If you were the Almighty Creator looking down upon a world that keeps falling farther and farther away from the ideals of Eden, wouldn't you be impressed to see someone trying to live their life and keep their body as close to the original perfection of Eden as possible? Of course you would and of course He does. Those people who strive to live their lives according to the Eden formula demonstrate a deeper wisdom that is sorely lacking in the world today. Ask yourself this. Was the world a better place during Eden or today? Why then would you opt for the modern world's way rather than God's Way? Are you deluding yourself by following Satan's philosophy of selfishness? Have you been placing your needs and appetites above God's wisdom? Perhaps it was our time that God was speaking about when He said to Daniel,

> "Many shall be purified, made white, and refined, but the wicked shall do wickedly; and none of the wicked shall understand, but <u>the wise shall understand</u>." (**Daniel 12:10**)

If you are one of those people who can't really see the connection between your diet and your physical **and** spiritual well being, let me remind you of something. The very first sin committed by human beings dealt with eating the wrong food and it led to their deaths and all of ours as well. So do you still think that what we eat isn't really all that important? It's about time you start reassessing your viewpoint. God outlined a specific diet for us in Eden and only altered it because of our weaknesses – not His.

> "For I am the LORD, I do not change." (**Malachi 3:6**) It is we who have changed. "Yet from the days of your fathers you have gone away from my ordinances and have not kept them." (**Malachi 3:7**)

No, you should never take the act of eating lightly. It is a most sacred event, consecrated and blessed by God Himself. It was God who formed us from the dust (chemical elements) of the earth, (**Genesis 2:7**) just as it was God who, in His infinite wisdom, connected us eternally to the earth by the food we eat. And just as a newborn baby feeds from its mother, so too do we feed from the earth that bore us. It is an unbreakable bond that extends from now straight into the Kingdom of God. Even Yahshua (Jesus) referenced this on the night before He died.

> "I will not drink of this fruit of the vine from now on until that day when I drink it new with you in My Father's kingdom." (**Matthew 26:29**)

All of the essential nutrients for life come to us from the earth and the food it provides. Protein, fat, carbohydrate, vitamins, minerals, enzymes, fiber, water. Yes, God has established a symbiotic relationship between us and the earth. And though our destiny may some day be among the stars, we will always be children of the earth. We are one with it and it is one with us. Now and forever.

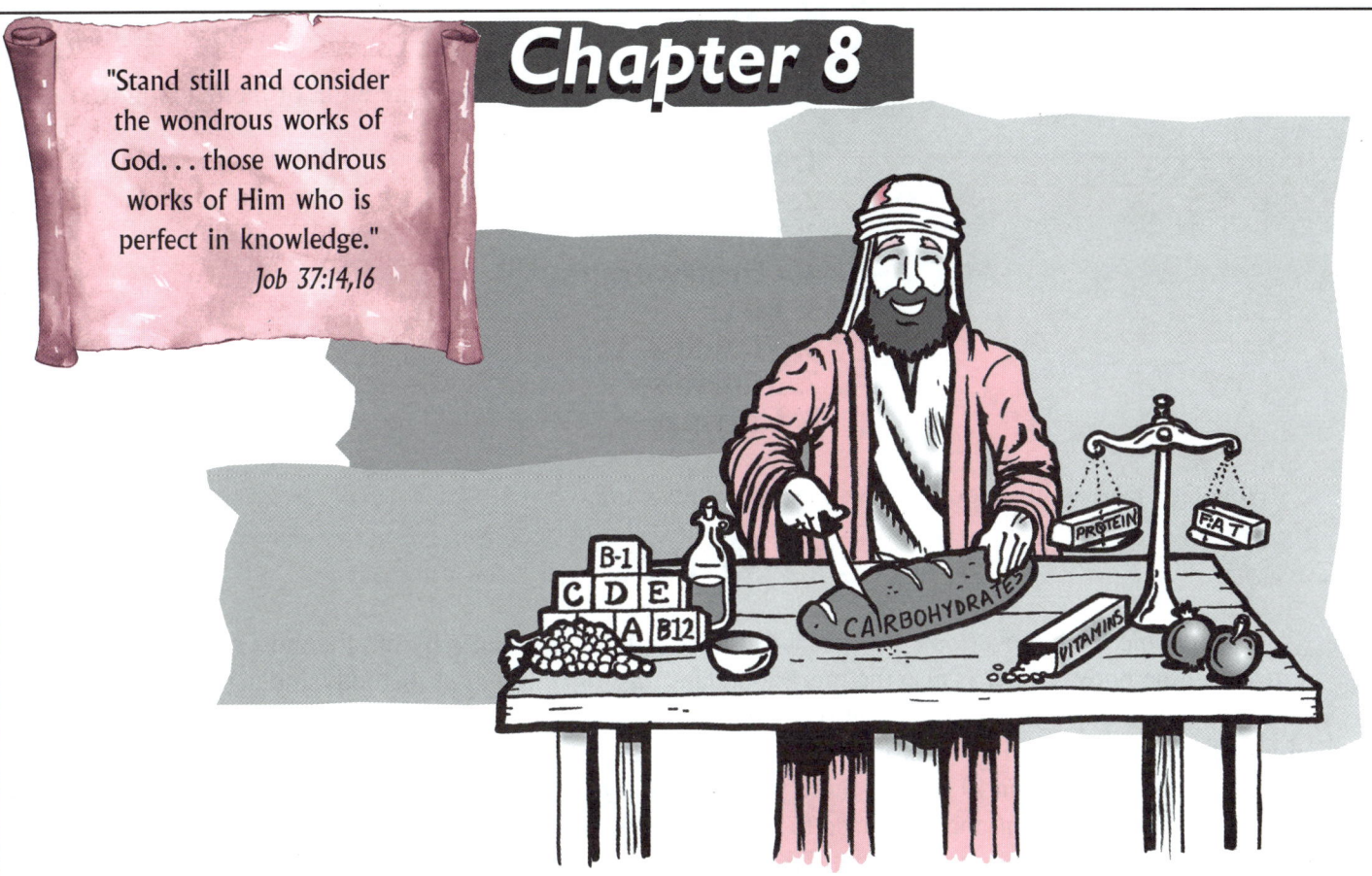

"Stand still and consider the wondrous works of God. . . those wondrous works of Him who is perfect in knowledge."
Job 37:14,16

Chapter 8

Behold How The LORD Has Made Our Food!

A Man Who Knows A Lot Is A Man Who Knows How Little He Really Knows.

Every diet and health book sooner or later gets into a discussion of the nutritional composition of food. That's things like protein, fat and carbohydrates (God's nutritional trinity), as well as vitamins, minerals, fiber, and enzymes. But just what are these wondrous components of God's food and how do they interrelate with each other to provide nourishment and health to the human body? That marvelous answer is subject matter for a complete book of its own. Nevertheless, in this chapter we will take a brief look at God's awe-inspiring genius work of food composition.

A BRIEF LOOK AT FOOD COMPONENTS

In order to understand how Biblical Nutrition can make you healthier, it is a good idea for you to have a basic familiarity with how nutrition works in your body. For the purposes of this book, we will define *nutrition* as the process of ingesting foods into the body and the assimilation and conversion of those foods into living tissue.

Nutrients are the main components or building blocks of food. There are eight of them as follows:

**1. Water
2. Protein
3. Fats
4. Carbohydrates
5. Fiber
6. Vitamins
7. Minerals
8. Enzymes**

Now let's take a closer look at how these nutrients work.

Water

Most people tend to overlook water as a food when, in fact, water is by far, the most important *nutrient* in the body. Water is also the most abundant *substance* found in the body and actually comprises the bulk of your bodyweight (65-75%). The average person's body contains up to 10 quarts of water. Body tissues are 75% or more water and blood is almost all water.

While you can live for 40 days or more without food, you will barely make seven days without water. It's the one nutrient that you need to consume each and every day. It's the first nutrient that, when it was in short supply, brought out the Israelites' wrath against Moses.

> *"And they went three days in the wilderness and found no water. Now when they came to Marah, they could not drink the waters of Marah, for they were bitter. . . And the people complained against Moses, saying, 'What shall we drink?' So he cried out to the LORD, and the LORD showed him a tree. When he cast it into the waters, the waters were made sweet."*
> **(Exodus 15:22-25)**

The average adult uses up to three quarts of water a day and it is important that this water be replaced. Using pure water to gain and maintain health is rooted in the most ancient systems of health building.

Pure water helps regulate your metabolism, hydrate your skin, replenish lost fluids, cool down your body after exertion and build healthy blood. Water also helps transport other nutrients to the cells of your body, assists in waste removal, helps chemicals and hormones react with one another, assists in the lubrication of bone joints, the eyes, and the digestive tract.

There is very little danger of consuming too much water since you will get rid of what you don't need through excretion, exhalation and perspiration. In fact, even when you cannot see it, water is continuously escaping through your breath and the pores of your skin. Instead, the more common worry is **dehydration** – your body not getting enough water to maintain good health. In fact, chronic dehydration can actually cause death.

It is a proven fact that most people just do not drink enough water every day. The average person should be drinking at least four to six glasses of water per day. People who exercise regularly should be drinking eight glasses or more since prolonged activity puts high demands on the body's need for water. If you are not adequately replenishing the water you are using, then both your health and your exercise program can ultimately suffer. But you must beware of certain liquids that can actually do you more damage than good. While such drinks do contain water, they actually act as diuretics – that is, they will make your body lose water. The chief offenders are coffee, tea, soft drinks and alcohol.

Even though I am urging you to drink plenty of water, I must issue you this one very important note of caution. **DO NOT DRINK TAP WATER!** The majority of sink (tap) water is over-chemicalized with chlorine, fluorine and other so-called purifying agents. The very chemicals that are supposed to protect you are actually very dangerous to your health. Therefore, the only way you can be certain you are getting good water is to drink bottled spring water. Carry a bottle with you at all times and learn to swig from it throughout the day, whether you are thirsty or not.

The Bible teaches that both Heaven and Earth were born from water.

> *"Then God said, 'Let there be a firmament in the midst of the waters, and let it divide the waters from the waters.'"* **(Genesis 1:6)**

Certainly then, pure, unadulterated spring water needs to be a principle part of all health-building diets.

Protein

If there's one nutrient that most people look upon as being the most important, it's protein. In fact, our English word protein is derived from the Greek word ***proteios*** and means *primary* or of *first importance*. This should give you a clue as to how important nutritionists view protein in the body. Protein is of first importance because it is found in just about all of the cells and tissues of the body. Here is a list of where protein is found and utilized in the body:

- muscles
- skin
- bone
- hair
- blood
- nails
- collagen tissue
- cartilage
- ligaments
- tendons
- glands
- hormones
- enzymes
- gums
- teeth
- eyes

As you can readily see, protein is found just about everywhere in the body. Next to water, it is the most abundant nutrient. But what exactly is it? Chemically speaking, protein is a very complex substance. It is actually made up of smaller components or building blocks known as ***amino acids***. There are 24 amino acids. To see how they work, think of the individual amino acids as the letters of the alphabet. Just as the 26 letters of the English alphabet can be joined together into hundreds of thousands of words, so too can the various amino acids be joined together into different types of proteins. So in a sense then, a protein is a combination of amino acids logically linked together just as letters are linked logically to form words.

Even though your body itself is composed of lots of different proteins, you must consume external forms of protein daily in your food in order to keep replenishing what your body is breaking down. When you eat a protein food, your digestive system breaks that protein down into its individual amino acids known as *free form amino acids*.

Next, your body rearranges these free form amino acids into human protein tissues. If you do not consume adequate amounts of protein, your body will break down its own protein tissues to be rearranged into other proteins where they are most needed. What this means then, is that people on extremely low protein diets will actually start digesting their own bodies. Unfortunately, one of the first organs to be broken down under these conditions is the heart muscle. This is why so many people with anorexia eventually die from heart failure.

Furthermore, when your body demands energy at levels higher than the amount provided by your diet, then your body will actually start converting its own human protein tissue into energy. This too, over an extended period of time can lead to protein deficiencies and health problems. There is no doubt that adequate protein intake is crucial to the health of the body.

But what foods are high in protein and are some better than others? These are important questions especially since some of you may decide to give up meat eating as a result of reading this book. It has been claimed over and over again that vegetarians do not get enough protein. This is just not true. As a matter of fact numerous studies have been conducted which have found that vegetarians can and do get adequate amounts of protein from a non-meat diet. The whole key is to *properly combine* a variety of vegetarian foods. For example, here are some food combinations that can help provide you with adequate protein levels:

- Combine legumes (dried beans, peas, lentils, soybeans, garbanzo beans, etc.) with grains (barley, wheat, millet, rice, oats, rye).
- Combine legumes with nuts and seeds (almonds, cashews, pecans, walnuts, peanuts, pumpkin seeds, sesame seeds, sunflower seeds).

Of course, if you choose to use eggs and dairy products, you will have no trouble meeting your daily protein needs since these foods are very high in protein. And if you do choose to continue eating meat, two servings a day will easily fulfill your protein requirements. However, if you do eat meat, you need to select very low fat meats such as turkey or chicken or very lean cuts of beef. Pork foods should be avoided both because of their high fat content and their proscription in the Book of Leviticus.

"and the swine. . . is unclean to you." **(Leviticus 11:7)**

There is another very important question when it comes to protein and that is whether people who exercise need to consume more protein than the average person? While this has been a highly controversial topic through the years, modern researchers are finding out that, yes indeed, athletes need more protein than the sedentary person. According to the book **Sports Nutrition For The 90s**, by Jacqueline R. Berning and Suzanne Nelson Steen, numerous studies show decreased protein synthesis during and for some time after exercise, while other studies reveal increased protein catabolism (breakdown) during or after exercise. One study concluded that the protein needs of athletes are at least 50% higher than the current government Recommended Daily Allowance (RDA). Other investigators too, continue to find that athletics puts a higher demand on the body's protein requirements.

Fats

You have to be very careful when discussing fats these days since no other nutrient has gotten so much negative publicity. In fact, most people, when they hear the word "fat" think of globs of unwanted, squishy adipose tissue hanging loosely all over the body. Granted, this type of fat is undesirable. However, fat, as a nutrient, plays a vital role in producing a healthy body. So then, let's try to de-mystify the confusing world of fats.

The first and most important function of fat is to store energy for future needs of the body. This is evidenced by the amount of calories found in a single gram of fat (nine calories) compared to the amount of calories found in a single gram of protein or carbohydrate (four calories). It's as if your body is saving money (fat) in the bank (fat cells) to withdraw for a later emergency. This stored fat becomes important for a reserve to draw on over prolonged periods of exercise. Please note that a certain amount of body fat is needed to stay healthy and meet the demands of extended work or exercise.

But storing up calories for a rainy day is not the only purpose of body fat. Here are several other functions of body fat:

- Serves as insulation for the body.
- Offers protection to vital organs.
- Helps to maintain healthy skin and hair.
- Acts as a transport medium and storage location for the fat soluble vitamins (A,D,E,K).
- Assists in the production of hormones.
- Activates the flow of bile from the gall bladder.

But what exactly are fats? Fats (commonly referred to as *lipids* by nutritionists), are chemical compounds which are found in many types of foods. All fats are made up of various combinations of chemical compounds known as ***fatty acids***. Fatty acids are molecules made up primarily of carbon as a core and varying amounts of hydrogen atoms attached or linked to the carbon. The number of hydrogen atoms attached to the carbon determine whether a fat is ***saturated*** or ***unsaturated***.

This will be easier to understand if you imagine a fatty acid molecule as a bicycle wheel. At the hub or center is a carbon atom. Coming out from the carbon hub are numerous spokes. Hydrogen atoms have the ability to attach themselves to one, several or all of the spokes. If only one or just a few hydrogen atoms are attached to the spokes, then that fat is said to be either ***mono-unsaturated*** or ***poly-unsaturated***. When all of the spokes are filled with hydrogen, that fat is referred to as ***saturated fat***. It is interesting to note that all fatty acids are made up of varying combinations of unsaturated and saturated fats.

Mono and poly-unsaturated fats are found primarily in plant foods and these are the source of our various vegetable oils. Saturated fats, on the other hand, are found mostly in foods of animal origin. These include butter, milk fat and the fat in various meats. Two vegetable oils – coconut and palm oil – are also very high in saturated fats. The amount of saturation also helps determine whether a fat is liquid or solid. All fats are insoluble in water.

We now know that there are good fats and bad fats. Good fats are those that are high in mono and poly-unsaturates with olive oil ranking at the top of the list. This should come as no surprise to Bible students. Good fats are vital to the health of the cardiovascular, immune, reproductive and nervous systems. The regular use of good fats like olive oil and flax seed oil may actually help reduce body weight and stimulate the metabolism.

So now that you see just how important fats are to the body, the question is, how much fat should you consume each day? In answering this question, one thing is for certain. The problem most people face is not having too little fat in the diet. On the contrary, most people are consuming far too much fat in their diets – especially the highly saturated animal fats. Some of the most current research indicates that for optimum health, between 25-30 percent of your total daily calories should come from fat. Unfortunately, the average American diet is much higher in fat than this. Therefore, you need to be aware of the fat content of foods and strive to stay within this recommended range. Here is a surefire way to keep your daily fat calories under control. Eat more grains, fruits and vegetables and then almost by default you are going to be reducing your fat intake without having to count fat grams or calculate calorie percentages.

TIPS ON HOLDING FAT INTAKE AT 30%

- If you eat meat, use only lean cuts of meat and trim all visible fat.
- Avoid deep fried foods.
- Bake, broil or roast trimmed meats and poultry on a rack allowing for cooking fats to drain away.
- Select regular non-basted poultry over pre-basted or self-basting birds; the latter are made juicy with injections of fat.
- Do not eat poultry skins. They contain the most fat.
- Skim off the fat of broth, soups and gravies.
- After cooking, chill stews, soups, stocks and gravies and then skim off the hardened fat.
- Eat plenty of vegetables, legumes, beans, peas, lentils, whole grain breads and cereals, pasta and fruit.
- Use olive oil, vinegar and herbs for salad dressings.
- Use no-stick pans.
- Use low-fat yogurt for sour cream.

Carbohydrates

The next category of nutrient I want to examine with you is carbohydrates. Carbohydrates are God's energy foods. They are found primarily in fruits, vegetables, grains and sweeteners such as honey. It is the sugars and starches in carbohydrate foods that are converted into glucose, the body's main source of energy.

Nutritionists refer to carbohydrates as being either *simple* or *complex*. The difference is determined by the type of sugar molecules that the carbohydrate contains. Here are the three types of sugar molecules:

1. monosaccharides = have one sugar molecule
2. disaccharides   = have two sugar molecules
3. polysaccharides = have three or more sugar molecules

Mono and disaccharides are commonly called sugars or simple carbohydrates. White table sugar, high fructose corn syrups, honey, fruits and fruit juices are examples of simple carbohydrates.

Polysaccharides are called starches or complex carbohydrates. These are the types of carbohydrates found in bread, cereal, pasta, potatoes, vegetables, beans and rice. On the whole, complex carbohydrates tend to be the more nutritious and health building.

Your body is well capable of metabolizing all types of carbohydrates and it ultimately breaks them down into a simple sugar called **glucose**. Glucose is the body's main energy producer. Glucose is to your body what gasoline is to your car. It is the fuel that keeps everything running.

Carbohydrate foods convert into glucose at varying rates. (See accompanying story – **What Is The Glycemic Index**.) You may be thinking that the faster a carbohydrate food converts into glucose/energy the better it is and therefore the simple carbohydrates would be preferred. Actually, it's just the opposite. Since complex carbohydrates tend to be higher in fiber, their overall digestive rate and metabolism is slower and more even. This leads to more sustained energy and better nutritional absorption.

I want to strongly caution you here against the use of foods made with refined, over-processed carbohydrates such as white flour, white sugar and white rice. These refined carbohydrates have been stripped of all of their original God-given nutritional benefits. In their place, the manufacturers have added back a handful of synthetic vitamins and minerals. Such low nutrition, low fiber foods are simply going to give you lots of empty calories thus contributing to your weight problems.

Furthermore, these foods can also lead to wide swings in energy levels by causing rapid spikes and drops in blood glucose. When glucose is dumped into the bloodstream too quickly because of high refined carbohydrate consumption, the body goes into a defensive regulation mode. What happens is that a rush of glucose brings a rush of insulin and by the time the insulin is done doing its job, there may actually be less glucose circulating than originally. This is manifested by a sudden boost in energy followed by an equally sudden loss of energy. That's why you'll often feel drowsy an hour or so after consuming these foods.

Prolonged use of refined carbohydrates with their concomitant blood sugar swings can actually lead to health problems like hypoglycemia (low blood sugar) and diabetes (high blood sugar).

Since unprocessed complex carbohydrates break down much slower in the body than refined, over-processed carbohydrates, and since they provide such an abundance of vitamins, minerals, fiber and enzymes, you need to make them a regular part of your diet program. This will assure you not only the greatest levels of energy and stamina, but health and well being as well.

The question then is how much carbohydrate should be in the average diet? Nutritionists are all over the place on the answer to this question. But it is my belief that complex carbohydrates as found in many Bible foods should provide approximately 50 percent of your total daily calories in order to maintain optimum health and normal body weight. Sadly, too many people today are dropping their carbohydrate intake well below this level because of the low carbohydrate fad. This is very anti-biblical and can lead to serious health consequences. Please eat freely and often from God's most nutritious and delicious energy food – carbohydrates.

Fiber

Even though fiber is technically a type of carbohydrate, it is easier to understand its role in nutrition if we look at it as a completely separate food component category.

Fiber is the non-digestible part of carbohydrate foods. It can be either insoluble such as cellulose, hemicellulose and lignin, or soluble such as pectin and guar gum. Since fiber cannot be digested, it provides no energy or nutritional value to the body. What fiber does do is provide *roughage* to your system. This fiber-derived roughage helps soften the stool and assist in regular elimination of body wastes. Fiber also helps add bulk to the diet without adding extra calories. Very current research also indicates that people who eat a high fiber diet experience reduced rates of cardiovascular disease, colon cancer, and diabetes.

Now here's some good news for those of you who are trying to lose weight. High fiber diets have also proved to be very beneficial for weight loss programs. At least five studies over the past few years have shown that consistent fiber intake helps decrease body fat. Fiber also helps control hunger and helps regulate the metabolism of carbohydrates.

Based on some very impressive research with high fiber diets, researchers are now recommending at least two servings of high fiber cereal each day. They report that cereals with oat bran or wheat bran can help replace high fat foods and improve a person's overall health. "Encouraging people to eat fiber rich cereal may be a simple, yet effective strategy to produce global improvements in diet," says Brenda Davy, M.S. a Research Dietician in the department of food science and human nutrition at Colorado State University.

If your diet is high in complex carbohydrates as specified in the **Moses Diet & Health Program** and you eat figs regularly, then be assured that you are getting ample amounts of fiber in your diet.

Vitamins

Even though you need only small amounts of vitamins in your diet, don't make the mistake of thinking that they are unimportant. Vitamins in fact, play a major role in the health of your body. As a matter of fact, even as this book is being written, scientists are continuing to find more and more ways in which vitamins positively affect health.

But what exactly are vitamins? Vitamins are chemical compounds which, for the most part, cannot be manufactured by the body. Hence, they must be consumed in the diet as part of the foods that you eat. They received their name in 1912 from Dr. Casmir Funk who combined the word *vita*, meaning "life," with the word *amine*, a nitrogen-containing organic compound. When scientists later realized that not all vitamins are amines, they dropped the final *e* in *vitamine* and our modern term was born. Vitamins are measured in milligrams (mg) and micrograms (mcg) whereas proteins, fats and carbohydrates are measured in the much larger unit called the gram (gm).

All vitamins are essential to life and must be supplied externally by the foods we eat. They are not actually converted into human tissue, but instead assist the body in carrying out the chemical reactions of life. Vitamins play a crucial role in just about every activity performed by your body. Some, like the fat-soluble vitamins A, D, E, and K can be stored in the body's fatty tissue (see FATS above). Since they are stored in fat, they don't necessarily have to be consumed every day.

The rest of the vitamins (B-family, C) are water-soluble and hence are expelled from the body rather quickly. You must be sure to replenish these vitamins daily through a well balanced diet. You must also be aware of the fact, however, that growing methods, storage and preparation can all play a part in reducing the vitamin content of foods. To derive the highest vitamin content from your foods, be sure to eat them as fresh as possible and avoid overcooking. To assure that you are consuming adequate quantities of vitamins, especially while you are dieting, I suggest that you supplement your diet with **Back To The Garden**, a comprehensive vitamin and mineral food powder concentrate made exclusively from foods of the Bible. (See page 94 for more information on this potent supplement.)

Minerals

Considered unglamorous by some accounts, nevertheless, minerals play an equally important role as vitamins in the well being of your body. While the twenty minerals that are essential to the body account for only about five pounds of the average person's weight, this small amount works hand-in-hand with vitamins, enzymes, hormones and other substances to keep your body running smoothly.

Minerals play a number of important roles in your body. Some regulate fluid and electrolyte balances, others provide rigidity to the skeleton, and still others regulate muscle and nerve function. While most of the minerals in the earth are found in our bodies, a few – such as mercury and lead – can be potentially toxic.

Like vitamins, minerals too cannot be produced by the body and thus must be supplied by your diet. Unfortunately, study after study shows that most Americans fall far short in their intake of these essential nutrients. Some of the key minerals that are under supplied by the diet include calcium, magnesium, zinc, iron and chromium. These and other minerals are needed to build bones, release energy from food, transport oxygen and maintain a strong immune system. Even a slight deficiency of zinc can play havoc with your immune system, and thus lower your defenses against infections. If you fall below your daily requirements for calcium, you run the risk of bone and joint injury. It is quite apparent then, how important it is to get an adequate daily supply of minerals.

Prolonged sweating most definitely can contribute to the body's loss of minerals. Recent research has indicated that people who engage in hard physical activity have a higher risk of being deficient in calcium, iron, chromium, and zinc. To assure that your daily intake of minerals is adequate, you must eat a variety of foods from the various Bible food groups. Once again, for further assurance that you are getting adequate amounts of minerals, I would suggest that you supplement your diet with *Back To The Garden*.

What Is The Glycemic Index?

One term being heard more and more often these days in the diet world is glycemic index. For some people it has become the Holy Grail of dieting. But what exactly is the *glycemic index* and does this mysterious sounding phrase really hold the eternal secret to weight loss?

Before defining what it means, let me first demystify the word *glycemic*. Glycemic simply means sugar producing and it comes from the Greek root prefix *glyco* or *gluco* meaning sweet. The glycemic index then, is a food rating system designed to list how quickly the body converts various carbohydrate foods into blood sugar (glucose). Carbohydrate foods that convert quickly are assigned a high glycemic index with pure glucose being ranked at 100. Foods with a glycemic index of 50 or more are considered high glycemic. Proponents of using the glycemic index for weight control argue that eating too many high glycemic foods inhibits weight loss. Their claim is that the faster a carbohydrate converts to blood sugar, the quicker the body will try to regulate it by either driving it into muscles for energy or converting it to fat for later energy requirements. Are they right?

First of all, it is true that when extra glucose enters into the bloodstream the body sends out a chemical to regulate and prevent any glucose overload. This special glucose-burning chemical is called *insulin*. Please note, however, that before any excess glucose gets converted to fat, the body will store as much of it as possible as *glycogen* in the muscles and liver. If you exercise regularly, your body will have a greater capacity for glycogen storage thus making it less likely that you will convert excess carbohydrates to fat.

Furthermore, while the glycemic index does have some merit for monitoring diabetic diets and for ranking the speed of isolated carbohydrate food absorption, its connection to weight loss menu planning is not as clear cut. The main problem is that the glycemic index measures and classifies *individual* carbohydrate foods rather than food combinations. Studies have shown that protein, fat and fiber from other foods eaten along with carbohydrate foods can dramatically alter their glycemic index thus rendering it questionable as a fat deposit indicator.

Lastly, some of God's best Bible foods fall into the high glycemic category making them caution foods for proponents of this system. It's hard to believe God would make such nutritious foods as carrots, barley, wheat, apricots, oats, rice, potatoes, bananas, papayas, mangoes, honey, pinto beans and couscous off limits simply because they exceed 50 on the glycemic index scale.

Let me just say that by sticking with the types of Bible foods recommended in the *Moses Diet & Health Program*, as well as with its exercise and prayer recommendations, you are going to normalize your bodyweight and build a healthy body without having to concern yourself with questionable concepts such as the glycemic index.

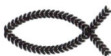

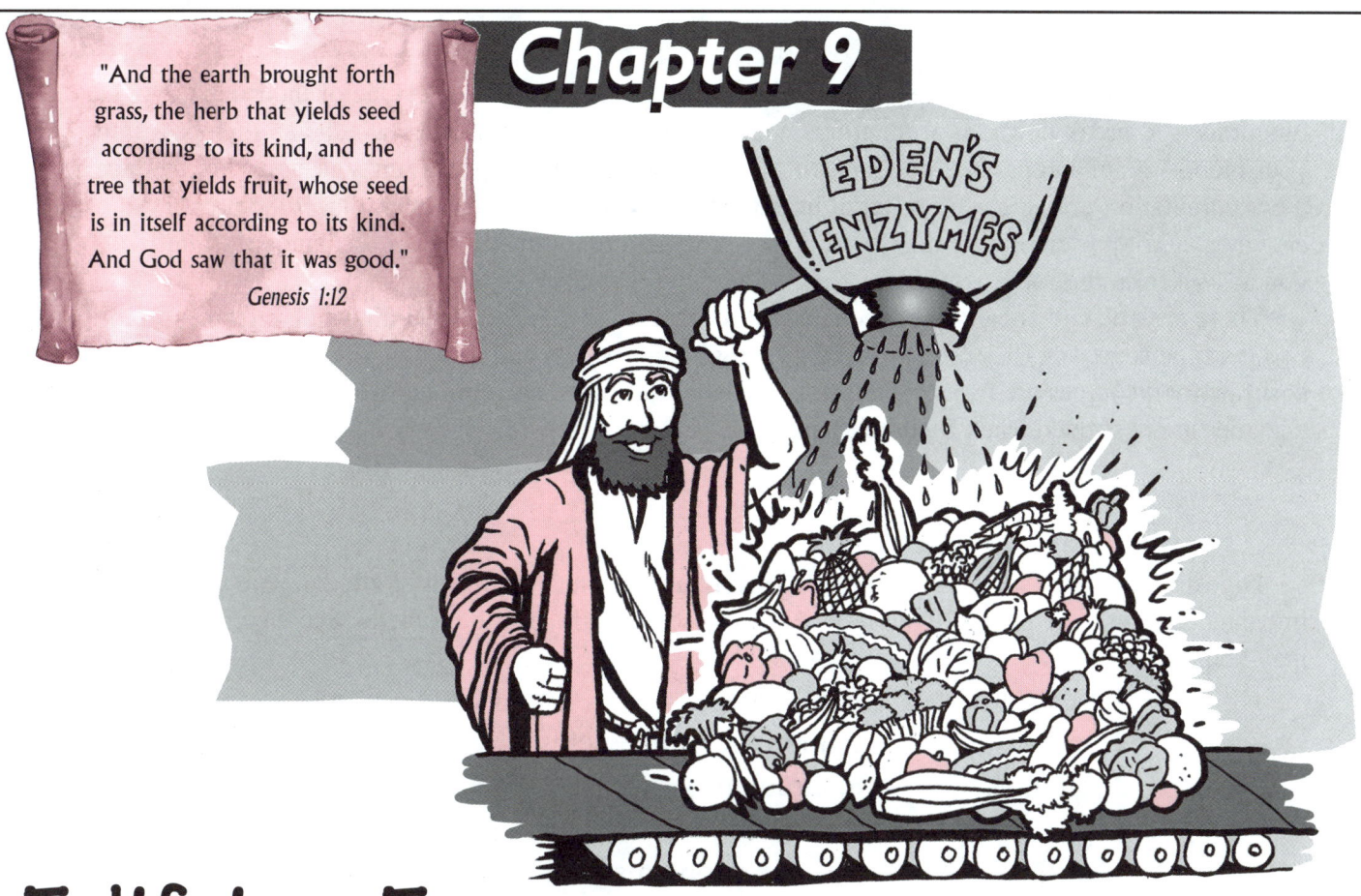

"And the earth brought forth grass, the herb that yields seed according to its kind, and the tree that yields fruit, whose seed is in itself according to its kind. And God saw that it was good."
Genesis 1:12

Chapter 9

Edifying Enzymes.

God Put These Special Messengers In All Of His Foods So That They Would Enable The "Life Essence" To Transfer To Our Bodies.

If there's one thing that nearly all Bible foods have in common, it's that they are loaded with powerful, nutrition-activating, digestion-promoting substances called *enzymes*. While there are many types of enzymes necessary for the health and well being of the body, our main concern in this chapter is with those enzymes that are necessary for food digestion. Unfortunately, such enzymes are rarely discussed in most articles on health and nutrition, and when they are, it is often in a cursory and brief manner. Consequently, very few people are aware of just how important these enzymes are to an effective health and nutrition program.

How important are they? Put it this way. **Without digestive enzymes, there is no life!** Even if you are getting all of the nutrients you need from your diet, if you are lacking in enzymes, you are going to get in trouble. That's because it's not just what you eat, it's what you absorb. Therefore, if you are to reap the highest benefits from the *Moses Diet & Health Program*, then you need to know about food digesting enzymes and how they work.

WHAT THEY ARE

Digestive enzymes are protein-based catalytic activators that are found in both raw foods and living organisms. They are made up of connected links (chains) of amino acids. The job of these special chemicals is to orchestrate and regulate biochemical reactions in the body. One of their main functions is to break down all of the foods you consume into tiny substrates which can then pass into your blood stream and provide nourishment to your body. In this capacity, enzymes also help reduce the accumulation of undigested material in the colon. Be cautioned, however, that if the proper enzymes aren't present during digestion, then you are going to greatly reduce the amount of nutrients you absorb from the foods you eat.

There are no synthetically produced enzymes. Instead, we get our food digesting enzymes from two possible sources. They are produced directly by our bodies and also contained in raw foods. The best raw food sources are fruits, vegetables, seeds, nuts, grains, and sprouts. However, please note that enzymes are destroyed when foods are heated above 120 degrees.

SOME OF THE THINGS THEY ARE GOOD FOR

Digestive enzymes serve a host of functions in the body and the result of any enzyme shortage or imbalance in the body is usually disease. Here are some of the health problems that enzyme therapy may help:

1. heartburn
2. indigestion
3. bloating
4. gas
5. arthritis
6. allergies
7. immune deficiencies
8. circulatory diseases
9. muscle injuries
10. skin problems
11. infections
12. inflammations
13. weight problems
14. premature aging
15. abnormal blood sugar

Billions of dollars are spent every year fighting these problems which in many cases can be helped simply by the addition of digestive enzymes.

THE PRINCIPLE DIGESTIVE ENZYMES

There are four key enzymes that are necessary for thorough food digestion.

1. Protease = helps break down proteins
2. Amylase = helps break down carbohydrates
3. Lipase = helps break down fats
4. Cellulase = helps break down fiber

The first three can all be produced by the body; but cellulase must come either from foods in the diet or from a good enzyme supplement (see page 58). Unfortunately, some supermarkets spray their vegetables with sulfite preservatives, which destroys the cellulase enzymes in them.

BEWARE OF THIS CATCH 22

Even though raw foods, including most of the Bible foods discussed in this book, are excellent sources of enzymes, God also put an enzyme-producing backup system in our bodies to ensure that we would never run short of these life-preserving substances. However, even with this body backup system, if you eat a diet of over-cooked, over-processed, enzyme deficient foods, you may soon find yourself caught up in a vicious Catch 22 downward cycle as follows.

By not eating enough raw, natural enzyme-carrying foods, you then force your body to carry the whole enzyme load by itself. But at the same time, your body needs the very nutrients contained in those raw, natural foods to manufacture its own digestive enzymes. And so, you now have begun a vicious cycle that will ultimately lead to enzyme depletion and a host of health problems. Surprisingly, most doctors never even consider enzyme deficiency as a possible culprit behind so many of their patients' health troubles.

ENZYME DESTROYERS

With so much riding on your getting plenty of enzymes from your diet, it's worth noting the kinds of things that can destroy or reduce the level of enzymes in food:

1. Growing with pesticides, herbicides and fungicides
2. Growing in nutrient-deficient soil
3. Chemical processing (additives, preservatives, etc.)
4. Irradiation
5. Drying
6. Pasteurization
7. Canning
8. Storing foods for long periods of time
9. Heating foods to over 120 degrees
10. Microwave cooking

OTHER ENZYME BENEFITS

In addition to the role they play in the digestion of foods, enzymes have also demonstrated *therapeutic* benefits for the body. Experts tell us that enzymes can help everything from immunity to metabolism. The reason for this is that in addition to their role in digestion, enzymes are also capable of being absorbed intact by the body, where they are then disseminated through the blood to areas where they are most needed.

Protease, the protein digesting enzyme, for example, has been shown to reduce both muscle and joint inflammations. In fact, some researchers believe that enzyme supplements with protease are as effective as ibuprofen and aspirin for soothing the pain of osteoarthritis. According to molecular geneticist Aftab Ahmed, Ph.D., "enzymes not only help control inflammation and pain, they neutralize the acidic molecules that attack and damage joint tissue." Taking an enzyme supplement three times daily, between meals, has been shown to alleviate joint pain within three weeks or less.

Nutrition specialist Lita Lee, Ph.D., another enzyme expert, claims that enzymes may also be effective at relieving chronic back pain and migraine headaches.

Protease also seems to work in conjunction with the immune system. For example, some very current research indicates that protease may assist in removing pathogens from the blood by bonding with alpha2-macroglobulin and then attacking those pathogens that have been targeted for destruction by the immune system.

Scientists also tell us that if sufficient amounts of the enzyme *lipase* are available when fatty foods are eaten, artery buildup of harmful fats such as cholesterol, triglycerides, and plaque may actually be inhibited. But beyond that, there is even evidence that lipase has the ability to travel into the blood and actually reduce existing fat buildup in the arteries.

(Please note that if you wish to use enzyme supplements for any of the above listed therapeutic benefits, it is important that you take the supplement either an hour and a half before or an hour and a half after a meal. This way, the enzymes will not compete with food and can be more readily absorbed into the blood stream.)

ENZYMES CAN HELP SPEED UP WEIGHT LOSS

Not very many people are aware that enzyme deficiency can be a big contributing factor to weight gain, especially as we age. As a matter of fact, the most common cause of enzyme depletion is aging. The body's enzyme levels start dropping in the 20's and continue to decrease quite dramatically with each passing decade. One study concluded that people 69 and over have 30 times less enzymes than they had in their 20's.

Might some of the weight gain we experience as we age be caused by this enzyme loss? Many nutritionists seem to think so. Some studies have shown that a drop in enzymes could be responsible for as much as a ten pound weight gain every decade. "Since enzymes help us burn calories for energy, weight problems are almost inevitable when we don't get enough," says Dr. Lee.

But no matter what age you are, I have some good news for you. You can overcome the problem of enzyme depletion simply by taking an enzyme supplement with each meal. But I can't stress enough to you how important it is that you choose a supplement that contains the four enzymes listed above. In addition, you should be aware that these enzymes can be derived from either animal or food sources. Of course, I strongly recommend that the enzyme tablets you use be vegetarian based.

ENZYME SUPPLEMENTS

As the use of enzyme supplements becomes more and more popular, there are still some nutritionists who will argue that taking supplementary digestive enzymes is unnecessary. Are they right? Perhaps under ideal dietary conditions. But with millions of Americans eating improperly, preparing foods improperly, and relying on overcooked and overprocessed foods, we are far from ideal conditions. Furthermore, as I just noted above, the most common contributor to enzyme depletion is aging. This means that no matter how well you eat, your enzyme production is going to decrease as you age. Therefore, I strongly recommend that you start using a digestive enzyme supplement.

If you do decide to use them, there are a variety of enzyme supplement formulas available in most health food stores. However, be sure to read the labels since these supplements come several different ways. Some, for instance, are animal derived, while others are totally vegetarian (plant based). Any enzyme supplement containing pancreatin is definitely animal based since the pancreatic enzymes are derived from the pancreas of either cows (bovine) or pigs (porcine). If you are an observer of the Bible's restrictions against pig products as discussed in the Book of Leviticus, I would strongly caution you against this type of enzyme supplement since the pancreatin source is not always disclosed on the label. Also, two other enzymes – *trypsin* and *chymotrypsin* are also derived exclusively from animal pancreas tissue so once again, be sure to read labels carefully.

While there are several acceptable digestive enzyme products on the market, none of them is exactly to my liking. Therefore, I felt the need to design a new enzyme formula especially for those of you who plan to follow the **Moses Diet & Health Program** as outlined in this book. I call this unique product *Eden's Enzymes* and I've made it according to all of the specifications that I've outlined here.

First of all, for several reasons, I believe that a plant derived enzyme formula is far superior to an animal based product. For one thing, not only do plant enzymes break down a wider variety of food components than animal-based enzymes, they also go to work the minute they enter the stomach whereas animal enzymes don't begin to do their job until they reach the intestines. Secondly, plant derived enzymes are available over a wider selection of foods and do not involve the taking of an animal's life. Thirdly, according to enzyme expert Daniel Crisafi, N.D., M.H., Ph.D., since animal-based enzymes are so much like our own, they may actually confuse our bodies and reduce our body's production of enzymes. Lastly, animal-derived enzymes have a much more limited pH range in which they are effective compared to plant enzymes.

Therefore, in light of this information, I decided to make *Eden's Enzymes* a one hundred percent vegetarian product. Please note too that not only are all of the ingredients in the product plant derived, but even the capsule shells themselves are vegetarian. (I used capsules instead of tablets for quicker breakdown and utilization.)

Next, *Eden's Enzymes* contain all three essential digestive enzymes produced by the body (protease, amylase and lipase) within physiological ratios similar to those produced in the human body. And in addition to that, I have also included the fourth crucial enzyme – *cellulase* – which, as noted above, is not produced by the body.

But even if *Eden's Enzymes* didn't contain another thing, they would still be an excellent formula. However, I didn't stop there. I also added *lactase* for those people who have difficulty digesting dairy products, as well as two other highly effective protein-digesting enzymes – *bromelain*, from pineapples, and *papain*, from papayas. Both of these enzymes are reported to boost the body's ability to overcome pain, infection and inflammation.

Finally, I blended the whole formula together into a base of herbal bitters of gentian, ginger, wormwood, goldenseal, barberry, dandelion and hops. These herbal bitters help stimulate the body's production of its own digestive enzymes, improve the muscle tone of the digestive tract and help restore regularity.

Eden's Enzymes are going to help you greatly increase your absorption of all food groups. They will also help you fight gas, bloat and indigestion and they are perfectly safe for everyone including pregnant and nursing women.

If you would like to try a bottle of *Eden's Enzymes*, they are available at select health food stores or they may be ordered directly from **Logia:** *Foods of the Bible*, at **1-800-537-7671**. (See the order form in back of the book for pricing and ordering information.)

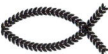

Chapter 10

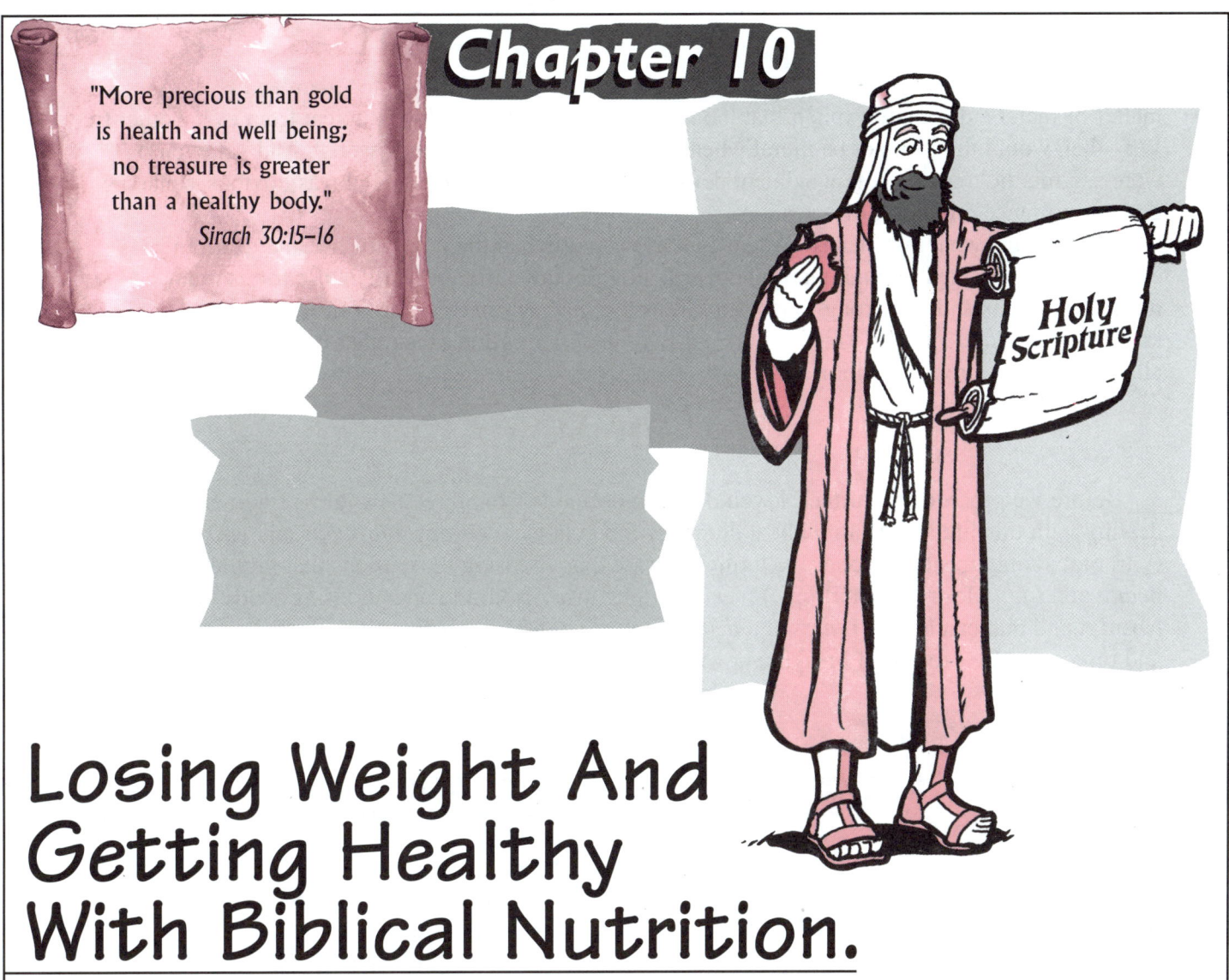

"More precious than gold is health and well being; no treasure is greater than a healthy body."
Sirach 30:15-16

Losing Weight And Getting Healthy With Biblical Nutrition.

The Two Best Times To Change Your Life Are 10 Years Ago And Right Now.

In this chapter I am going to introduce you to a highly beneficial, life-changing philosophy that I call **Biblical Nutrition**. Let's start with a basic definition. Biblical Nutrition is the study of the various foods of the Bible and how they can be used to build dynamic health, normalize bodyweight and even cure some illnesses. Biblical Nutrition is based on the premise that God gave mankind a perfect diet to follow in the Garden of Eden **(Genesis 1:29)** and that after Adam and Eve sinned, the human race drifted from this perfect diet prescription.

As I noted earlier in this book, God definitely put a connection between eating the proper foods and eternal life. In fact, He was quite explicit in His very first commandment:

> "And the LORD God <u>commanded</u> the man, saying, 'Of every tree of the garden <u>you may freely eat</u>; but of the tree of the knowledge of good and evil <u>you shall not eat</u>, for in the day that you eat of it <u>you shall surely die</u>.'" **(Genesis 2:16)**

Bible scholars have debated for millennia as to what the fruit of this tree might have been, and if, in fact, there even was a literal tree of good and evil. As a 30-year student of the Bible, it is my belief that there most definitely was a literal tree whose fruit God put off limits to Adam and Eve. As a matter of fact, God is quite explicit that the man and woman were allowed to eat from every other tree. Why then would this tree not be literal when all the other ones obviously were? And yet even if it were a symbolic tree, the commandment definitely uses the word *eat* so God was obviously placing great importance on the act of ingestion.

Just imagine what this means! Adam and Eve actually had the power of life and death in everything that passed through their mouths. Is it really any different with eating for us today? Bad nutritional habits and the wrong foods can kill us too, just as surely as the fruit from the tree of the knowledge of good and evil killed Adam and Eve. Don't you think then, that it behooves us to learn all we can about proper nutrition?

CHOOSE LIFE – NOT DEATH

Before we proceed any further, I would like to define for you three new terms I will employ for dealing with this life and death biblical drama of food choices: ***vitropy, mortropy*** and ***entropy***. Vitropy (vitropic) simply means selecting, or turning towards, or choosing those foods that promote *good health* and *life*. Mortropy (mortropic) means turning away from life and choosing foods that are harmful and that can lead to *illness* and *death*. Entropy (entropic) is the gradual diminution of health and represents the process of breaking down or passing from life to death.

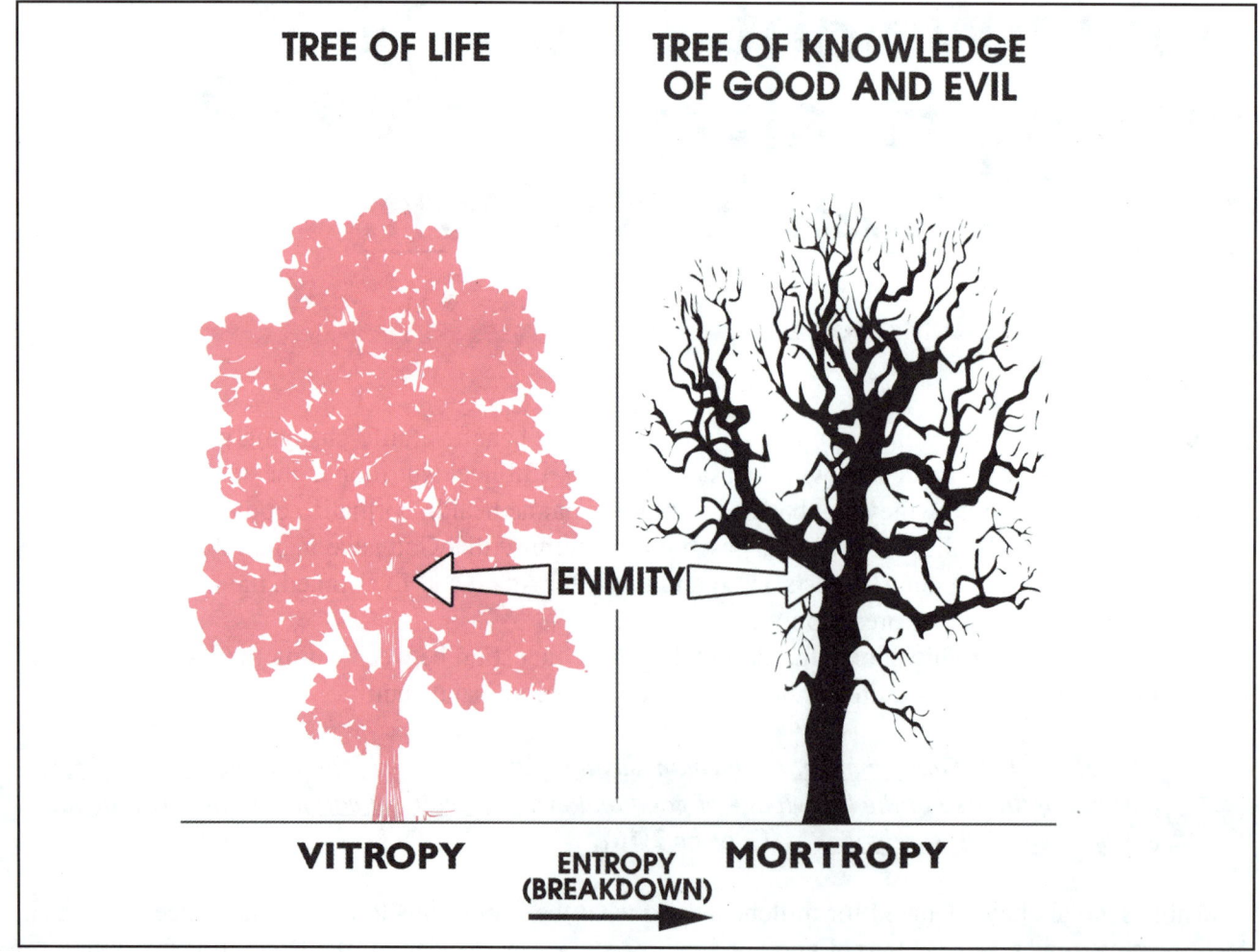

Unfortunately, the majority of Americans are making mortropic rather than vitropic food choices because of their lack of good, solid nutritional information.

> "*My people are destroyed for lack of knowledge.*" **(Hosea 4:6)**

A study in the *American Journal of Clinical Nutrition* found that 27 percent of the average American's total daily caloric intake comes from junk foods with an additional 4 percent coming from alcoholic beverages.

God was explicit right from the beginning that man's diet had to be vitropic *only*. In fact, by the very laws of logic, vitropy and mortropy are mutually exclusive terms (enmity). Therefore, any attempt to "mix" them ultimately must lead to confusion (mixing=babel=Babylon) and death. Therefore, Adam and Eve would die (entropy) as much from *consequence* as they would from *punishment* when they ate from the tree of knowledge of good and evil.

God has not changed His mind today. He hasn't reluctantly granted us permission to eat both vitropic and mortropic foods. That would be a breach of the laws of logic and God never breaks the laws of logic since He is Logic. (***Logos*** is the Greek word for "word." See **John 1:1-2**.) His food commandment remains the same today as it always has been. Eat only those foods that are vitropic. That's why you absolutely must learn the difference between vitropic and mortropic foods and never attempt to mix them in your diet. For obvious reasons, Satan does not want you to know the difference.

> "*I have set before you life and death, blessing and cursing; therefore choose life, that both you and your descendants may live, that you may love the LORD your God, that you may obey His voice, and that you may cling to Him, for He is your life and the length of your days.*"
> **(Deuteronomy 31:19-20)**

IMPORTANT QUESTION: Those of you who feel you cannot give up eating meat should ask yourself the following question. How can the consumption of dead animal flesh (mortropy) contribute to the long life and health (vitropy) of the body? Isn't meat eating then a form of illogical nutrition? Just something to think about.

CATEGORIZING THE FOODS OF EDEN

So what types of foods are considered Bible foods? If we use the original Eden diet as defined in **Genesis 1:29** as our guideline, then the following food categories would all fall within the parameters of that scripture. Any and all foods you eat from these food groups would therefore be, by God's own direction, most definitely vitropic:

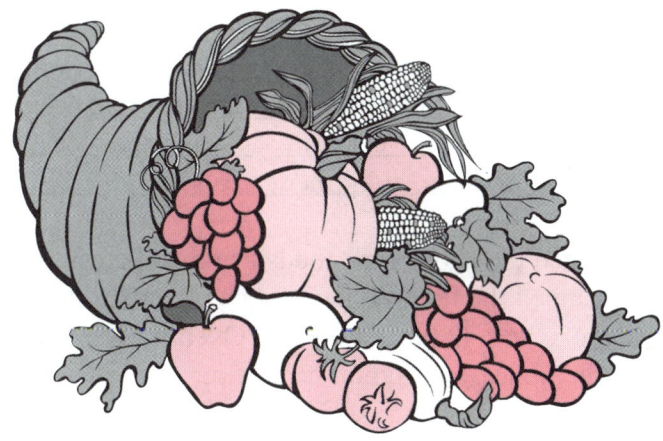

- **fruits**
- **vegetables**
- **legumes**
- **beans**
- **grains (cereal grasses)**
- **nuts**
- **seeds**
- **herbs**
- **spices**
- **sprouts**

Please note that based on God's Biblical description of the Promised Land as a land flowing with *milk* and *honey* **(Exodus 3:8)**, I am also going to include these two foods in the Bible food list and I will discuss my reasons and their attributes more extensively in the next chapter.

A BIBLE FOOD DIET IS A HEALTHY DIET

Just how healthy (vitropic) are these foods? Study after study continues to show immense health benefits to be gained from eating a diet high in these biblical foods. Here are just a few examples.

Some of the earliest research that pointed to the benefits of a Biblical Nutrition diet was performed by a researcher named Ancel Keys, Ph.D. way back in the 1960s. Keys compared the diet of people who reside in countries bordering the Mediterranean (very much a biblically based diet) with that of people living in northern Europe, the United States and Japan. His research found that Mediterranean people lived healthier and longer lives than people in these other regions. Diet seemed to be the main contributor. <u>The Mediterranean diet is high in fruits, vegetables and grains, with very low meat consumption. In addition, olive oil usage is very high</u> (see benefits of olive oil in Chapter 12). Lower incidences of heart disease, diabetes, obesity and cancer were noted among the Mediterranean population as compared to the other regions.

The Mediterranean diet was described by Henry Blackburn, professor emeritus at the University of Minnesota and co-researcher with Keys in this way. The typical Mediterranean's midday main meal "is of eggplant with large mushrooms, crisp vegetables and country bread dipped in olive oil. Other meals are hot dishes of legumes seasoned with meat and condiments. The main dish is followed by a tangy salad, then by dates, Turkish sweets, nuts, or fresh fruits. A sharp local wine completes the meal." Blackburn also noted that limited amounts of lamb, chicken and fish are also consumed.

Not surprisingly, when this Mediterranean (biblical) type of diet was recommended by an organization titled *Oldways Preservation and Trust* together with the World Health Organization and the Harvard School of Public Health in 1994, it came in for severe criticism from the beef and dairy industries. They charged that such a diet was too expensive and could only be followed by the wealthy. (Go figure!)

A study conducted by the University Hospital of Lausanne in Switzerland produced evidence that *whole grain cereals* may have a protective effect against cancer of the upper digestive and respiratory tracts. Even more significantly, the study showed **a link between eating refined grains and these same cancers**. Researchers studied 156 cases of cancers of the oral cavity and pharynx, 101 of the esophagus, 40 of the larynx and 349 control subjects admitted for a wide range of acute non-cancerous conditions.

In a more recent study reported in the April 2000 issue of the *Journal of the American Medical Association*, researcher Ashima K. Kant, Ph.D., from Queens College, City University of New York in Flushing compared the effect of eating habits and health in an eight year study of over 40,000 women. Participants were asked to monitor the amounts of the following foods they consumed weekly: <u>apples, pears, cantaloupes, oranges, grapefruit, orange or grapefruit juice, other fruit juices, dried beans, tomatoes, broccoli, spinach, other greens, green salad, carrots, sweet potatoes, yams, potatoes, non-fried poultry, non-fried fish, whole grain breads, corn products, high fiber cereals, milk (2%, 1%, skim)</u>.

The study found that women who most consumed the above type foods had a 40 percent lower chance of dying from cancer than those who consumed the least of these foods. In addition, risk of heart disease was 33 percent lower and risk of stroke was 42 percent lower. Overall, their death rate from all causes was 30 percent lower than those in the least consumption group.

In a study of 34,492 postmenopausal women ranging in age from 55 to 69 who participated in the Iowa Women's Health Study, it was reported that there is a clear inverse association between eating whole grain foods (a Bible food category) and the risk of death from ischemic heart disease. Nutritionists theorize that the benefits are derived from the plant nutrients (phyto-chemicals), fiber, antioxidants and vitamin E contained in the whole grains.

Even the US Government is finally starting to acknowledge the benefits of Biblical Nutrition. Here's what they recommend in their most recent year 2000 *Dietary Guidelines For Americans*. "Choose a variety of grains daily, especially whole grains. Choose a variety of fruits and vegetables daily."

A recent study conducted by the Institute of Public Health in Barcelona, Spain found that eating a variety of vegetables lowers the risk of developing colon and rectal cancer. According to the study, eating a variety of vegetables lowered the risk of these cancers by 35 percent in men and 15 percent in women.

A study in the November 15th 2000 issue of the *International Journal of Cancer* reported that heavy consumption of meat, animal fat and salt was associated with an increased risk of esophageal cancer. The study went on to say that eating plenty of fruits, vegetables and cereals and drinking green tea was found to be protective. Regular fruit consumption, for example, appears to lower the risk of cancer by 63 percent according to the researchers.

And it just goes on and on like this. Suffice it to say that there now is a plethora of research supporting the health building benefits of a biblically based diet. In fact, I could fill up a book just on these types of studies alone. (As hard as I looked, however, I could not find a single study that gives this kind of health endorsement to eating meat of any kind. Kind of makes you wonder, doesn't it?)

PRINCIPLES OF BIBLICAL NUTRITION

Biblical Nutrition goes beyond simply eating Bible foods. It embraces a total dietary protocol that you must follow consistently in order to reap the rewards of better health and fitness. Here is the ten-point protocol of Biblical Nutrition:

1. Choose as many of your foods as possible from the **Bible food categories** listed above.
2. Eat a *variety* of biblical foods daily.
3. Try to consume many of these Bible foods in a *raw* state.
4. Eat the Bible foods as *close to harvest* as possible.
5. Do not eat when you are anxious or stressed.
6. Avoid processed, adulterated, over-chemicalized, man-made foods.
7. Avoid over-eating.
8. Greatly limit or eliminate completely all meat.
9. Drink copious amounts of natural spring *water* throughout the day.
10. Consume two tablespoons of *olive oil* daily.

WHAT BIBLICAL NUTRITION CAN DO FOR YOU

"So you shall serve the LORD your God, and He will bless your bread and your water. And I will take sickness away from the midst of you. No one shall suffer miscarriage or be barren in your land; I will fulfill the number of your days." **(Exodus 23:25-26)**

Biblical Nutrition is such a powerful concept that I have to wonder why more people don't chose this manner of eating. Bible foods have cleansing, healing and health-building properties that make them nothing short of miraculous. They are chock-full of vitamins, minerals, unsaturated fatty acids (the good ones), complex carbohydrates, enzymes, fiber, and natural proteins, thus making them the perfect diet food. As a matter of fact, there are so many benefits to Bible foods that they may rightly be called **God's Perfect Health Foods**. Here now, is a list of just some of the many benefits you can derive from following the principles of Biblical Nutrition:

1. Helps keep you lean and fit.
2. Strengthens the immune system.
3. Promotes healthy skin and hair.
4. Promotes quicker illness recovery.
5. Provides more energy.
6. Helps relieve depression and mood swings.
7. Helps normalize blood sugar (diabetes, hypoglycemia).
8. Helps regulate cholesterol and other blood fats.
9. Helps lower and regulate blood pressure.
10. Promotes bowel regularity.
11. Reduces risk of heart disease.
12. Reduces risk of cancer.
13. Helps purify the blood.
14. Purifies the body-Temple.
15. Increases chance for longer life.

WHAT ARE YOU WAITING FOR?

If you haven't been following a biblically based diet, what are you waiting for? There isn't a pill or a drug, a diet program, or health book that will ever compare to the wisdom of God and His Eden food program. His foods will make you whole both **physically** and **spiritually**. They are God's perfect "medicine," His natural healers, His gift to mankind. Are you ready to accept God's gift to you? Are you ready to feast on His nutritional masterpieces every day of your life?

Yahshua (Jesus) Himself said,

"Behold, I stand at the door and knock. If anyone hears My voice and opens the door, I will come in to him and dine with him, and he with Me." **(Revelation 3:20)**

Have you any idea what you are going to feed Him when He sits at your table?

Chapter 11

> "But while the meat was still between their teeth, before it was chewed, the wrath of the LORD was aroused against the people, and the LORD struck the people with a very great plague."
> Numbers 11:33

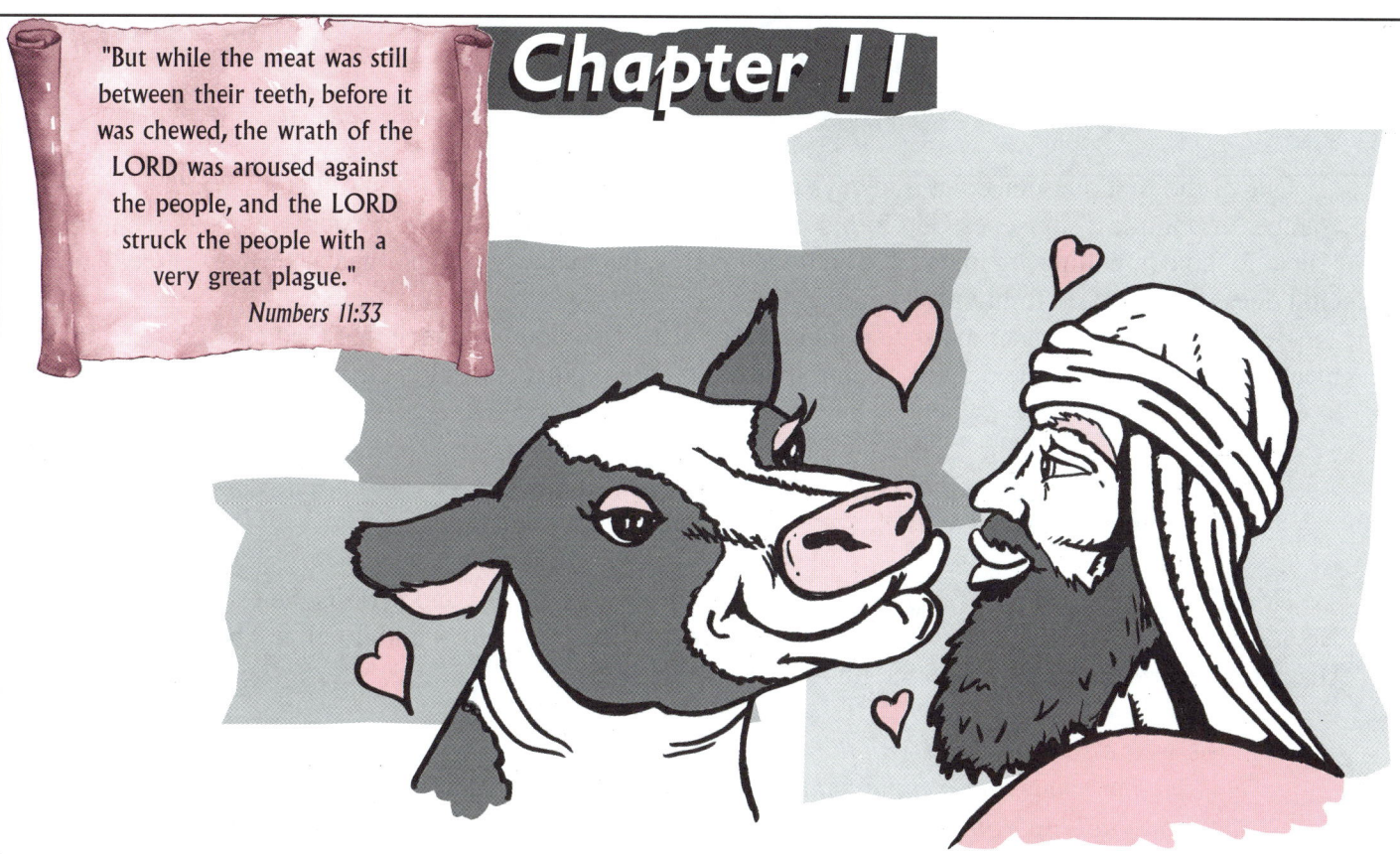

To Eat Meat Or Not To Eat Meat- That Is The Question?

You Change People's Minds With Knowledge And Not With Guilt.

WARNING: This chapter contains graphic descriptions of animal slaughtering procedures. If you find this type of material upsetting, please skip to the next chapter.

We human beings seem to have no reservations when it comes to our choices of food. We are known to eat the *dead* flesh of just about anything that moves – either on land or in the water.

In the last chapter, I discussed God's perfect diet for man before the fall in the Garden of Eden. I also mentioned the fact that animal products were *not* part of that original perfect menu. Does this mean then, that we should not now be eating meat or other animal derived foods such as eggs, milk, cheese and so forth? A closer examination of these issues is now in order.

IS IT A MORAL ISSUE?

One of the first questions that is always raised during a religious discussion of eating meat is whether or not it is a sin – does God forbid it? I have researched this question extensively and, while I have found compelling arguments for both viewpoints, the majority of theologians seem to agree that God does not expressly forbid meat eating.

Before going on then, let me state right up front that I also do *not* believe that God classifies eating meat as a sin. After all, He did tell Noah right after the Flood that it would be permissible henceforth to eat meat.

> *"Every <u>moving thing</u> that lives shall be food for you. I have given you all things even as the green herbs."* **(Genesis 9:3)**

However, as I theorized in the previous chapter, while God tolerates and permits the eating of meat – He doesn't like it – it wasn't the way He made the world to be originally – and it will not be the way His perfect world is going to be in the future.

> *"The wolf also shall dwell with the lamb, the leopard shall lie down with the young goat, the calf and the young lion and the fatling together; and a little child shall lead them, the cow and the bear shall graze; their young ones shall lie down together; and the lion shall eat straw like the ox, the nursing child shall play by the cobra's hole, and the weaned child shall put his hand into the viper's den."* **(Isaiah 11:6-8)**

> *"In that day I shall make a covenant for them with the beasts of the field, with the birds of the air, and with all creeping things of the ground. Bow and sword of battle I will shatter from the earth, to make them lie down safely."* **(Hosea 2:18)**

So if you like meat and don't believe you could ever give it up, most Bible scholars will tell you that it's okay. But before you go toss your steaks on the grill. . . you might better keep reading. There's a lot more to discuss about this issue.

NOT A SIN BUT DEFINITELY A SHAME

So if eating meat is not a sin, why would anyone ever want to give it up? Because it's **inhumane**, **unhealthy**, **barbaric** and **wasteful** – that's why! Now let me prove my point.

I realize that what I am about to share with you is not a pleasant subject and some of you may find it offensive. If so, then perhaps you should skip over this whole chapter. However, I have set out in this book to teach you biblical principles of health. Therefore, I feel it is my duty to give you all of the facts – as unpleasant or upsetting as they might be. I know that I will also upset some of the big boys in the meat business who don't want you to know what I am about to tell you. But as I said before, I will have to answer to God someday for this book. To omit this chapter would be a travesty. Perhaps it's time you heard a truth that can really set you free.

Moral issues aside, there are plenty of environmental, health and sanitation issues which condemn the current practices of the meat production industry. Meat production is a huge multi-billion dollar business. Meat has become a staple in our diets and is usually the main food around which we plan the rest of our meals. Have you ever pondered how many cows and chickens must be slaughtered each and every day just to keep the local burger and chicken franchises operating? Let me give you the shocking figures of just how many animals we butcher in the United States alone each year. *Ninety-three million pigs are slaughtered; thirty-seven million cattle; two million calves; six million horses, goats and sheep; and eight **billion** chickens and turkeys.*

Beyond that, have you ever considered how much grain must be fed to a single cow during its lifetime just so that it can be carved up and eaten *once*? For most people, eating meat means simply enjoying the end product without giving much forethought as to where it came from. Most grocery shoppers think that meat is something that comes neatly wrapped in clear packaging out of the store's coolers and freezers. Hardly anyone views it as the dead flesh of a recently living animal.

TWO AUTHORS WITH COURAGE TO SPEAK OUT

Few people ever want to go farther than the kitchen table or the grocery store to find out where their favorite meat is coming from. If they did, it might change their whole outlook on meat eating. *Moses Wasn't Fat* is a book on getting healthy. Therefore, you not only have a need but an obligation to know about the horrors of the meat production industry. There's plenty of information out there for those who are willing to take the time to look. In this chapter I will be quoting extensively from two books that I highly recommend you read:

> ### Classifying Vegetarians
> While most people think of all vegetarians as one in the same, there are actually three different classifications:
> - **Lacto Vegetarian.** Someone who abstains from all animal flesh but will eat dairy products.
> - **Lacto-Ovo Vegetarian.** Someone who abstains from all animal flesh but will eat dairy products and eggs.
> - **Vegan.** Vegans are vegetarians of the strictest form. They abstain from all forms of animal products including all dairy products, eggs and even honey, as well as condiments derived from or containing animal products.
> - **Pesco Vegetarian**. Someone who believes that not eating meat but still eating fish makes them a vegetarian. It's a stretch.
> - **Partial Vegetarian.** Someone who believes that giving up red meat but still eating poultry and fish makes them a vegetarian. Nice try but there's no such thing.

(1) Mad Cowboy – Plain Truth From The Cattle Rancher Who Won't Eat Meat, by Howard F. Lyman. Published by Scribner, New York, NY. (Available for $24, plus $2.95 postage, from Axion Publishers, 731 Kirkman Road, Orlando, FL 32811, 1-800-537-7671). It was Lyman's appearance on *The Oprah Winfrey Show* in 1996 that led to a highly publicized and unsuccessful lawsuit against Winfrey and Lyman by the beef industry. Lyman was once a very successful cattle rancher from Montana until he walked away from it all after learning the truth about the meat production industry. His excellent book is a startling expose of the entire livestock industry from hoof to the table.

(2) Slaughterhouse – The Shocking Story of Greed, Neglect, and Inhumane Treatment Inside the U.S. Meat Industry, by Gail A. Eisnitz. Prometheus Books, Amherst, NY. (Available for $28, plus $2.95 postage, from Axion Publishers, 731 Kirkman Road, Orlando, FL 32811, 1-800-537-7671). What started out with a single complaint about a Florida slaughterhouse turned into a tale of intrigue and suspense as Eisnitz uncovered even more startling information about the meat and poultry industries. The book takes you on a journey from one problematic slaughterhouse to another throughout the country. It is a most unpleasant and unsettling trip.

In reading both books, you will quickly see how the story goes from bad to worse as the gruesome and gory facts unfold. Are you aware, for example, that cattle which God made herbivorous, are actually forced to eat the ground-up flesh of other animals like horses, dogs, cats, pigs, chickens, turkeys, as well as blood and fecal material of their own species? As a matter of fact, until the FDA

Health Benefits of Vegetarianism

(1) Live longer
(2) Lower incidence of heart disease
(3) Lower incidence of cancer
(4) Less obesity
(5) Less digestive and elimination problems
(6) Lower risk of high blood pressure
(7) Lower risk of diabetes
(8) Lower incidence of gall stones
(9) Overall better health and energy levels

issued a prohibitive regulation in 1997, cattle were even forced to eat the dead flesh of other cows (cannibalism). This alphabet soup of dead animal body parts is euphemistically referred to as **protein concentrates** and then used as an additive in almost all pet food and livestock feed. Here's how Lyman describes this horror.

"When a cow is slaughtered, about half of it by weight is not eaten by humans: the intestines and their contents, the head, hooves, and horns, as well as bones and blood. These are dumped into giant grinders at rendering plants, as are the entire bodies of cows and other farm animals known to be diseased. Rendering is a $2.4 billion a year industry, processing forty billion pounds of dead animals a year. There is simply no such thing in America as an animal too ravaged by disease, too cancerous, or too putrid to be welcomed by the all-embracing arms of the renderer. Another staple of the renderer's diet, in addition to farm animals, is euthanized pets – six or seven million dogs and cats that are killed in animal shelters every year. Added to the blend are the euthanized catch of animal control agencies, and roadkill. When this gruesome mix is ground and steam-cooked, the lighter, fatty material floating to the top gets refined for use in such products as cosmetics, lubricants, soaps, candles, and waxes. The heavier protein material is dried and pulverized into a brown powder – about a quarter of which is fecal material. . . I used to feed tons of the stuff to my own livestock."

Lyman goes on to say that animal excrement itself is also used to "enrich" these feed concentrates. He sites Arkansas as an example where the average cattle farmer feeds over fifty tons of chicken litter to cattle every year. "One Arkansas cattle farmer was quoted in *U.S. News & World Report* as having recently purchased 745 tons of litter collected from the floors of local chicken-raising operations. After mixing it with small amounts of soy bran, he then feeds it to his eight hundred head of cattle, making them, in his words, 'fat as butterballs.'"

Now if you are wondering whether this practice, other than sounding completely nauseating and revolting, can possibly be harmful to your health as a meat eater, the answer appears to be yes. Have you heard about Mad Cow disease which is now afflicting Great Britain? Some investigators believe that it originated with the feeding of ground-up, disease infected sheep to cows. The sheep disease is called scrapie, because intense itching makes sheep scrape off virtually all of their wool. Scrapie apparently manifests itself in cows as **bovine spongiform encephalopathy** (BSE), commonly referred to as Mad Cow disease.

The disturbing question is whether people who eat meat from such infected cows can suffer any health problems? While the British government has been busy assuring its citizens that Mad Cow disease is not transmutable to human beings, not everyone is convinced. Several researchers theorize that it is now appearing in humans as a slowly progressing brain disorder called **Creutzfeldt-Jakob disease** (CJD). At present, there is no treatment for CJD and no test for its presence other than a biopsy of brain material at an autopsy.

According to Lyman's book, the American rendering industry in 1989 *voluntarily* banned the use of sheep heads at rendering plants. An FDA survey three years later found that 15 of 19 inspected plants were not observing this voluntary ban, and six of them were using the rendered sheep protein in cattle feed. "Unenforced safety regulations can do little more than lull us into a false sense of security," Lyman states.

So how about you? Are you still willing to play Russian roulette with the health of yourself and your family? Irrespective of Mad Cow disease and CJD, do you really want to eat meat from animals that have been fed such a witch's brew? Before you answer, you had better keep reading. Our story doesn't end here. There are still other health problems for you to be concerned about from eating meat.

In his book *Mad Cowboy*, Lyman articulately describes how so much of the meat in America is contaminated with carcinogenic pesticides such as dioxin. One reason for this is that crops grown as cattle feed are permitted to have far higher levels of pesticides than crops grown for human consumption. Another reason is that, since pesticides are stored in animal fat and cattle are fed other animals, they are getting a double dose of carcinogens. Now guess who sits at the top of this food chain? That's right! You do! So all of these potentially health-damaging toxins end up in your steak dinner.

And what about heart disease? Are you aware that saturated fats as found primarily in animal products are one of the main contributors to heart attacks. I just love the following line from Lyman's book. "Heart attacks are never caused by corn, broccoli, or cauliflower; they are not the work of pears, plums, or peaches; they are never brought on by rice, barley, or lentils." It sounds to me like Howard Lyman would make a good advocate for Biblical Nutrition.

Another strong point against meat eating in Lyman's book is the impact that cattle raising has on the environment. "To be an environmentalist who happens to eat meat is like being a philanthropist who doesn't happen to give to charity," is how he puts it.

According to Dr. Michael W. Fox in his book *Agricide*, "An estimated eighty-five percent of all U.S. agricultural land is used in the production of animal foods, which in turn is linked with deforestation, destruction of wildlife species, extinction of species, loss of soil productivity through mineral depletion and erosion, water pollution and depletion, overgrazing, and desertification."

And have you ever thought about what happens to all of that cow waste? On a typical feedlot with ten thousand head of cattle, as much as half a million pounds of cow dung is produced ***daily!*** As a matter of fact, livestock waste exceeds human waste in tonnage nationwide by a factor of one hundred and thirty. The ammonia, nitrates and bacteria generated by this waste inevitably ends up polluting rivers, streams and wells.

Lyman convincingly argues further that it takes tremendous amounts of water to raise large herds of cattle. "We often hear about water shortages in areas such as Southern California, where citizens are recurrently requested not to wash their cars, not to over-water their lawns, and to use low-flow showers and toilets. Good ideas all. But you never hear city, county, or state officials combating drought by urging their citizens to cut down on meat consumption, even though the water required to produce *just ten pounds of steak* equals the water consumption of the average household for a year."

Now if you think that Lyman's book *Mad Cowboy* is pretty intense and that it covers most of the reasons for not eating meat, "you ain't seen nothing yet." Yes, it gets worse. Gail Eisnitz' book *Slaughterhouse* is even more horrifying.

SLAUGHTER OF THE INNOCENT

What Howard Lyman's book does to blow the lid off of the cattle raising industry, Eisnitz' book does to the slaughterhouse, meat packing industry. In her book, Eisnitz takes the reader on a behind-the-scenes examination of the revolting and horrifying goings-on in the slaughterhouses of America. It is a very upsetting and life-changing book to read.

The impetus for Eisnitz' book came when she was tipped off that the largest beef slaughterhouse in Florida was actually skinning cattle while they were still alive. Her investigative search would soon reveal that this was only the tip of the iceberg. Just about everything inhumane that could be done to animals led to slaughter was being done. Even when done according to approved procedures, slaughtering is disgusting. Here's the whole gruesome process as described by Eisnitz.

"The stun operator, or 'knocker,' shoots each animal in the forehead with a compressed-air gun that drives a steel bolt into the cow's skull and then retracts it. If the knocking gun is sufficiently powered, well maintained, and properly used by the operator, it knocks the cow unconscious or kills the animal on the spot.

"The next man on the line, the 'shackler,' wraps a chain around one of the stunned cow's hind legs. Once shackled, the animal is automatically lifted onto a moving overhead rail. The cow, now hanging upside down by a leg, is sent to the 'sticker,' the worker who cuts the throat – more precisely, the carotid arteries and a jugular vein in the neck. . .

"Next the cow travels along the 'bleed rail' and is given several minutes to bleed out. The carcass then proceeds to the head-skinners, the leggers, and on down the line where it is completely skinned, eviscerated, and split in half."

Eisnitz did indeed substantiate that there are many instances of cattle being skinned alive – kicking wildly and frantically in a futile effort to save their lives. But pity the poor pigs. They don't fare any better. They're often immersed in a scalding tank and boiled alive. Sadly, government watchdog agencies appear to be looking the other way on this type of barbarism as well as a whole litany of other offenses.

A talkative sticker from a hog processing plant willingly shared his experiences with Eisnitz. Unfortunately, the troubles start for the pigs the minute they arrive at the plant. "Two or three drivers chase the hogs up (the chute). They prod them a lot because the hogs don't want to go. When hogs smell blood, they don't want to go. I've seen hogs beaten, whipped, kicked in the head to get them up to the restrainer. One night I saw a driver get so angry at a hog he broke its back with a piece of board. I've seen hog drivers take their prod and shove it up the hog's (behind) to get them to move."

The situation doesn't get much better once inside the plant after the hogs have been "killed." The informer continues, "I was kicked, bitten, stabbed in the forearm, had a tooth knocked out, an eardrum punctured, and finally got my face slashed. And that was *after* I complained about live hogs to almost every level of management. . ."

America's demand for animal flesh is so high that the slaughterhouses are often forced to work at breakneck speed just to keep up with it. Sadly, this leads to all kinds of atrocities in order to keep up the efficiency rate. Those unfortunate cows that get their heads stuck between a fence gate, for instance, are often beheaded on the spot. Slow moving cattle are kept moving with whips, chains, boards, shovels and hoes. Cows that get hurt during the transport or slaughter process are hooked up to an electric winch at any convenient spot on their bodies and then dragged quickly through the so-called kill alley. Birthing cows often have their calves yanked right out of their bodies so as not to slow things down. One worker reports that "it's nothing to have a cow hanging up in front of you and see the calf inside (the uterus) kicking, trying to get out."

In her book, Eisnitz exposes blatant slaughterhouse infractions of USDA regulations whereby horsemeat is mixed with cow's meat and then sold as pure beef. She cites another instance where a hog worker told her how hog body parts such as stomach, intestines, testicles and feet were being sold to restaurants out the back door of his slaughterhouse.

In case you're thinking of switching to chicken in hopes that things might be better, they're not! Eisnitz relates her first visit to a chicken farm this way. "Inside, the air was thick with ammonia and dust. Through watering, stinging eyes I saw. . . a sea of forty thousand chickens packed together so tightly in one giant shed they could hardly move, pecking around in their own droppings on the floor. I wasn't surprised when I noticed that here and there a chicken was lying on its back, motionless." Her tour guide informed her that genetic alteration and growth stimulants now made chickens grow very rapidly. The ones who couldn't handle such rapid growth died from a heart attack at the ripe old age of one month. Eisnitz also noted that she saw behind the warehouse a huge pile of dead chickens swarming with flies and filling the air with the smell of rot.

Twenty five to thirty million chickens are slaughtered every single *day*. Eisnitz book vividly describes this sickening process. Chickens are dumped from their overcrowded storage cages and shackled upside down to an overhead conveyor. Rather than being stunned as are cattle and hogs, the chickens are mildly electrocuted into a state of paralysis. A conveyor then carries thousands per hour of the shocked and paralyzed birds through a high-speed circular blade that slits their throats. After a one-minute bleed-out, the birds are then dunked into a scald tank to loosen their feathers.

"After their heads and feet are removed and they've been washed, the chickens are re-hung on an evisceration line where machines automatically cut them open and pull their guts out. Thanks to automation in the industry, poultry plants. . . can kill and process as many as 340,000 birds per day."

Eisnitz details how one ex-chicken plant worker reported to a Congressional hearing that the floors of her facility were covered with grease, fat, sand and roaches. Workers were instructed by supervisors to take chickens that dropped to the floor and send them back down the line. Bugs were all over the walls, flies were everywhere and the roaches were up to five inches long. There was so much fecal material on the floor that it kept getting into one worker's boots and burned his feet so badly he lost his toenails. To make matters worse, many of the employees were chewing and spitting out snuff and tobacco on the floor.

Another worker reported on conditions at his plant as follows. "I saw black chicken, green chicken, chicken that stank, and chicken with feces on it. Chicken like this is supposed to be thrown away but instead it would be sent down the line to be processed."

Maggots show up everywhere and some chicken plant workers have even reported seeing them get ground up right along with the meat into chicken franks. Still another worker noted how "rotten chicken meat is mixed with fresh meat and sold for baby food. We are asked to mix it with the fresh food, and this is the way it is sold. You can see the worms inside the meat."

CONTAMINATED MEAT

If the inhumane treatment of these animals were the end of the story, that would be bad enough, but it's not the end of the story. There are also numerous contamination problems that put both your health and your life at risk. Eisnitz quotes USDA meat inspector David Carney who gives a very graphic description of the problem. "We used to trim the s_ _ t off the meat. Then we washed the s_ _ t off the meat. Now the consumer eats the s_ _t off the meat."

Food poisoning is now a common occurrence in America with animal foods being a major cause. Two of the most harmful and deadly food poisoning bacteria are **E. coli** and **salmonella**. According to Eisnitz, most deaths from these pathogens are erroneously ascribed to other ailments like cardiac or pulmonary arrest, stroke or secondary illnesses resulting from bacterial invasion. Sloppy, high-speed slaughter operations are known contributing factors to E coli contamination and its most vulnerable victims are children and the elderly.

"With one hamburger containing meat from as many as one hundred different animals, one infected animal can cross-contaminate sixteen tons of beef. And because the grinding process creates a much larger surface area for bacteria to inhabit than a cut of beef, they find hamburger meet especially hospitable."

With the advent of high-speed chicken processing plants, there has been a dramatic increase in contaminated birds. In the scald tanks, "fecal contamination on skin and feathers gets inhaled by live birds, and hot water opens birds' pores allowing pathogens to seep in. The pounding action of the defeathering machines creates an aerosol of feces-contaminated water which is then beaten into the birds." One official told Eisnitz that immersing clean, healthy birds in the same tank with dirty ones practically assures cross-contamination.

IT JUST GETS WORSE AND WORSE

And this type of disgusting detail goes on and on and on. What I have excerpted here from these two books only scratches the surface. I assure you that there is much more of this horror story to report but I think by now you've gotten the message. However, I strongly urge you to purchase both books and read them and then share this tragic information with the people you love.

I'd like to let the words of Gail Eisnitz close out this chapter for me. "Animals, by virtue of their existence, have value unto themselves and certain inalienable rights. If humankind is so grandiose in its dominion over animals as to overlook even the most basic freedoms during life, surely we can't be so insensitive as to think that beating, maiming, and strangling animals is an acceptable precursor to death. That being boiled, skinned, and dismembered alive is an acceptable way to die.

"And now, at last, after all this time and all the obstacles my slaughter investigation faced, it feels wonderful to finally put these words on paper in black and white, knowing that people will finally read about what's really taking place behind the closed doors of America's slaughterhouses. The more a person learns about what's really going on out there, the more he or she wants to tell the whole world, in the hopes that society will see and, more importantly, want to do something about it. And now I am telling the world. I feel a colossal sense of relief knowing that the responsibility for ending these atrocities does not fall entirely on my shoulders alone. Now you know, and you can help make the changes."

I couldn't have said it better.

Daniel The Vegetarian Stands His Ground

Does the Bible ever promote vegetarianism? Most definitely it does. Are you familiar with Holy Scripture's most famous vegetarian story from the Book of Daniel? Daniel and his three companions, Hananiah, Mishael and Azariah – better known as Shadrach, Meshach and Abed-Nego – were all taken captive to Babylon where they were conscripted to serve in the king's palace. When told they would have to eat the rich meat dishes of the king, Daniel and his companions protested, preferring to stick with their usual vegetarian diet. Let's pick up the story from the Bible.

"And the king appointed for them a daily provision of the king's delicacies (meat) and of the wine which he drank. . . so that all of them might serve before the king. But Daniel purposed in his heart that he would not defile himself with the portion of the king's delicacies (meat), nor with the wine which he drank; therefore he requested of the chief of the eunuchs that he might not defile himself.

Now God had brought Daniel into the favor and good will of the chief of the eunuchs. And the chief of the eunuchs said to Daniel, 'I fear my lord the king, who has appointed your food and drink. For why should he see your faces looking worse than the young men who are your age? Then you would endanger my head before the king.'

So Daniel said to the steward whom the chief of the eunuchs had set over Daniel, Hananiah, Mishael and Azariah, 'Please test your servants for ten days, and let them give us vegetables to eat and water to drink. Then let our appearance be examined before you, and the appearance of the young men who eat the portion of the king's delicacies (meat); and as you see fit, so deal with your servants.'

So he consented with them in this matter and tested them ten days. And at the end of ten days their features appeared better and fatter (fuller) in flesh than all the young men who ate the portion of the king's delicacies (meat).

Thus the steward took away their portion of delicacies (meat) and the wine that they were to drink, and gave them vegetables." **(Daniel 1:5-16)**

75

Late Breaking News

I wish I could report that things in the meat industry were getting better but unfortunately, as this book was getting ready to go to print several new disturbing stories were breaking.

• First of all, evidence continued to mount that the human form of Mad Cow disease – Creutzfeldt-Jakob disease (CJD) – may actually be transmittable via milk and dairy products as well as by blood, much like HIV and hepatitis C. If the later were true, there is grave concern that CJD may have been making the rounds in the nation's medical blood supply for years. (As of the fall of 2000, the American government continued to claim no cases of Mad Cow disease in this country.) Since Mad Cow/CJD takes years to show up, some researchers are theorizing that there's a time bomb ticking away in this country and that there will be a future day of reckoning.

• Also in late summer of 2000, the U.S. Department of Agriculture was considering new rules that would classify animal carcasses with cancers, tumors and open sores as safe for human consumption. Such conditions would simply be classified as aesthetic problems and thus no longer be an obstacle to receiving the USDA purple seal of approval. The USDA acknowledged that it had already been implementing the new regulations in 24 slaughterhouses since October of 1999.

Delmer Jones of Renlap, Alabama, a federal food inspector for 41 years, said he's so revolted by the government's lowering of food wholesomeness that he won't buy meat at the supermarket anymore. Jones, president of the 7000 member National Joint Council of Meat Inspectors Locals, said he is also trying to discourage family members from eating meat. Jones verified what was reported in this chapter when he cited the huge increase in the number of birds an inspector is expected to examine. "When I started inspecting, inspectors were looking at 13 birds a minute, then 40, and now it's 91 birds a minute with three inspectors. You cannot do your job with 91 birds a minute," Jones commented.

In another change in policy, the USDA said that inspectors would spend more time examining and monitoring plant processing *procedures* rather than actual meat *inspecting*. So now federal inspectors spend more time checking paperwork than potential food. Karen Henderson of the USDA's division of field operations admitted that defective carcasses are being approved for human consumption under this pilot program.

Felicia Nestor, director of the Government Accountability Project (GAP), a Washington watchdog group, reported that under the new inspection procedure, chickens were found with higher levels of fecal and other contamination than in the traditional inspection methods. "A lot of diseased animals are going out," she said.

• In a report called **The Jungle 2000**, GAP and another Washington-based consumer group called Public Citizen, examined conditions at 92 percent of America's meat processing plants. The report claims that the various inspection changes begun by the Clinton administration in 1995 under its "Hazard Analysis and Critical Control Program" have actually weakened the USDA's authority by giving the meat packing industry a larger role in monitoring meat safety. Disturbingly, the report noted that 210 inspectors acknowledged that under the new procedures they had not taken any direct action against meat contaminated with feces, vomit and metal shards whereas they would have under the former system.

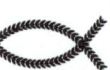

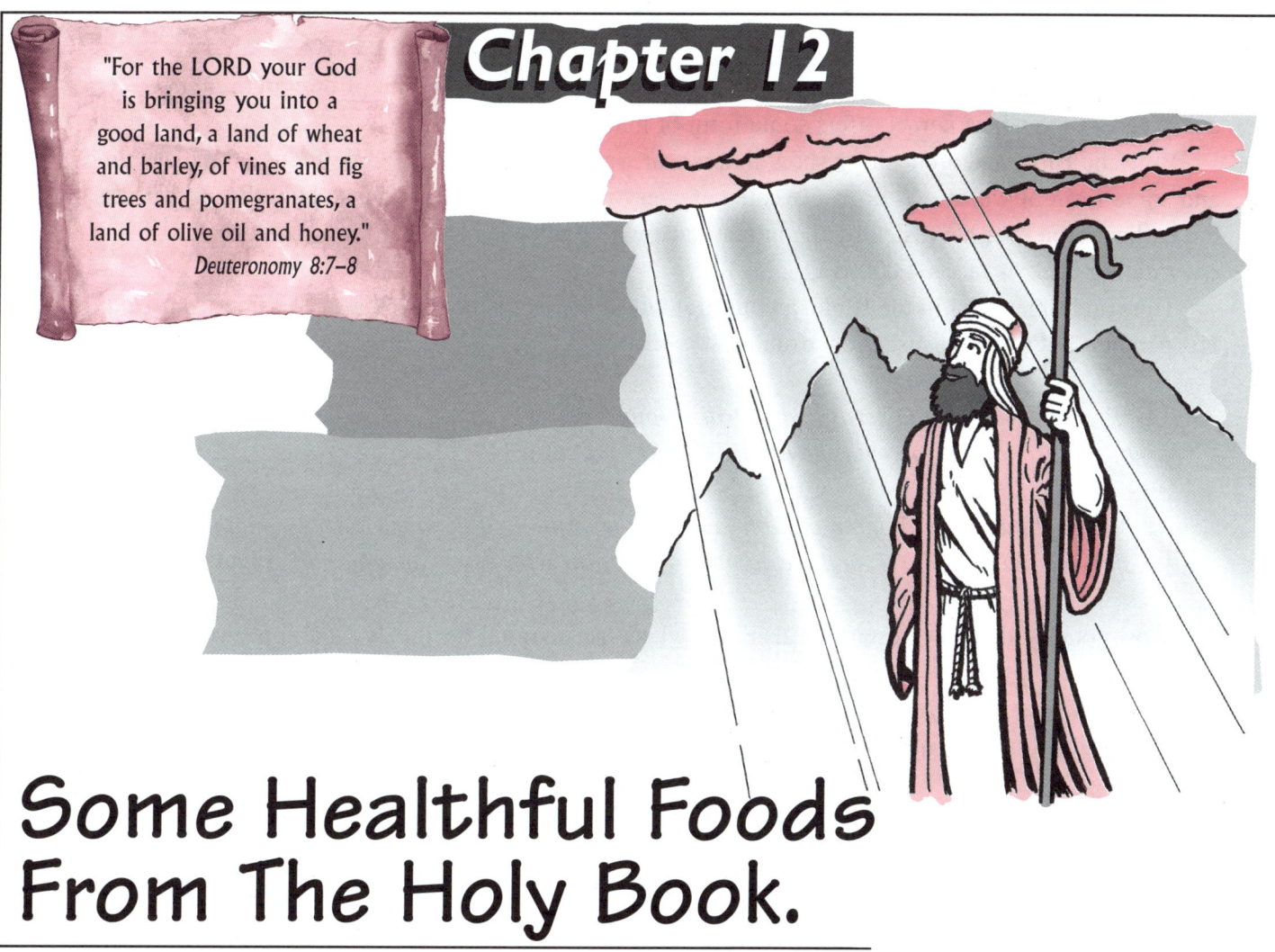

"For the LORD your God is bringing you into a good land, a land of wheat and barley, of vines and fig trees and pomegranates, a land of olive oil and honey."
Deuteronomy 8:7–8

Chapter 12

Some Healthful Foods From The Holy Book.

Some Days You Drink The Wine And Some Days You Squeeze The Grapes.

Most people hardly give a second thought to the Bible's references to food and drink, yet food is mentioned in some way in many of the books of the Bible. Some foods are even mentioned by name. Should you be consuming these special Bible foods on a regular basis? Might these foods have a beneficial effect on your health and well being? I think that after reading their impressive attributes you will want to make them all a regular part of your diet.

WHEAT

Of all the foods mentioned in the Bible, assuredly none holds a higher position of importance than wheat – the staff of life. Nearly 50 percent of all the foods we consume contain some form of wheat. It is a nearly perfect food with all of its important nutrients distributed throughout the entire kernel or wheat berry as it is called. Wheat contains a well-balanced array of protein, fat and complex carbohydrates as well as a variety of vitamins, minerals and enzymes. The germ portion of the wheat is an excellent source of vitamin E and essential fatty acids. Wheat bran is one of the best sources of dietary fiber and some researchers believe that vitamin E may actually lower the incidences of heart diseases and cancer. Just a half a cup of wheat germ contains four times the amount of protein of an egg. Yes, every part of the wheat kernel offers some form of nutritional benefit.

Both the Bible and archeology show that wheat was one of the main staple foods of ancient times and some form of wheat was probably eaten at every meal. In fact, historians claim that wheat was the earliest crop ever harvested by the human race with evidence of wheat farming along the Nile river dating back as far as 4,000 B.C.

Time and time again in the Bible, a bountiful wheat harvest is portrayed as a blessing from God to His people. Let's look at just a few examples.

> *"Praise the LORD, O Jerusalem! Praise your God, O Zion! . . . He makes peace within your borders, and fills you with the finest WHEAT."* **(Psalm 147:12-14)**

> *"Be glad then, you children of Zion, and rejoice in the LORD your God; . . . the threshing floors shall be full of WHEAT, and the vats shall overflow with new wine and oil."* **(Joel 2:23-24)**

Most notably, the New Testament also uses wheat as a symbol for the dying and resurrected Savior.

> *"Unless a grain of WHEAT falls into the ground and dies, it remains alone; but if it dies, it produces much grain."* **(John 12:24)**

Further proof of the link of wheat to salvation is the fact that Yahshua (Jesus) used unleavened wheat bread at the Last Supper as a symbol for His body.

The 13th Chapter of the book of Matthew may well be called the **wheat chapter** as Yahshua (Jesus) cites two parables in this chapter where wheat is used as a symbol for God's children.

The Biblical feast day of Pentecost, also known as the **Festival of Weeks**, or **Shavuot** was held in celebration of the spring wheat harvest. This same wheat festival was the day in the New Testament when the Holy Spirit descended upon the Apostles.

Truly wheat is a special gift from God and rightfully deserves to be first on our list of Bible foods. Use it only in its whole grain form – never white, bleached and enriched. It is available commercially as wheat berries, wheat flakes (rolled wheat), wheat flour, wheat germ and wheat greens.

BARLEY

Barley, like wheat, is a highly nutritious grain and is mentioned close to 40 times in the Bible. In ancient Israel, its growing season and harvest actually came before wheat and it was the first crop of the year. Symbolically, then, barley is representative of the prophet or the one who comes first to announce the Messiah. Hence, some Bible scholars compare barley to John the Baptist and wheat to Yahshua (Jesus).

To the Hebrews, the first green barley shoots springing forth out of the ground were a sign for them to begin their new calendar year. They called this month *Abib* which means tender or green. Symbolically then, barley also represents a new beginning or a fresh start.

While barley was never considered to be quite as versatile or prized as wheat, nevertheless, it played an important role in the diet of the Israelites. It was plentiful and inexpensive making it highly accessible to the masses. Besides its usage as human food, it was also used to feed animals.

According to the books ***Healing Foods From The Bible***, and ***Foods and Nutrition Encyclopedia***, barley is reputed to improve potency, vigor and strength. Ancient Greek athletes would often eat an easily digested barley-mash while in training. Roman gladiators were sometimes called ***hordearii***, meaning "barley eaters," because the grain was added to their diet to give them bursts of strength before their contests. Barley was also a common rendering on ancient Greek coins.

Like wheat, barley is also an excellent source of protein, fat, carbohydrates, vitamins, minerals and enzymes. It is also high in beta carotene, vitamins C, E, B-1, B-2, B-3, B-6 as well as 19 amino acids. Furthermore, some recent studies seem to indicate that barley may actually help lower cholesterol.

It is available commercially as barley grain, barley flakes, barley malt powder, barley syrup, pearled barley and barley greens.

GRAPES

Of all the foods mentioned in the Bible, grapes – also referred to as the fruit of the vine – are one of the most frequently discussed. As a matter of fact, the Bible makes literally hundreds of references to grapes, vines, and vineyards. Of course, since grapes are also used to make alcoholic wine, they are a Bible food that can be used for both good and evil.

The first mention of grape cultivation in the Bible is in **Genesis 9:20** where we are told that one of the first things Noah did after the flood was to plant a vineyard. This makes grapes one of the oldest cultivated foods on earth.

Apparently, the grapes that grew in ancient Israel were enormous as noted in the Book of Numbers.

> *"And they came unto the brook of Eshcol, and cut down from thence a branch with one cluster of GRAPES, and they bare it between two upon a staff;"* **(Numbers 13:23)**

Grape juice and wine are used throughout the Bible as symbols for blood. Even Yahshua (Jesus) uses this symbolism at the Last Supper where He refers to the juice of the grape as His blood.
(Matthew 26:27-29; Mark 14:23-25; Luke 22:17-18)

Grapes were also a symbol of fruitfulness, and the grape harvest was a time of great festivity.
(Genesis 40:9-11; Psalm 105:33; Zechariah 3:10)

The grapes of the Middle East during Biblical times were sweet and either dark purple or green. They were eaten fresh and also sun dried into raisins. They were also squeezed and drunk as grape juice or wine. A less expensive form of wine vinegar was also made from the grapes and used by the poorer people. The grape leaves were also eaten and the stalks and vines were used in feeding the animals.

The nutritional and health value of grapes has been intensely explored over the past few years. According to a University of Wisconsin Medical School study, a glass of purple grape juice daily may be good for your heart. Grape juice makes blood platelets less sticky and therefore, they are less likely to clump and form clots. In an impressive study cited in the journal *Circulation*, 15 patients with confirmed coronary artery disease drank purple grape juice for 14 days. After just two weeks, the subjects showed a significant improvement in both artery pressure and the good blood cholesterol.

Grape skins are also another source of rich nutritional value. *Resveratrol* is a bioflavonoid found in grape skins that scientists now believe may be helpful in the prevention and treatment of cancer. Resveratrol is a powerful antioxidant that seems to have the power not only to prevent tumor formation but to actually inhibit the spread of cancer. In addition to resveratrol, grapes also contain *ellagic acid, glucaric acid, phenols* and other antioxidants that help protect cellular DNA from damage.

Another product from grapes – grape seed extract – has also recently been shown to be beneficial for the heart. Grape seeds are a rich source of biologically active *bioflavonoids*. These are potent antioxidants which help fight harmful free radicals in the body. The bioflavonoids from grape seeds are 50 times more potent than vitamin E and 20 times more potent than vitamin C.

Two other components of grapes are *polyphenols* and *tannins*, both of which show promise as antiviral and anti-tumor compounds.

FIGS

The fig is another one of those Bible foods that is referenced with both good and evil associations. Of course we all know the story of Adam and Eve sewing fig leaves together to cover their nakedness **(Genesis 3:7)** and how Yahshua (Jesus) cursed the fig tree **(Matt 21:19, Mark 11:13, Luke 13:6)**. These references are interesting not in their condemnation of figs – which they do not do – but in the inability of the fig tree to be used *properly*. Adam and Eve, rather than eat and partake of the nutritional blessing of the fig, instead used the leaves to cover their sin. Yahshua (Jesus), in cursing the fig tree, was not implying that figs were bad but that the fig tree out of season was a direct tieback to Adam and Eve's use of the fig leaf when they too were out of season so to speak.

Other references in the Bible definitely show that figs that reach maturity (just as Adam and Eve should have), are indeed a good food. Here are just some of the many positive biblical references to the fig tree in addition to **Deuteronomy 8:8** quoted at the beginning of this chapter.

> "And Judah and Israel dwelt safely, each man under his vine and his FIG TREE." **(1Kings 4:25)**

> "The FIG TREE puts forth her green figs, and the vines with the tender grapes give a good smell." **(Song of Solomon 2:13)**

> "Do not be afraid, you beasts of the field; for the open pastures are springing up, and the tree bears its fruit; the FIG TREE and the vine yield their strength." **(Joel 2:22)**

> "But everyone shall sit under his vine and under his FIG TREE, and no one shall make them afraid; for the mouth of the LORD of hosts has spoken." **(Micah 4:4)**

> "'In that day,' says the LORD of hosts, 'everyone will invite his neighbor under his vine and under his FIG TREE'." **(Zechariah 3:10)**

Notice here that both figs and grapes together are a sign of peace and rest. Along this same mythology, an image of a man sitting under a fig tree is always a symbol of rest, peace and tranquility in the land.

Fig trees can thrive equally as well on the rocky slopes of Greece as on the sandy shores of North Africa. Because fig trees grow so easily and abundantly in the Mediterranean countries, figs became known as "the poor man's food."

Nutritionally, figs are an excellent food. They have been highly valued throughout history both in their fresh or dried form. As with barley, figs too were popular among Greek and Roman athletes to improve their performance.

Figs are an excellent source of potassium and other minerals and are also very high in fiber. As a matter of fact, figs contain all of the five types of fiber (see page 51) and are particularly high in pectin. Figs help promote weight loss and therefore make an excellent addition to a diet program.

According to the book **Healing Foods From The Bible**, figs were associated for centuries with healing power for cancer, constipation, scurvy, hemorrhoids, gangrene, liver troubles and boils. Figs are also good detoxifiers, they aid in the health of the stomach, spleen and large intestines, and help reduce inflammation and swelling. Fig juice made from soaking figs in spring water makes an excellent laxative and is also good for sore throats, coughs and stomach ulcers. There are a variety of figs available commercially.

POMEGRANATES

While the pomegranate definitely played an important nutritional role in the diets of biblical peoples, its main usage in the Bible seems to be more for its symbolic meaning. The pomegranate is given the unique distinction of being closely linked to the House of God – not once, but twice. The first time is when the Tabernacle is set up under Moses' direction in the wilderness. The second time is at the building of King Solomon's Temple. Other than the olive (see next page), no other food anywhere in the Bible gets this kind of special treatment. Here are some specific examples from the Bible.

When Moses is given instructions in the wilderness on how to prepare the vestments of the High Priest (a foreshadowing of Yahshua (Jesus)), he is told to decorate them with pomegranates.

> *"And upon its hem you shall make POMEGRANATES of blue, purple, and scarlet, all around its hem, and bells of gold between them all around."* **(Exodus 28:33-34)**

Then later, when Solomon is building the first, and what most Bible scholars consider to be the most magnificent house of the LORD ever, the pomegranate once again plays a significant role. The two main pillars at the entrance to God's house (named *Jachin* and *Boaz*), are heavily decorated with pomegranates.

> *"The capitals on the two pillars also had POMEGRANATES above, by the convex surface which was next to the network; and there were two hundred such pomegranates in rows on each of the capitals all around."* **(1 Kings 7:20)**

The question Bible scholars need to ask then, is what is it about the pomegranate that makes it so closely linked to God's Temple? The answer is that the pomegranate is a symbol for eternal life and fertility because of its many seeds. So what exactly is God trying to tell us here? His first commission to Adam and Eve was to be fruitful and multiply and fill the earth. Furthermore, whenever His blessings are upon Israel, they are always manifested by fruitfulness and abundance of the crops. Our God is a God of ever expanding *life* and the pomegranate is the symbol He has chosen to represent this.

Pomegranate fruit grows on a small, semi-tropical tree or bush which apparently was indigenous to Persia where it was known to grow in the Hanging Gardens of Babylon. From there, it appears to have spread throughout the Middle East. The tree was also cultivated in Egypt and as **Deuteronomy 8:8** notes it was already flourishing in Canaan prior to the arrival of the Israelites.

The pomegranate tree yields a leathery, hard skinned, reddish-purple fruit. The thin rinds inside contain many seeds, each in a pulp sack filled with a tangy, sweet amethyst-colored juice. Although it is a relatively small tree giving little shade, its refreshing fruit more than compensated tired Bible travelers such as King Saul who rested under it **(1 Samuel 14:2)**. While the fruit was used to quench thirst, the rind was used to make medicine and red dye. Pomegranates are low in calories yet high in fiber, vitamins and minerals, particularly potassium and vitamin C. The pomegranate has a cleansing and cooling effect on the body and is also a good blood purifier.

In an impressive study conducted in May of 2000, a team of Israeli researchers found that drinking pomegranate juice daily may significantly reduce the risk of atherosclerosis and heart disease. I was so impressed by this pomegranate information that I wanted to add pomegranates to my diet immediately. I spent many days in my local area searching out grocery stores, gift shops, gourmet stores and flea markets looking for any form of pomegranates I could find. All to no avail. Finally, out of complete frustration, I knew that the only way I was ever going to be able to reap the benefits of the pomegranate was to bring something out under my own brand. I am pleased to tell you that **Logia**: *Foods of the Bible* now offers what I think is the most delicious pomegranate concentrate you will ever find. (For more information, check out page 97.)

OLIVES & OLIVE OIL

If the seven foods of **Deuteronomy 8:8** appear to be God's favorite of all foods, then perhaps the olive, judging by its special usage in the Bible, may well be called God's *favorite of favorites*. Judging by the many holy references to olives and olive oil in the Bible, we would have to say that the olive is truly a fruit of singular symbolic religious importance. Nearly every mention of olives and olive oil in the Bible ties into a deeper, religious or spiritual meaning. To understand this usage, we have to understand what that symbolism is.

The olive is a symbol for long life and in fact, everlasting life. Olive trees live longer than any other living organism on earth. It has been claimed by some that an olive tree can live for up to four thousand years or more. Some Bible scholars theorize that perhaps a few of the olive trees currently growing on the Mount of Olives in Israel were actually alive at the time of Yahshua (Jesus).

You may recall also that when Noah sent out a dove from the ark to check the weather conditions, it returned with an olive leaf in its mouth. **(Genesis 8:11)** The dove with an olive leaf or branch in its mouth has thus become nearly a universal symbol for peace. (Could the olive tree that the dove broke the leaf off of still be alive today? Might this be another way for God to show continuity from the Great Flood up to our times, much like the rainbow?)

Olive oil was always used in lighting the Temple Menorah (lamp stand) which stood in front of the Ark of the Covenant in the Temple's Holy of Holies. The symbolism here is that God's Law is everlasting.

> "And you shall command the children of Israel that they bring you pure OIL OF PRESSED OLIVES for the light, to cause the lamp to burn continually." **(Exodus 27:20)**

Olive oil was also used to anoint both the King and High Priest in ancient Israel. Our English word Messiah comes from the Hebrew word ***mashiyach*** which simply means to smear with olive oil. The Greek word "Christ" has the same meaning. And so, Christ the Messiah is the one who is anointed or smeared with olive oil. This certainly shows the importance God has given to this fruit.

Olive oil was a dietary staple in the ancient Middle East and used for a multitude of dietary purposes. Hundreds of ancient olive presses have been found by archeologists throughout the region. Olive oil was spread on bread, used in cooking, and mixed with flour to make bread. Apparently, the olive industry was a huge trade in biblical times.

But perhaps the most amazing thing of all about the olive is the fact that today, thousands of years after the Bible was written, researchers are finding out just what a miracle food this really is. For instance, olive oil has been shown to help in the prevention of cardiovascular disease, aid in digestive problems, while protecting against everything from arthritis to diabetes to constipation to cancer. Let me caution you here that there are several different grades of olive oil on the market. The best one to buy for the health benefits is **100 percent extra virgin olive oil**. Extra virgin olive oil is particularly high in *phenolic antioxidants* as well as *squalene* and *oleic acid*.

Researchers in Greece recently reported that consuming olive oil regularly might reduce the risk of arthritis. Using a test base of 333 people, researchers found that those people who regularly consumed olive oil had a 62 percent lower risk of getting rheumatoid arthritis than those who ate it infrequently or never. The head of the research team, Athena Linos, M.D., theorized that it is the oleic acid in olive oil which acts as a joint lubricator and anti-inflammatory.

Other researchers have shown that oils high in mono-unsaturated fats, of which olive oil ranks the highest, are excellent for protecting the arteries against heart attacks. Olive oil is 77 percent mono-unsaturated.

Olive oil also assists the body in regulating cholesterol production, keeping the Low Density Lipoproteins (LDLs) low while encouraging the production of the good cholesterol known as High Density Lipoproteins (HDL). Olive oil also helps protect the body against harmful free radicals.

In a recent book entitled ***Your Miracle Brain*** (HarperCollins), author Jean Carper reports that olive oil, garlic and vinegar (all Bible foods) can help keep your mind sharp and improve your memory. Carper claims that eating just three tablespoons of olive oil every day with food can help prevent memory loss. "Studies at the University of Bari in Italy, led by Dr. Anthony Carpuso, showed that southern Italians who eat the most olive oil, cut their memory loss by one third," States Carper.

Certainly, in light of these impressive spiritual and nutritional attributes, olives and olive oil most definitely belong near the top in Bible food ranking.

HONEY

Honey is another food that is mentioned extensively in the Bible. Since the dawn of history, man has used honey in countless ways. Ancient scrolls dating over 3,000 years ago have been found that list the reputed benefits of honey. Through the ages, honey has been used for a variety of purposes including sweetening, flavoring, cosmetic, health food, aphrodisiac, medicine, religious symbol, energy food, athletic performance booster, embalmer, and even as money. Both honey and salt were mankind's earliest preservatives.

Both the Assyrians and the Babylonians poured honey on the foundation stones and walls of their temples in order to insure the good favor of their gods. Curiously, honey was also considered a symbol for resurrection. Hence, it was not uncommon to find honey jars in the tombs of Egyptian kings. Ancient societies also used honey as part of their wedding ceremonies. Bee keeping was a major industry of the Roman Empire and the honey harvest was a time of wild celebration and merry-making. Even today, honey plays an important part in the sacred holidays of many of the world's religions.

Since sugar was unknown during bible times, honey was the primary sweetener. In the Bible, honey is used as a symbol of abundance and blessings and is mentioned over 50 times.

> "*I will bring you up out of the affliction of Egypt. . . to a land flowing with milk and HONEY.*"
> **(Exodus 3:17)**

Honey was considered to be a special gift of friendship. Jacob exhorted his sons to take honey as a present to the Pharoah of Egypt, along with balm, spices, myrrh, nuts and almonds. **(Genesis 43:11)**

Some Bible scholars even suggest that manna, God's miracle food that fell from heaven, may actually have been a combination of wheat and honey. Judging by the way the Israelites described its taste as "*wafers made with HONEY,*" **(Exodus 16:31)**, this speculation may not be that far fetched.

Psalm 81:16 tells us that if God's enemies would have submitted themselves to Him, He would "*have fed them also with the finest of wheat; and with HONEY from the rock.*" Yes, golden honey, just like golden wheat, is one of God's most precious foods in the Bible.

Honey is as popular a food today as it was in Bible times and the bees produce it exactly the same way now as they did then. Bees make honey from the nectar and pollen of flowers. Even modern man with all of his science and technology, cannot duplicate what God's bees can do. The only thing man needs to do is separate the honey from the comb and then to package it.

The sugars in honey are predigested by the bees so that honey requires little or no digestion as do other sugars. Honey is a nutrition powerhouse and is loaded with enzymes, B vitamins, natural sugars and essential minerals.

Honey has several reputed health benefits. It is a natural antibiotic, aids in the rapid healing of wounds and burns, helps alleviate arthritis symptoms (vinegar and honey), helps ease sore throats, colds and coughs, aids in intestinal distress and helps relieve allergies.

Yes, honey rightfully deserves to be called a miracle food and it is obvious why God would include it in His description of the Promised Land.

Logia: *Foods of the Bible* now offers a variety of honeys and other hive related products including pollen, propolis and royal jelly. (For more information see page 95.)

LENTILS

Lentils are considered by many nutritionists to be the most nutritious legumes on earth. Perhaps that's why Esau was so willing to sell his birthright for some bread and lentil stew.

> "*And Jacob gave Esau bread and stew of LENTILS; then he ate and drank, arose, and went his way. Thus Esau despised his birthright.*" **(Genesis 25:34)**

They were also prepared and brought to David and his weary troops to renew their strength. **(2 Samuel 17:28-29)**

Curiously, David won an impressive battle while defending a lentil field.

> "*The Philistines had gathered together into a troop where there was a piece of ground full of LENTILS. So the people fled from the Philistines. But he (David) stationed himself in the middle of the field, defended it, and killed the Philistines. <u>So the LORD brought about a great victory</u>.*" **(2 Samuel 23:11-12)**

Lentils have been cultivated for food for thousands of years and are still today one of the staples of Mediterranean and Middle Eastern diets. They are inexpensive and can be used in soups, stews, stuffing, dips, salads and sauces. They have a mild flavor and can be enhanced with many herbs, spices and seasonings.

Lentils are extremely high in protein, fiber and complex carbohydrates. They are also a good source of iron, B vitamins, phosphorus and potassium. **Logia**: *Foods of the Bible* now offers hard-to-find organic lentils. (For more information, see page 99.)

ALMONDS

The almond tree is the first tree to bloom in the Holy Land, blooming in late January. Because of this, it is used in the Bible as a sign of new hope, new birth (born again) and possibly resurrection. When God gave Moses instructions on how to build the first Menorah lamp stand **(Exodus 25:33)**, He requested almond blossoms at various locations on the stand. These were obviously to be a symbol of new birth just as the Menorah was a symbol of everlasting life (and light).

When the authority of Moses and his brother Aaron was challenged by a rebellious group of Israelites, it was Aaron's budding staff that served as a sign of God's approval of the two brothers.

> *"Now it came to pass on the next day that Moses went into the tabernacle of witness, and behold, the rod of Aaron, of the house of Levi, had sprouted and put forth buds, had produced blossoms and yielded ripe ALMONDS."* **(Numbers 17:8)**

These Bible references to the almond show just how favorably God views this food. With that kind of endorsement, don't you think you should eat a handful of almonds every day?

Raw almonds are an excellent source of unsaturated fatty acids. They also contain protein, fiber, iron, potassium, calcium and phosphorus. Almonds make a delicious substitute for candy and junk snacks and may be used in baking and with fruit and vegetable salads. Stay away from salted almonds. The unsalted ones taste just as good if not better.

Other Foods Mentioned In The Bible

Here are some of the other foods mentioned in the Bible.

- Cucumbers
- Milk
- Garlic
- Spelt
- Mulberry Juice
- Cinnamon
- Millet
- Beans
- Onions
- Vinegar
- Flax
- Anise
- Cummin
- Mint
- Leeks
- Cheese
- Pistachio nuts
- Melons
- Bitter Herbs
- Hyssop
- Mustard Seeds

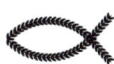

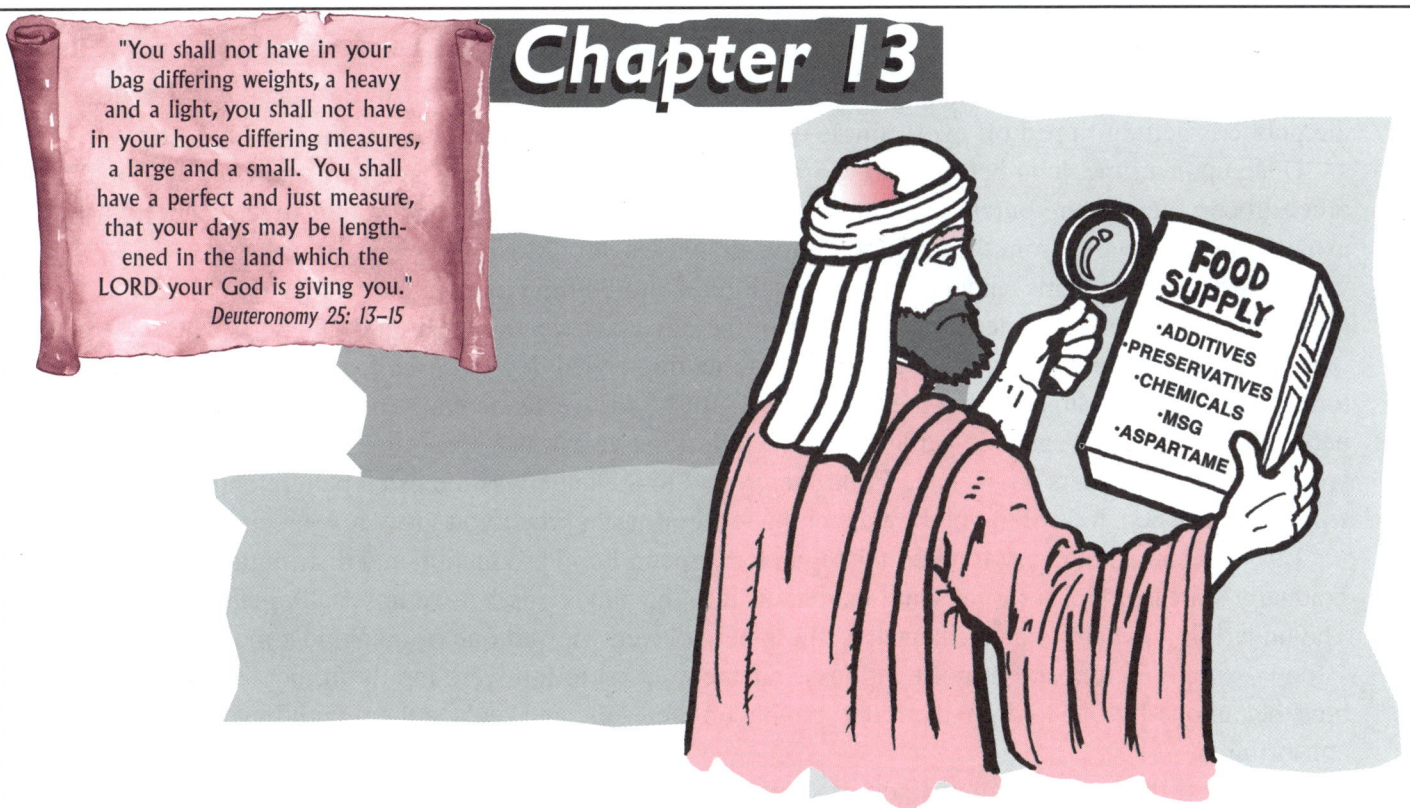

"You shall not have in your bag differing weights, a heavy and a light, you shall not have in your house differing measures, a large and a small. You shall have a perfect and just measure, that your days may be lengthened in the land which the LORD your God is giving you."
Deuteronomy 25: 13-15

Food. . . Lies. . . And The World of Big Business.

**You Can Fool Some Of The People All Of The Time,
And You Can Fool All Of The People Some Of The Time,
But You Can't Fool All Of The People All Of The Time.**

Wouldn't it be great if every business ran according to the laws of God? Wouldn't it be nice to know that when you spent your hard-earned dollars on a purchase that you were getting the highest quality product at a fair and reasonable price? And wouldn't it be wonderful if you could explicitly trust everyone you did business with?

Well that's exactly how things are supposed to work in an ideal world. But since this is not yet an ideal world, unfortunately the old adage "buyer beware" still holds true. And no place is it more true than in the food and nutritional supplements businesses. In this chapter, I am going to take you behind the scenes and tell you some things you've probably never been told before. I am going to lift the veil on all of the shenanigans and show you the hidden and dirty side of these businesses.

MONEY MAKES THE WORLD GO 'ROUND

I might as well state it right up front – and I'm sure it comes as no surprise to you – money and the quest for huge profits makes the world go around. Not honesty, not integrity, not love, not compassion.

Just pure, unadulterated **greed!** After more than 30 years in business, I am still hurt deeply to see how the public is getting ripped off every single day. For starters, let's take a look at the food industry.

Once upon a time, long before there were supermarkets, hypermarkets and megamarkets, food and other grocery items were purchased either at the local neighborhood store or from a street vendor who usually plied his wares from the back of a horse-drawn wagon. Most likely the various fruits, vegetables and meat items came from farms within a 25 to 50 mile radius. No one gave a thought to preservatives because freshness was the order of the day. If it weren't fresh, it didn't sell. There were even some stores that made their living selling something called **day-old bread**, a strange concept in today's world where supermarket breads can stay "fresh" for weeks on end. In those days, many people had their own vegetable gardens and the fall of the year was a great time for tomatoes, peas, corn, squash, cucumbers and beans. From the ground to the table was the usual pattern and you will still hear gardeners today tell you how much better food tastes when you grow it yourself.

But then something very foreboding began to happen. Food production and distribution started to gradually shift from local farmers and merchants into the hands of what we now call **agribusiness**. The underlying dynamics also changed as these new players viewed one of mankind's most basic needs – food – simply in terms of a profit and loss statement. First to fall were family farmers as the big boys began one-by-one to drive them out, gobble up their land and replace them with huge farming consortiums.

Next went the corner mom and pop grocery stores and neighborhood street vendors as vast food processing plants and gigantic supermarket chains began to make their appearance across the land.

Fresh, wholesome natural foods had a hard time surviving in this new, bottom line oriented infrastructure. Profits demanded long product shelf life and that gave rise to the chemicalization of our food supply. Thus were born *preservatives, antioxidants, emulsifiers, thickeners, stabilizers, anti-mold agents, anti-caking agents, artificial colorants*, and what has now grown into an endless list of chemical food additives.

Highly toxic herbicides and pesticides were indiscriminately sprayed across hundreds of thousands of acres of American farmland, leading to extensive loss of wildlife and increased levels of cancer in the population. An unaware nation was rudely awakened when the shocking book **Silent Spring** by environmentalist crusader Rachel Carson documented the terrible damage to nature of the toxic pesticide DDT. In typical fashion, the chemical companies dismissed her efforts to warn us as "unfair, one-sided and hysterically overemphatic." Of course, time proved her right.

With brave whistle blowers like Carson and others sounding the alarm, it was inevitable that the indiscriminate use of herbicides, pesticides and chemicals would cause a backlash in the nation. Thus the 50s and 60s saw the rise of numerous consumer activist groups as well as a whole new, albeit small struggling industry called "health foods."

But things kept getting worse. Artificial fertilizers forced tired soil to continue producing crops year after year with no rest. Of course this is totally against God's law.

> *"Six years you shall sow your field, and six years you shall prune your vineyard, and gather its fruit; but in the seventh year there shall be a sabbath of solemn rest for the land, a sabbath to the LORD. You shall neither sow your field nor prune your vineyard. What grows of its own accord of your harvest you shall not reap, nor gather the grapes of your untended vine, <u>for it is a year of rest for the land</u>."* **(Leviticus 25: 3-5)**

God was so insistent on this law of rest for the land that He warned the Israelites that if they did not rest their land, He would let their enemies carry them away captive, thus forcing a rest on the land.

"I will scatter you among the nations and draw out a sword after you; your land shall be desolate and your cities waste. <u>Then the land shall enjoy its sabbaths</u>." **(Leviticus 26: 33-34)**

Do we really think that we, in the United States, are somehow immune from God's agricultural laws? If He is true to His words – and He is – then a day of reckoning is coming to our land. God will not be mocked.

A CLOSER LOOK AT TODAY'S "FOODS"

Much of what we pass off as food in the supermarket today is nothing more than worthless "junk food." Granted, it may look appealing and nutritious in its fancy packaging, but this is all part of the charade. In many cases, the packaging costs more than the worthless food product inside. I'll never forget the "advice" I was once given by a top food industry executive. "Spend 10¢ of every dollar on your product and the other 90¢ on marketing and advertising." Does that sound like godly advice? I'll let you decide.

Labels are designed to fool and mislead you. Take fruit juice, for example. Products labeled "juice cocktails" or "juice drinks" are simply disguise terms to make you think you are buying 100 percent juice. In reality you are getting sugar flavored, artificially colored water with just a smidgen of real juice. Sure, the labels look like the real thing with pretty pictures of fruit all over them, but the fact is that you are purchasing a man-made liquid beverage that costs pennies to manufacture. Your health is the last concern for most of these drink bottling companies.

The agribusiness giants learned early on that highly processed foods lasted much longer on the store shelf. That opened the door for bleached white flour, white bread, white sugar and white rice. These products aren't much better than eating plaster of Paris yet they have now become staples in many people's diets.

And don't be fooled by words like "vitamin enriched" and "vitamin fortified." All this means is that the manufacturers have put back in their products a few artificial nutrients to replace the ones they processed out in the first place. "Enriched white flour" for instance, simply means that a handful of man-made vitamins and minerals are put back into the flour in a meager attempt to compensate for the 22 God-given nutrients that are removed from the whole wheat during the milling process. Thus, the original nutritional spectrum of many foods as designed by God has long since been broken up and rearranged by man – for money.

No food exemplifies the type of tampering I'm talking about more than today's bread – what once was called the staff of life. First of all, let me ask you a question. Have you ever heard of something called the ***Code of Federal Regulations: Title 21*** or the ***Standard of Identity***? I'll bet you haven't. Yet, because of this Code and the Standard of Identity, many of today's food labels do *not* have to list all of the ingredients they contain. How's that, you say? Well according to this Code, the ingredients of many commonly used foods, like bread for instance, are standardized by the Federal Food, Drug, and Cosmetic Act and the Fair Packaging and Labeling Act. A "standard of identity" is then established for each food which names mandatory and optional ingredients to be used in preparing these foods, while prohibiting the use of any non-standardized ingredients. The Code also provides guidelines for package labeling and sets standards for container fill.

Now here's the catch. Since the details of these regulations are published in the Code, foods which are standardized are thus exempt from certain labeling requirements, under the assumption that you are free to consult the Code should you want to know the ingredients. How many of you carry the Standard of Identity Code around with you when you go grocery shopping?

Back to bread. Since bread falls under the Standard of Identity Code, many of its ingredients do *not* have to be listed on its label. In case you're curious, the regulations define bread as being "prepared by baking a kneaded yeast-leavened dough, made by moistening flour with water" along with one or all of seventeen *categories* of optional ingredients. Consequently, besides listing flour, yeast and salt on the label, the bread you buy may also contain more than a hundred other food and chemical additives that are not listed – things like shortening, sugar, dough conditioners, emulsifiers, anti-mold agents, yeast nutrients and fresheners. And all this because of something called **Standard of Identity**.

And one final note of caution. If the label says simply *flour* or *wheat flour*, it is more than likely bleached white flour. This means that the bread is very low in biblical nutritional value. This is why you need to read your food labels closely.

Here is my rule of thumb on label reading. The majority of food product labels are written in a prevaricating way to make you believe that you are getting your money's worth when in reality, it is the manufacturers who are getting their money's worth. **Buyer Beware!**

THE NIGHTMARE OF GENETICALLY ALTERED FOODS

Just when I thought that the food processing problems couldn't get any worse, along come **genetically altered foods** – the so-called "Frankenfoods." If you thought tampering with foods chemically was bad enough, what do you think about the altering of foods genetically? Ask yourself this important question. Does God want us to pull certain genes out of one food and mix them with another? Or worse yet, how about mixing animal and plant genes? Yes, that's being done even as I right this book. Is this type of science within the domain of man or are we dangerously treading on ground where we do not belong?

Of course, the big food companies are telling us that these new foods are perfectly safe and for our own and the world's betterment. They're even fighting for the right to not have to label foods as genetically modified. In other words, they want to force these frankenfoods down your throat without your even knowing about it. How do you like that idea?

And what about the short and long-term health effects from eating such altered foods? I don't even need to do the research to know that this is insanity! The whole theme of this book is that God set up a natural order of life that included our eating His natural foods. To deviate from His perfect plan by eating genetically altered foods is to invite a disaster upon ourselves of unknown magnitude.

By the way, if you're wondering what God's law says about so-called transgenic research, let me remind you that He has been quite explicit as to His feelings about mixing different substances. Just read what He has to say.

"You shall not let your livestock breed with another kind. You shall not sow your field with mixed seed. Nor shall a garment of mixed linen and wool come upon you." **(Leviticus 19:19)**

"You shall not sow your vineyard with different kinds of seed, lest the yield of the seed which you have sown and the fruit of your vineyard be defiled. You shall not plow with an ox and a donkey together. You shall not wear a garment of differing sorts, such as wool and linen mixed together." **(Deuteronomy 22:10-11)**

Now I ask you. Do you really think that the same God who gave us these explicit rules about mixing, would possibly condone the cross-mixing of genes of different species? This is obviously an abomination in His sight and there is going to be a great retribution for such actions.

WHAT ABOUT THE HEALTH FOOD INDUSTRY?

I said earlier that it was all of this food tampering that gave rise to the health food industry in America. After all, it was only natural that once people began to realize what was being done to their food supply that some of them would start demanding better choices. Thus, a cottage industry of mom and pop health food stores began to spring up across America back in the 1950s. Their goal was to offer pure, natural, unadulterated foods and food supplements – and for the most part, they continue to do just that. But over the last few years, even the idealistic health food stores have begun showing some cracks as some questionable items are now appearing on their shelves.

With this increase in popularity of health foods, many new *manufacturers* are now coming into this marketplace. Unfortunately, some of them do not have the same standards as their predecessors. Most of the problems are coming from these Johnny-come-lately manufacturers who are sacrificing quality and integrity for quick profits.

One of their approaches is to find some health angle for a food product or supplement and then promote that heavily while underplaying or ignoring the questionable ingredients that their products also contain. This is quite apparent in the new breed of nutritional bars that are now popular. It seems as long as they are high in protein or low in carbohydrates, nothing else seems to matter. Thus you will find a wide range of not so healthy ingredients in many of these so-called *health bars*.

And what about the aspartame scandal? One of the most toxic substances ever to be approved by the FDA can now be found in many of the protein powders and low carbohydrate bars now being sold as health food. I must admit that a few years ago, I too used aspartame in a protein product that we manufactured until a very concerned consumer advocate named Betty Martini made me aware of its dangers. That was all I needed to hear. Once I saw how dangerous this man-made artificial sweetener really is, I couldn't yank it from my product fast enough. I encourage other manufacturers and storeowners to do the same thing.

But now here's the rub. Several clever manufacturers who are aware of the aspartame controversy have begun substituting another controversial and under-tested sweetener called **acesulfame-K** for the aspartame. While their advertising and product labels proudly state "no aspartame," they fail to tell you about the use of this other unproven sweetener. And just recently I saw one company list acesulfame-K on their product as ascesulfame-*potassium* in a further effort to mislead its customers. What deception from businesses who purport to care about your health.

WHAT ABOUT SUPPLEMENTS?

Well at least they're not playing games with our food supplements. Right? Sure they're not! There's probably more deception going on here than anywhere else in the health food industry. That's because there are huge profits to be made in food and dietary supplements. Please don't misunderstand me. Most of the manufacturers and storeowners in the health food industry are honest and caring people who truly want to give you healthy alternatives. But unfortunately, a few bad eggs are making it bad for the whole industry.

There are so many ways you are being deceived that I almost don't know where to start. Let me give it a try. One of the most blatant deceptions is simply to *not* put everything in a product that's listed on the label. Shorting is as old as the human race. Just read the Bible quote at the start of this chapter. The reason companies can get away with this is because no authority monitors this part of the supplements industry. Thus, potency variances are being found in many products. There are a few good private watchdog sites starting to spring up on the Internet and they too have been substantiating a very serious potency shortage problem throughout the industry.

Let me demonstrate to you why this is such a temptation for some of these unscrupulous companies. Let's imagine that Company X is selling 50,000 bottles a week of its most popular nutritional supplement. (Not an unrealistic number.) Now someone in the company figures out that by shaving 20¢ worth of raw materials off of the formula without changing the label, Company X will now make an extra $10,000 a week (50,000 times 20¢) or **$520,000 extra profit** a year. Imagine that! An extra half million more dollars just by cheating the public by 20¢ per bottle. It's being done every single day and you have no way of knowing it.

Then there are the raw materials scams. Both the suppliers and the manufacturers are complicit in this deception. So many inferior raw materials are being pushed on manufacturers today that it's pathetic. Take herbs, for instance. It's common practice for some unscrupulous suppliers to mix the very cheapest parts of the plant with its more desirable and more costly parts and then sell the diluted combination at the higher ingredient price. Raw materials suppliers are able to get away with this since they know that many manufacturers shop for raw materials simply on the basis of price. Furthermore, many of the smaller companies will never assay or test what they purchase for potency. This is why there's a good chance that some of those expensive herbal formulas you're buying at the health store or pharmacy have very little active ingredients in them. But once again, unless you have good reason to trust the company you are purchasing from, you have no way of knowing what you are getting.

Next I'd like to share with you the shady procedures some of these companies follow when they set out to design a new nutritional supplement. Wouldn't it seem that the logical place to start would be to determine the desired results someone will get by using the product? And once that's decided, shouldn't the next step be to determine which are the best ingredients to use to achieve those results? Not so with these fast buck companies.

First of all, the unscrupulous manufacturer starts, not with the desired end result, but with the *price* he wishes to pay to get his product manufactured. Let's say for instance that Company Y decides to market a new "weight loss" pill. What they will do is start out with a retail price – say $39.95 – and then pick a low target manufacturing price – say $2.75 per bottle. (Not unlikely numbers.) Of course the usual popular "weight loss" ingredients must be in the formula *but the quantity really doesn't matter*. What does matter is that the product gets produced for $2.75 a bottle. As I write this book, some of the most popular weight loss products on the market today are guilty of this exact scenario. Unfortunately, you have no way of knowing which ones.

Several years ago, a popular sports supplement kit hit the marketplace at well over one hundred dollars. It was very popular and sold like hotcakes. The whole kit cost well under $10 to produce and contained little of any substance. I am appalled by this kind of marketing. Obviously, this company bought into the strategy of 10¢ on product and 90¢ on marketing. Yet, rather than be castigated for such unscrupulous practices, instead companies like this are held up as role models by other companies who seek to pull off the same sort of scam. Just remember this. While it is true that a really high quality nutritional food supplement is always going to cost more, it is not always true that an expensive food supplement is always a high quality product.

Then there's that old trick of naming a dietary supplement brand to sound like it's an *all-natural* line of products. I know you've seen them. **"Nature's. . . this & that."** The label graphics will often continue the charade by showing beautiful pictures of outdoor scenes, or fruits and vegetables. But worse yet, other unscrupulous manufacturers will use deceptive words on their labels to make it seem like their products contain all natural ingredients when in fact, there are little or no naturally derived materials present. This happens routinely, for example, with so-called "natural vitamin C" tablets where 90 percent or more of them are made from synthetic *ascorbic acid* while words like **natural rose hips** or **natural acerola** appear on the front of their labels. What they fail to tell you is that there is only a miniscule amount of the natural ingredient present in the formula base just so they can use the natural description on their labels. Once again – **Buyer Beware!**

If these types of practices are not stopped, then there's no doubt in my mind that the entire health food industry will be facing a growing crisis of credibility. As word of these deceptions and hoaxes continues to leak out, more and more people are coming to distrust the whole field. This is sad since the majority of people in the health food industry are very honest and dedicated people. What is now desperately needed is a way to restore consumer confidence – a way for you to buy products that are not long on marketing and short on nutritional value. I would like to encourage other manufacturers to follow our example.

IS THERE NO WAY OUT OF THIS DILEMMA?

I imagine by now that you are probably wringing your hands in frustration and anger. Well don't despair just yet. I do have some good news for you. Studying the Bible and writing this book have given me the impetus to develop the world's first line of high quality, Bible-based foods and food supplements. As I have stressed over and over again in this book, I truly believe that our bodies are meant to be God's Temple and therefore, we have a moral obligation to keep them as healthy as possible. Since eating properly plays such an important role in staying healthy, I am now committing all of my energy, talents and financial resources to the goal of bringing you the purest, most natural and healthiest foods and food supplements humanly possible.

Because of the importance of what this endeavor stands for and because it's the right thing to do, I pledge to God and to you that I will do all in my power to make this new brand the very best that I possibly can. I promise you that there will be no game playing, no shaving ingredients, no undeclared substitutions, no skimping on raw materials and no price gouging.

In addition, all products will always be biblically based and made from the highest grade and best foods and raw materials in the world – including organic foods whenever possible. No food additives or artificial ingredients will ever be used in this product line.

My goal is to bring you nutrition as pure and as healthful as God intended it to be in the Book of Genesis. I have established this line based on the following seven biblical nutrition principles:

(1) All foods should be eaten as close to their natural state as possible.
(2) The more food is processed, the less biblical it is.
(3) Eating and drinking should always be done in moderation.
(4) Artificial, man-made chemicals and additives should never be added to foods.
(5) All foods should be grown organically whenever possible.
(6) Fresh fruits, vegetables, seeds, grains, nuts, herbs constitute the principle categories of Bible foods.
(7) The Bible mentions several foods by name. We should strive to eat as many of these foods as possible on a regular basis.

I have named this new product line **Logia** (pronounced Low-Jah), an unusual word that means the words and sayings of Yahshua (Jesus). I assure you that any product that bears this name will always come with the highest integrity behind it.

I see this endeavor as a mission for God. It is my humble effort to raise the health awareness among His children and to help build stronger body temples for His Spirit. Consequently, every product in the **Logia** line will always come with my pledge of your total satisfaction. If for any reason, at any time, you are dissatisfied with any **Logia** product, you may return it for a full refund of your purchase price – no questions asked.

I am hoping that you will share my vision for a stronger, healthier, holier country and I look forward to your help, support and feedback. Together we can make a difference.

A CLOSER LOOK AT SOME LOGIA PRODUCTS

I would like to take a few minutes at the close of this chapter to introduce you to some of the great Bible-based products that are already available from **Logia**. Should you wish to purchase any of them, they are on sale at select health food and religious bookstores around the country. If they are not yet available in your area, you may order them directly from **Logia**. (See price list and order form in the back of this book.)

BACK TO THE GARDEN

I must confess that I get excited about each and every product that we develop at **Logia**, but formulating this particular food concentrate really got my juices boiling. I guess the reason is that it represents just about everything I've talked about in this book – a comprehensive product containing fruits, vegetables, herbs, fiber and enzymes. I knew as I was writing *Moses Wasn't Fat* that there would be some people with busy lifestyles who would have a difficult time trying to consume five servings of fruits and vegetables every day as recommended by nutritionists. That's when I realized that there was a true need for a convenient, all-in-one source of these great Bible foods. Since there was no such Bible oriented product currently on the market, I knew I would have to develop my own formula. And that's how **Back To The Garden** was born.

I wanted **Back To The Garden** to be as complete a Bible-type meal supplement as possible. That's why I insisted that it had to contain plenty of fruits, vegetables and herbs – as a matter of fact, it has over 60. In addition, I wanted it to also be a good source of the popular, health-promoting green foods such as barley grass and wheat grass. I'm proud to say that our mission was accomplished. **Back To The Garden** is a virtual cornucopia of Bible-based natural foods in a concentrated, delicious and easy-to-use supplement powder.

So forget taking daily vitamin pills. **Back To The Garden** contains your full daily supply of nutrients in a complete natural food base. Its loaded with vitamins, minerals, enzymes, trace elements, phytonutrients, fiber and nutritional support co-factors just as they are found in the wholesome, unspoiled foods of nature. You could even say it's the next best thing to eating fresh fruits and vegetables.

In addition to that, **Back To The Garden** is also a good source of protein, fat and carbohydrates, making it an ideal meal choice for breakfast, lunch or dinner. With its high nutrition, low calorie profile it makes an excellent supplement for dieters. It's also perfect for athletes as a pre- or post-workout drink. Vegetarians are going to love it too since it is totally free of animal products. Mothers, it's also a great product to give to your children.

Back To The Garden comes in individually packaged meal servings. Nothing could be easier. Simply tear one open, mix it in your favorite drink, and you've got yourself a fantastic Bible food meal or in between snack.

Here's what it contains: barley grass, wheat grass, alfalfa grass, tomato concentrate, brown rice powder, broccoli, Jerusalem artichoke, spinach, celery, grapefruit, parsley, green pea, cabbage, kale, onion, pineapple, papaya, cranberry concentrate, garlic, apricot, beet juice powder, elderberry extract, grape skin extract, red wine extract, cayenne pepper, apple, orange, blueberry, whole grape, lemon/lime, plum, raspberry, strawberry, watermelon, cantaloupe, cherry, peach, pear, carrot, Brussels sprouts, cauliflower, radish, leek/yellow pepper, aloe vera, flaxseed, myrrh resin, ginger root, hyssop, olive leaf, sage leaf, spearmint leaf, nettle leaf, oat straw, almond, black walnut, coriander seed, sunflower seed, fig, date, astragalus, acerola berry, oat bran.

SACRED NECTAR

Honey truly is a Bible food seeing that it is mentioned over 60 times in the Holy Scriptures. In fact, God even uses honey as a descriptor for the Promised Land which He calls "a land flowing with milk and honey." Consequently, **Logia** has plans for introducing several exciting honey-based products over the months ahead.

But the good news is that our premier honey product called *Sacred Nectar* is available right now. *Sacred Nectar* is a one-of-a-kind combination containing three of nature's most powerful and precious substances – *raw honey, pollen* and *royal jelly*. Each 24-ounce jar contains 75,000 milligrams of pure royal jelly and 68,000 milligrams of pollen mixed in a base of raw, granulated pure honey.

Our honey comes from the high, dry Arizona desert – a near-perfect environment for the honeybee and one very similar to the Judeaen wilderness area of the Holy Land. Bees flourish amid this desert vegetation which is free of both pollution and pesticides. Honey is a symbol for the word of God and also serves as a natural antibiotic.

For millennia, beekeepers have known of the nearly supernatural power of royal jelly. This mysterious substance is made exclusively by bees and utilized within the hive. Because it is so nutrient dense, it is fed to all bees in their early growth period. Furthermore, it is the only food fed to the queen bee during the duration of her reign, who incidentally, is the longest lived and largest of all the bees in the hive. Some people speculate that there are unknown factors in this highly concentrated substance that are extremely beneficial for human beings. What we do know is that royal jelly is one of the best natural sources of pantothenic acid and the other B vitamins as well as all eight essential amino acids. It also contains vitamins A, C, D and E, biotin and folic acid.

One of the most amazing things about pollen is that it cannot be duplicated in a laboratory since there are still certain components of this dynamic food that science cannot identify. It is often referred to as *nature's perfect food* since it contains nearly every ingredient required for sustaining life, including amino acids, more than a dozen vitamins, 28 minerals and 11 enzymes and co-enzymes. It makes a perfect compliment to the honey and royal jelly of our *Sacred Nectar*.

We've included a beautiful prayer on the label of *Sacred Nectar* which we suggest you recite when using this wonderful Bible food.

DA' UDDER MILK

It's a cute name for a very serious product. As noted above, God routinely describes the Promised Land as "a land flowing with milk and honey." This has led some Bible scholars to believe that milk should have a special place at God's table. However, there's one serious problem. Much of the milk today comes from cows that have been injected with antibiotics, fed pesticide-laden grasses, and worse yet, injected with a genetically engineered hormone called rBGH every two weeks to increase their milk production. So consuming this food of the Bible in a pure, unadulterated state has not been an easy task.

Well now you no longer have to worry about using their milk because we've got *Da' Udder Milk* – an organic, non-fat, wholesome milk powder. As you may have already guessed, because of economics, it isn't easy finding dairy farmers who are willing to raise their cattle according to biblical standards. We scouted everywhere for a worthy dairy source for this product. Fortunately, we found one who shares our beliefs about biblical nutrition and the sanctity of animal life. They were more than happy to supply us with all the powdered milk we wanted.

Thus, it gives me great pleasure to tell you that *Da' Udder Milk* comes from cows that are not treated with antibiotics or hormones, never receive any form of animal by-products in their diet, and no pesticides, herbicides or chemical fertilizers are ever used on their feed. This Grade A, non-fat milk powder is certified organic by Quality Assurance International.

So if you've been hesitant to use milk because of all of the health scares and warnings, it's time you tried *Da' Udder Milk*. It's a dairy product as pure and nutritious as anything from Bible days.

THOROUGHLY CLEANSED

One of the first things I recommend that you do when you make the switch to a biblically based health and fitness lifestyle is to go on a detoxification program. This is a procedure whereby you attempt to rid your body of all of the pollutants, toxins, contaminants and metabolites which have been deposited in your various tissues and organs. This is usually done by fasting and the use of various cleansing herbs.

To assist you in your detoxification program, **Logia** has formulated a fantastic supplement comprised of a variety of biblical herbs. We call it *Thoroughly Cleansed* and for a very special reason. In Hebrew, the word for cleansing and purification is *tohorah*. Hebrew scholars will quickly note that the consonant base of this word is **THRH** from which we have derived the name *Thoroughly Cleansed*.

Thoroughly Cleansed is a carefully selected blend of several Bible-based herbs noted for their cleansing and purifying qualities. It is all natural and totally safe to use. It is ideally recommended for:
- people wishing to cleanse their bodies of stored environmental and nutritional toxins
- people beginning a weight loss program
- chemotherapy patients
- people recovering from alcohol and substance abuse
- cigarette smokers
- athletes who have quit using anabolic steroids and other bodybuilding drugs

In addition, I strongly recommend that if you are going to follow the **Moses Diet & Health Program**, you begin your program with a 14-day detoxification plan using **Thoroughly Cleansed**.

OLIVE OIL CAPSULES

You will notice in the menu portion of this book (see Appendix F), that I have recommended the use of olive oil or olive oil capsules with several of the meal plans. Olive oil is readily available at every grocery store but olive oil capsules are difficult, if not impossible to find. That's why **Logia** has developed a convenient-to-use, 500-milligram 100 percent extra virgin olive oil capsule. There are few olive oil capsules being sold today. We're happy to report that our **Olive Oil** capsules are now available for shipping. There is no better olive oil capsule on the market. What an easy way to add this great Bible health food to your diet.

OLIVE LEAF CAPSULES

The wonders of the olive tree never seem to cease. It appears that God has designed numerous health benefits into this often-mentioned Bible food. Just when you think that science has found the last of the health-building properties of the olive tree, along comes olive leaf extract. Its therapeutic value is so high we might well call the olive leaf "God's natural medicine." Two factors seem to account for this – ***oleuropein*** and ***calcium elenolate***. Oleuropein protects the olive tree against nearly every insect and bacterial predator and calcium elenolate is a powerful compound that is capable of killing pathogenic microbes. Olive leaf is credited with the ability to destroy viruses, bacteria, fungi, parasites and other microorganisms while not harming the beneficial ones. I can't help recalling a pertinent passage from the Book of Revelation.

"The leaves of the tree were for the healing of the nations." **(Revelation 22:2)**

If you would like to use a Bible-based product to protect your body from harmful microscopic invaders, then **Olive Leaf** capsules are your answer. Each capsule contains 250 milligrams of olive leaf and 250 milligrams of olive leaf extract in an all vegetarian capsule.

POMEGRANATE JUICE

Here's another **Logia** first-of-a-kind product – **Pomegranate Juice** concentrate. When I began researching Bible foods, the pomegranate immediately caught my attention. As I've noted elsewhere in this book, this ancient fruit has great symbolism attached to it. (See page 81) What puzzled me was that I was unable to find any research that demonstrated any specific health-imparting qualities for this Bible food which God calls good. I knew it had to be there but where was it?

Then, as if right on cue, a story appeared in the May 2000 issue of the *American Journal of Clinical Nutrition*. I could hardly believe my eyes. A group of scientists in Israel had made an incredible discovery. Pomegranate juice is a powerful anti-oxidant capable of both reducing the amount of harmful cholesterol in the arteries while neutralizing its bad effects. The research team demonstrated the substantial antioxidant capacity of the juice to scavenge free radicals. They noted that pomegranates are a good source of *polyphenols*, a potent antioxidant also found in grape skins.

Alas, I had my answer. I knew that God called the pomegranate good for a reason. But now I had another dilemma on my hands. There were virtually no pomegranate products available in America. No juice, no preserves, no concentrates, nothing! I knew this would have to change and I knew that **Logia** was the perfect company to make that change.

So we set out scouring the world for sources of pomegranates. We discovered that much of the pomegranate production was coming from the Middle East. We also found out that Americans use very little of this great Bible food and the little we grow in this country gets shipped overseas almost immediately. The few suppliers we did manage to locate told us that we were wasting our time. Americans would never develop a taste for this product.

I'm betting that they're wrong. I think that once people like you come to understand the great health benefits of the pomegranate as well as its important biblical significance, you will gladly add it to your diet. And why not? It's one of God's most delicious fruits and makes a very satisfying and thirst quenching juice.

Fortunately, we have been able to locate a supplier out of California who produces a fabulous pomegranate juice concentrate. We're now bottling this great concentrate with spring water and raw honey to make one of the most delightful and healthy Bible juices you will ever taste. I believe pomegranate juice is destined to become one of the most sought after foods of the Bible.

POMEGRANATE CAPSULES

In addition to using our **Pomegranate Juice**, here's another great option for getting a steady supply of the antioxidant and numerous other health benefits of the pomegranate. Our all-vegetarian **Pomegranate** capsules contain 150 milligrams of pomegranate fruit extract in each capsule. We are proud to announce that these are also another first on the market.

GRAPE DUET

The grape is another Bible food whose natural healing properties continue to amaze researchers. Two of its miraculous components are *grape seeds* and *grape skins*. We've combined both of them in this unique supplement.

Grape seed extract has been demonstrated to help a variety of ailments including allergies, arthritis, diabetes, cardiovascular problems, varicose veins and vision problems. While relatively new to the United States, grape seed extract is popular in Europe where it is regularly prescribed by physicians.

Grape skins are also a great natural healer. *Resveratrol* is a bioflavonoid found in the grape skin which scientists now believe may be helpful in the prevention and treatment of cancer. Like the pomegranate, it is a powerful antioxidant that seems to have the power to prevent tumor formation and actually inhibit the spread of cancer. Each **Grape Duet** all-vegetarian capsule contains 100 milligrams of grape skin extract and 50 milligrams of grape seed extract.

BIBLE GRANOLA

This **Logia** product is based on the same principle as the **Bible Bar** in that it contains the seven foods of **Deuteronomy 8:8** that the Lord calls *good*. Once again these foods are: wheat, barley, raisins (grapes), figs, pomegranates, olive oil and honey. As I've noted elsewhere in this book, I firmly believe that God had a purpose for naming these seven foods and that He wants us to consume them regularly. That now becomes an easy task with two great products like the **Bible Bar** and **Bible Granola**. Both are all natural with no additives or preservatives.

Way back in the 70s when I owned a health food store in upstate New York, granola was one of my best selling cereal items. It was a great product and all of us "health nuts" just loved it. Gradually, the mass marketers also discovered the popularity of this cereal and it was just a matter of time before they took it to the general public. In the process, they worked their usual processing tricks and this once healthy cereal became just another junk food. As we were working on **Bible Granola**, I checked out every granola that was being sold in the supermarkets. I couldn't find one that was satisfactory. That's why I am now so glad to bring you **Bible Granola** – a granola cereal in the tradition of the original health food movement, with one slight improvement. It is now made from God's seven special foods. I am so anxious for you to try it and don't forget – we have a 100 percent satisfaction guarantee or your money back. But I think you're going to really like this cereal.

HYSSOP

Hyssop is mentioned 12 times in the Bible, often in reference to cleansing and purifying.

> *"Purge me with hyssop and I shall be clean."* **(Psalm 51:7)**

It is hyssop which is used to spread the blood of the lamb on the door lintels at the first Passover. **(Exodus 12:22)** And it is hyssop which is dipped into the vinegar and offered to the crucified Messiah, the Passover Lamb of God **(John 19:29)**. Hyssop is a blood cleanser that is also good for colds and flu symptoms. Our high potency **Hyssop** formula contains 300 milligrams of pure hyssop extract in each all-vegetarian capsule.

ORGANIC LENTILS

Here's one of the most versatile and nutritious foods of the Bible and quite possibly the food that cost Esau his birthright.

> *"And Jacob gave Esau bread and stew of LENTILS; then he ate and drank, arose, and went his way. Thus Esau despised his birthright."* **(Genesis 25:34)**

Lentils are legumes that have been cultivated for food since the earliest Bible days. They are extremely high in protein and an excellent source of dietary fiber and iron. They are also low in sodium, fat and calories and contain no cholesterol. Lentils are easy to prepare, require no pre-soaking and have a shorter cooking time than any other dry legumes. They can be used in soups, stews, stuffing, meat, dips, salads and sauces. They have a mild flavor and can be enhanced with various herbs, spices and seasonings.

If this book has convinced you to cut back on your meat consumption – and I hope that it has – then lentils, with their high protein content, will make the perfect meat replacement. Because of their high nutritional value, I felt that they were a must for the **Logia** line of Bible foods. Our organic lentils are the very best on the market.

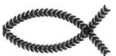

Chapter 14

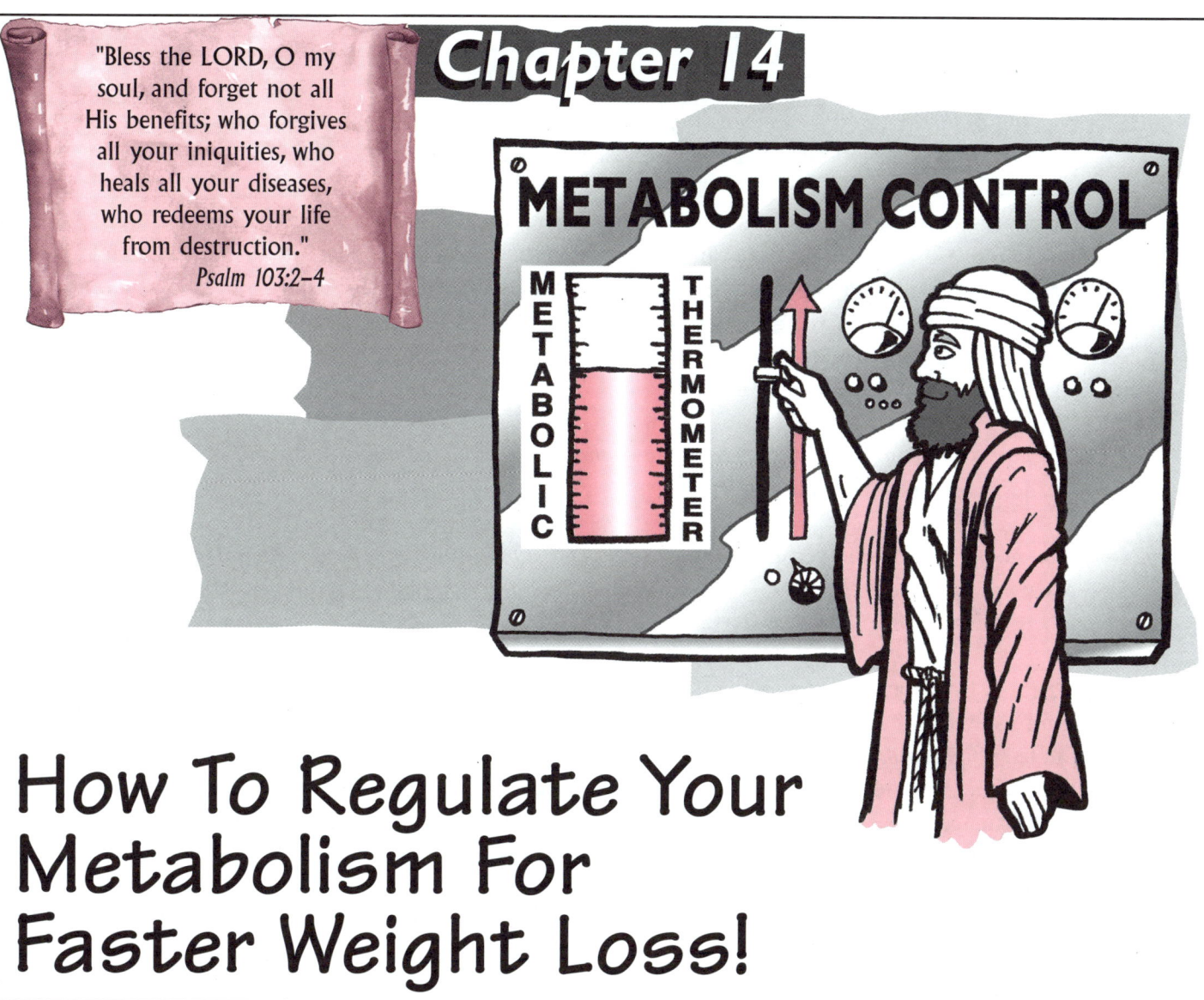

"Bless the LORD, O my soul, and forget not all His benefits; who forgives all your iniquities, who heals all your diseases, who redeems your life from destruction."
Psalm 103:2-4

How To Regulate Your Metabolism For Faster Weight Loss!

A Successful Life Is Made Up Of A Series Of Successful Days.

Your body is like a huge manufacturing plant that never shuts down – three shifts a day, seven days a week, 365 days a year. The product it turns out is something very precious called *life*. From the moment you were conceived in your mother's womb until the day you draw your last breath, your body-factory is busy producing and converting energy into life – that special and holy gift from our Creator. This process of turning energy into life is called *metabolism*. And while modern science has come to a good understanding of the dynamics of metabolism, there remains hidden deeply in its processes the very mysteries of the Kingdom of God. Yes we know basically how it works and even how to control it to some degree, but the question remains to be asked, why did God even design us to eat food several times a day? Couldn't He just as easily have created us self-sustaining, never needing to take external substances into our bodies? I am of the firm belief that everything is the way it is in creation because God determined that this is the best way and the most perfect way and the *only* way it all works. Therefore, the question remains, why do we have to eat to stay alive?

As I have mentioned several times already in this book, eating the proper foods is so important in the eyes of God that He addressed this issue almost immediately in the Garden of Eden.

"And the LORD God commanded the man saying, 'Of every tree of the garden you may freely eat; but of the tree of the knowledge of good and evil you shall not eat, for in the day that you shall eat of it you shall surely die.'" **(Genesis: 2:16-17)**

Furthermore, there are several Bible scriptures which indicate that we will still be eating in the Kingdom of God. At the Last Supper, Yahshua (Jesus) tells His apostles that He will indeed drink the fruit of the vine with them again in the Kingdom of God **(Matthew 26:29)**. And just a few days later, after His resurrection <u>in His glorified body</u>, one of the first things He requests is for something to eat **(Luke 24:41)**. The Book of Revelation makes several mentions of eating again in the Kingdom of God.

"<u>To him</u> who overcomes I will give <u>to eat</u> of the Tree of Life, which is in the midst of the Paradise of God." **(Revelation 2:7)**

And how about this powerful scripture, *"Behold I stand at the door and knock. If anyone hears My voice and opens the door, I will come in to him <u>and dine with him</u>, and he with me."* **(Revelation 3:20)** See also **Revelation 2:17; 22:2**.

We've eaten from the very beginning and obviously, we will be eating forever in Paradise. But once again I ask why? Let me offer one possible explanation.

As I noted above, *food* – *energy* – and *life* are all interconnected. The main source of energy on this planet comes from the sun. Without sunlight there would be no life. Plants have a miraculous way of using a substance called chlorophyll to convert sunlight energy into carbohydrates and other food substances. We call this process **photosynthesis** which means interestingly enough, to synthesize light. The only other thing needed to make this whole wonderful process work is water. Therefore, since God is the Light of the world as well as the Living Waters, He uses plants (all of the grasses and herbs that yield seed according to their kind, **Genesis 1:12**) to convert His very essence (Holy Spirit) into a material form of food. Therefore, when we eat the correct, wholesome biblical-type foods described in this book, we become one with God. And then His essence becomes our essence as we take His Light and Water into our bodies through food and convert them into our living tissue. Can you see now how important it is that we eat properly and why God put so much emphasis on the rules of eating way back in the beginning?

METABOLISM – CONVERTING GOD'S ESSENCE INTO LIVING ORGANISMS

And so now we come back to the main topic of this chapter – metabolism. Scientists define metabolism as "the sum of the physical and chemical processes in an organism by which protoplasm is produced, maintained and destroyed and by which energy is made available for its functioning." While this definition is certainly adequate by scientific standards, I would amend it slightly based on its deeper aspects as I discussed above. Here then is my definition.

Metabolism is the sum of the physical, chemical and *spiritual* processes in all living organisms whereby the essence of the Living God, through the transference of eternal energy, is mysteriously and wonderfully converted into living tissue.

If you need further proof that metabolism is of divine origin, ask yourself these questions. Can you do anything to consciously control the metabolic processes in your body after you eat a meal? Do you tell your stomach to secrete hydrochloric acid and digestive enzymes in just the right amounts? Do you break down the foods you've eaten into their various nutritional components and then guide them into your blood stream? Do you actively control anything about your digestive processes other than just the fun part of eating?

The answer is obvious. Once food enters your body, it begins the spiritual metabolic process that I've just described. Therefore, it is the eternal wisdom of God our Creator that watches over and directs this very important part of life. (I cannot help commenting here just how ridiculous it is to believe that random evolution could possibly have produced this kind of intrinsic wisdom. What an insult evolution is to an All-Wise Creator.)

WORKING WITH GOD FOR A PERFECT METABOLISM

Since the purpose of this book is to teach you how to build health and fitness through biblical principles, and since metabolism has such a spiritual significance, it is imperative then, that you learn as much as possible about how metabolism works. Then you will be able to work in conjunction with God's intrinsic wisdom to maintain a well-functioning, healthy body.

When your metabolism is working properly, you will be operating at peak efficiency. And by the same token, a faulty metabolism can lead to all sorts of health problems. Before going on, let's define a few other terms that pop up when discussing metabolism.

- **BASAL METABOLISM – BASAL METABOLIC RATE (BMR):** Basal means at the lowest or base level. Therefore, basal metabolism is the amount of energy the body expends for all of its various processes at its base or least level of activity. These processes include: digestion, circulation, respiration, gland and internal organ function, as well as body temperature maintenance and muscle activity. The actual unit of energy measurement is the *calorie* and the total amount of calories burned per hour by the body in a basal state is known as the basal metabolic rate (BMR). BMR can vary extensively based on age, weight, gender, illness, growth rate, body size, body composition, pregnancy, dieting history and so forth.

- **ANABOLISM:** This refers to all of those metabolic processes in the body that deal with growth, repair and tissue synthesis.

- **CATABOLISM:** This refers to all of those metabolic processes in the body that deal with the destruction or breaking down of tissue.

A Rule Of Thumb Way To Generally Determine Your Basal Metabolic Rate

As I noted above, there are many variables that help determine your basal metabolic rate. However, here's a rule of thumb formula that will at least get you in the ballpark in determining your rate. According to this formula, your body requires one calorie per kilogram of bodyweight per hour of the day to maintain your BMR. (To convert your bodyweight from pounds to kilograms, simply divide it by 2.2.)

Here's an example of how it works. Before accounting for any additional activity, a person weighing 150 lbs. (68 kilograms) would require 1 calorie (times) 68 kilograms (times) 24 hours = 1,632 calories to maintain BMR. Remember – this is a ballpark number of the calories your body needs at rest and does not account for activity level and other variables.

The first thing you can do to assure yourself optimum metabolism is to eat a well-balanced diet of biblically based foods. That of course, is one of the main purposes of this book. Therefore, if you effectively follow the *Moses Diet & Health Program* as outlined herein, you will already have begun to optimize your metabolism. The natural vitamins, minerals, enzymes, fiber and macro nutrients (protein, fat, carbohydrate) that are found in abundance in these types of God-ordained foods will help regulate a sluggish metabolism and slow down a too rapid metabolism. Conversely, a diet high in processed, non-nutritive, chemically laced junk foods sooner or later is going to play havoc with the metabolism.

When you are at optimum metabolism, you will be deriving the most nutritional benefit from your foods, your energy levels will stay high and constant and your immune system will be maximized. Certainly, these are all worthwhile benefits.

METABOLISM, CALORIES AND WEIGHT CONTROL

There is still another aspect of metabolism that concerns many people today and that is its relationship to weight control. The majority of metabolism articles appearing in the popular consumer magazines deal with its role in dieting and weight management. Unquestionably, there is a body fat connection between the amount of calories consumed, the food sources of the calories consumed and the time of day when they are eaten. A plethora of theories have been expounded, proposing a number of ways to vary calorie consumption for weight control. Before examining some of them in detail, let's take a look at what we do know.

First of all, gaining and losing weight is definitely linked to the metabolism of the calories in our food. Simply stated, if we consume more calories than our body needs to sustain its basic energy needs (metabolic rate), we will store the excess calories as body fat. And if our body's energy requirement is higher than the amount of calories we take in, then we will burn stored body fat to make up the energy difference. Nearly every nutrition and health book will tell you that a pound of body fat yields 3,500 calories and therefore every time you put 3,500 aggregate calories into your body beyond what you need for your normal metabolism, you will store an additional pound of body fat. However, it is not that simple. It is your own personal metabolic rate that will determine how quickly you will either store or burn excess calories and therefore, how quickly you will gain or lose weight.

Secondly, research has conclusively proven that our metabolism begins to slow down in our mid-20s and continues to slow down with each passing decade. Another way of putting it is that the older we get, the less food we need. This also means that the older we get, the more carefully we must watch our food consumption. Unfortunately, most people actually eat more as they get older thus compounding their problem.

Thirdly, exercise has a direct, positive and immediate impact on metabolic rate. People who exercise regularly tend to maintain an optimum metabolism and have less trouble keeping their bodyweight in check. Exercise is a big part of the *Moses Diet & Health Program* and is discussed at length in Chapter 17.

OTHER PROPOSED WAYS OF ALTERING METABOLISM TO LOSE WEIGHT. DO THEY WORK?

There are several techniques making the rounds these days that purport to alter the body's metabolism and lead to weight loss. Do any of them have merit? Let's take a look at some of the more popular ones.

- **EAT MORE**. This almost sounds contradictory doesn't it? The premise is that many raw foods such as carrots, lettuce, peppers, celery, apples, oranges and so forth are so low in calories that you can eat a large amount of them throughout the day without gaining weight. Furthermore, this technique stresses that by eating more of these foods throughout the day, you prevent your body from going into a starvation protection mode which it tends to do when you drastically reduce your calories. Also, because of the high bulk content of the raw fruits and vegetables, it takes time and energy for your body to digest them so that you may actually be burning up more calories in digestion than you are taking in from the foods (this is known as ***thermogenesis***).

  This concept has a lot of evidence going for it. There is much good to be said for eating raw, low calorie, high bulk foods throughout the day. They indeed are loaded with vitamins, minerals, enzymes and fiber and they do tend to be very low calorie. And yes, in many cases, they may actually require more calories for your body to burn than they contain. I highly endorse this technique.

- **STARVATION**. Unfortunately, this is the first thing that comes to most people's minds when they think of dieting. After all, food makes us fat so very low calorie eating will make us thin – right? Wrong! This is the worst thing you can do when trying to lose weight. First of all, it is very unhealthy to restrict calories for extended periods of time. This causes nutrient deficits that can lead to illness. Secondly, when you starve your body repeatedly, it sets up a defensive mechanism against future starvation periods. What this means is that when you start to eat normally again, your body will actually store extra fat to protect it from any further periods of starvation. Intermittent periods of starvation dieting are very counterproductive and will lead to what is known as the yo-yo syndrome. I want to strongly discourage you from starvation dieting.

- **EAT OFTEN**. Also called grazing, this is one of the more recent dieting techniques to come into vogue. The basic idea is to eat smaller meals more often. The principle behind it is that by eating smaller meals more often – say five or six times a day – your body's metabolism will tend to be more regular, not experiencing the hunger pangs and highs and lows of a few large meals. Furthermore, nutritionists tell us that smaller meals tend to be better digested than larger ones.

  In an interesting study conducted with female athletes at Georgia State University, energy intake and expenditures were measured hour-by-hour for 24 hours of a typical training day. Those athletes whose energy deficits dropped by 300 calories or more at various times during the day tended to have a higher percentage of body fat. This supports the belief that the kind of caloric balance resulting from frequent eating helps reduce body fat. I am a great believer in the grazing technique and I highly recommend it.

- **EAT SOME PROTEIN WITH EACH MEAL**. Some studies have shown that protein foods can stimulate metabolism by as much as 30 percent. Hence, the idea that protein should be included with each meal as a good way to stimulate your metabolic rate. This is a good idea especially for athletes and very active people. But a word of caution. If you are following a grazing type of diet, you do not have to eat protein every time you eat a mini-meal. You would be better off having protein with two or three of your main meals and using the raw foods as suggested in the **EAT MORE** paragraph above.

• **ALTERNATING LOW CALORIE – HIGH CALORIE PERIODS**. The idea here is that your body tends to adapt to a low calorie regimen over a period of time and once it does, it will then resist losing any more weight no matter how hard you try. Therefore, it is reasoned, you can fool your body into believing it is not on a prolonged diet by mixing in intermittent high calorie periods. There are various ways to set up calorie variation cycles. Here are some of them:

(1) Diet 3 days; have a high calorie day every 4th day.
(2) Diet 6 days; have a high calorie day every 7th day.
(3) Diet 2 weeks; have a high calorie week every third week.
(4) Diet 3 weeks; have a high calorie week every fourth week.

There is much to be said for this concept and it often helps dieters who have been deadlocked at a plateau. I recommend that you experiment with the various suggestions above until you find the one that works for you.

• **EATING THERMOGENIC FOODS AND SUPPLEMENTS**. This concept was discussed briefly above under the first heading **EAT MORE**. The belief is that certain foods, herbs and spices actually require more calories to digest than they contain. Therefore, your body will actually lose weight if you eat enough of them. Supplement companies have really capitalized on this idea and consequently, thermogenesis is the main selling point behind many of today's most popular diet pills.

While it is true that certain high fiber foods as mentioned above and some spices such as capsicum, ginger, mustard and others require more calories to digest than they contain, the caloric deficits such foods contain are negligible in the big picture of weight loss. In other words, thermogenesis sounds nice on paper but it's pretty much an exercise in futility. It's a lot like looking for a perpetual motion machine. For long term success in your weight control program, stick to the more valid dieting principles as discussed in this book.

But there is some good news to report. Some exciting things have been happening recently in food product development that may at long last hold great promise for dieters. Indeed there has been a major nutritional breakthrough in the area of metabolism and appetite regulation and not surprisingly, it comes from the Bible. And that's the subject of our next chapter.

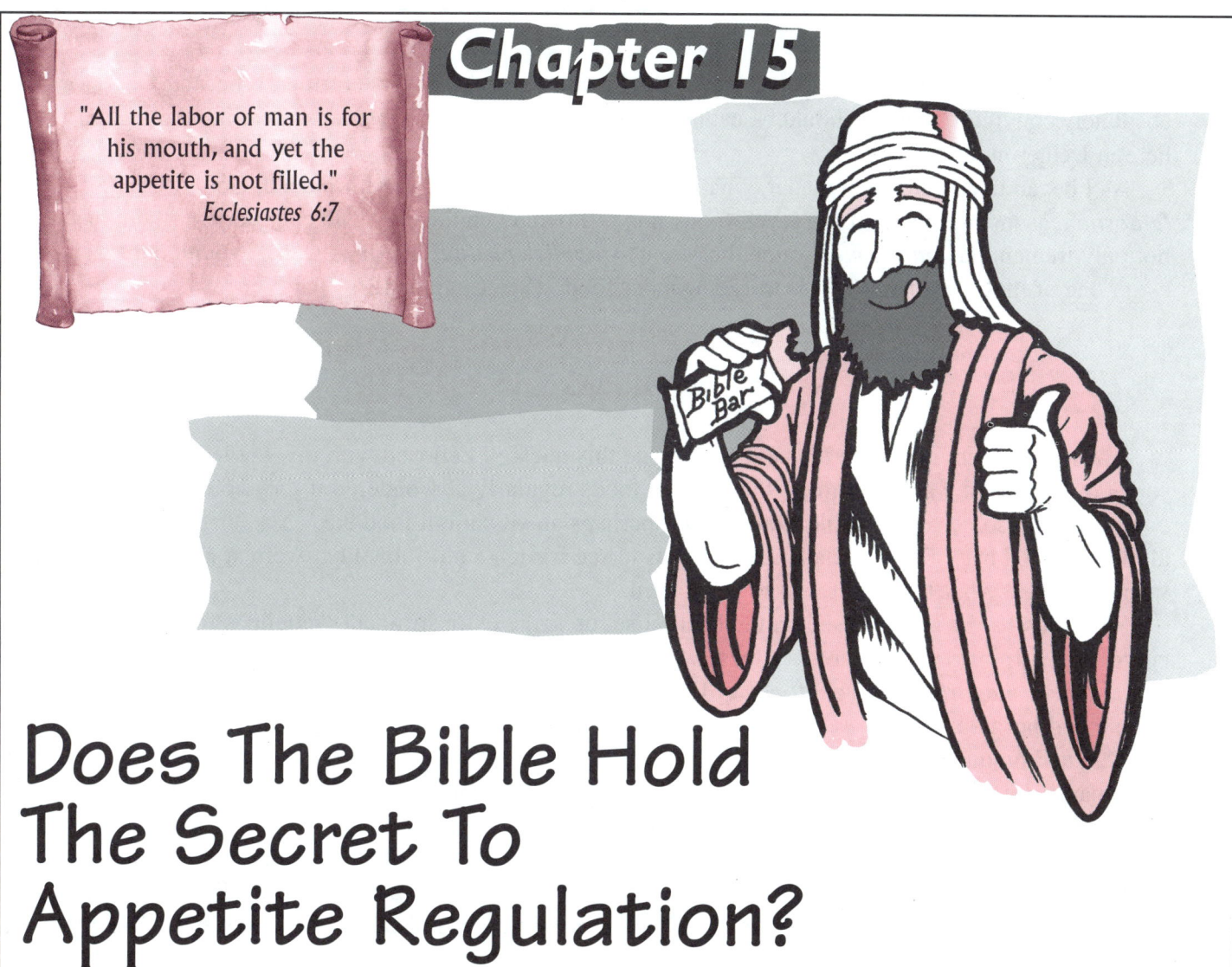

Chapter 15

"All the labor of man is for his mouth, and yet the appetite is not filled."
Ecclesiastes 6:7

Does The Bible Hold The Secret To Appetite Regulation?

Once You Start From Scratch, Always Remember To Keep On Scratching.

I want to share with you now a most unusual and interesting story – a story about how a Bible verse accidentally led to the discovery of a highly effective weight control food product. Little did I know when this all began that I was stumbling into an area of nutrition that was destined to change the lives of thousands of struggling and frustrated overweight people. Here's how it happened.

A few years ago, while I was reading the Book of Deuteronomy, I stopped dead in my tracks after reading the following verse:

> *"For the LORD your God is bringing you into a good land, a land of wheat and barley, of vines and fig trees and pomegranates, a land of olive oil and honey."* **(Deuteronomy 8:7-8)**

I thought to myself – "Wow! What an interesting list of foods! Why did God list them here? Could they possibly have a deeper meaning? What was so special about these seven foods?"

I found it quite astonishing that of all the possible ways the Lord could have selected to describe the goodness of the Promised Land, He picked food as His main choice. Something told me there was more to this scripture than first meets the eye. As I contemplated this verse further, I became absolutely convinced that we should be eating these foods regularly since God was calling them *good* here in Deuteronomy.

As I began to research this matter, what I found out truly amazed me for indeed, God did have *fantastic* reasons for calling these seven foods good. Lo and behold, each and every one of them has not only tremendous **nutritional** value, but great **symbolic/spiritual** merit as well. I found out that every one of these seven foods was truly a wonder food. (See Chapter 12.)

I WAS MORE EXCITED NOW THAN EVER TO KEEP EXPLORING THIS MATTER

I was convinced now more than ever to pursue this quest. I believed with my whole heart that somehow, the Lord wanted us to eat these seven foods regularly. I wondered if they couldn't be combined into some sort of Bible **super food** – perhaps an all natural food bar? Yes, that was it – an all natural food bar! But my challenge now was to see if such a nutritional bar were at all possible. It wouldn't be easy but I couldn't wait to get started.

Since this bar had to be based on the Bible, I set up some extra stringent guidelines for myself. It could be no ordinary candy bar since these were no ordinary ingredients. Not only did it need to contain these **magnificent seven** foods of Deuteronomy, but these foods also had to be of the highest quality and purity available. A cheaply made bar would never do. This bar had to represent all of the holiness and uniqueness that God Himself had given to these foods. It had to be as absolutely perfect as humanly possible. I would accept nothing less. It could contain no additives, preservatives or anything else artificial. This truly had to be a Bible bar.

It took many hours of research, experimentation, and trial and error to get things right. Finally, after months of testing, I was satisfied that we had done it. The **Bible Bar** was born! By the spring of 2000, my new company **Logia** began distributing the Bible Bar in health food stores and religious bookstores throughout America.

What happened next can only be called a miracle. Within just a few months, several thousand stores were enthusiastically stocking the bar. We began working frantically just to keep up with the demand. Never in my 30 years of distributing nutritional products had I seen anything this well received. I never anticipated that the Bible Bar would generate this kind of response so fast.

THEN THE UNEXPECTED HAPPENED

And then something very unusual began to happen. Things started to snowball in a way I had never even imagined. People began reporting back to us that they were using the Bible Bar as a diet aid. Hardly a day went by that we didn't hear from all kinds of people how the Bible Bar was helping them lose weight. Honestly, I had never even given weight control a thought when I began designing this bar. In my mind, it would just be a very convenient and nutritious way for spiritually minded people to eat these fantastic Bible foods from the Book of Deuteronomy. Weight control came as a complete surprise to me.

I immediately began to ask customers how they were using the Bible Bar for weight loss. I found a consistent pattern in their answers. The Bible Bar was helping them regulate their appetite and control their hunger pangs. They were eating it either in place of a meal or as a between meal snack. All were reporting impressive results in weight loss. I now realized that not only was the Bible Bar healthy and nutritious, it was also a fantastic aid to weight control. It didn't take me too long to figure out why.

BIBLE BARS MAKE THE PERFECT BETWEEN MEAL APPETITE REGULATOR

As we learned in the last chapter, metabolism plays an important part in weight control. We also learned that eating smaller meals more often is a great way to regulate the metabolism and thus help you to lose weight. Because of the nutritional composition of the Bible Bar, it helps to reduce hunger and food cravings. This makes it an ideal between meal snack and appetite/metabolism regulator. One of the main reasons it works this way is because of the complex carbohydrates found in the wheat and barley. Each Bible Bar contains 53 grams of carbohydrates and while it isn't fashionable these days to be eating lots of carbohydrates, they may be the very thing you need in abundance to regulate your metabolism and appetite. Numerous studies have shown that complex carbohydrates, when combined with other nutritionally balanced foods such as found in the Bible Bar, help significantly in a weight loss program. Evidently, diets high in complex carbohydrates make weight *gain* harder and weight *loss* easier.

In one study conducted by the Director of the Clinical Research Center at the University of Vermont, test subjects were fed equal amounts of excess calories from protein, fat and carbohydrate. Those people consuming the excess protein and fat foods gained weight much more quickly than those fed carbohydrates.

In another pro-carbohydrate study, researchers at the Institute of Nutrition Science in Germany found that moderately overweight subjects who ate up to ten slices of whole grain bread daily lost an average of 13 pounds in just four weeks. Interestingly, there are still people who feel that they must give up bread when they go on a diet when apparently just the opposite is true.

Still other scientific studies have shown that people on a diet high in complex carbohydrates have up to three times more endurance than those on high protein or high fat diets. This means that you get a double benefit from a high carbohydrate weight loss plan. Not only will you lose weight faster, but you'll also have lots of energy in the process.

CARBOHYDRATES ARE UNDER ATTACK

With so much going for them, you have to wonder why carbohydrates are constantly being disparaged by so many diet programs and diet counselors. For instance, one recent advertisement for a high protein snack shouts out in its headline: **"Why Settle For Low Carbs When You Can Have No Carbs!"** Another reads: **"Lose Your Carb Craving, Lose Your Weight."**

At any given time, low carbohydrate diet books rank near the top of the best seller list. The shelves of health food and grocery stores are bursting with all of the latest low carb and no carb diet products.

Get into a discussion with a group of people on the most effective ways to lose weight and chances are more than half of them will start telling you how wonderful low carbohydrate diets are.

There's no doubt about it. There's a war going on today against carbohydrates. Could there be a deeper reason for this? Might it have anything to do with the fact that carbohydrates are the primary nutrients found in the Bible food sources as described in Genesis.

> *"And the earth brought forth grass, the herb that yields seed according to its kind, and the tree that yields fruit, whose seed is in itself according to its kind. <u>And God saw that it was good</u>."*
> **(Genesis 1:12)**

So many of God's excellent Bible foods are naturally high in carbohydrates that it makes you stop and wonder why so many of the popular diets are bad mouthing this vital nutrient. Nevertheless, despite this unwarranted attack, I am recommending that you consume generous amounts of natural and complex carbohydrates in your daily diet, be they from the Bible Bar or others of the great Bible foods. Carbohydrates are not your enemy. They are an essential part of any health building and weight loss program. You have nothing to fear when you eat them regularly and in abundance. So eat freely from foods like bread, pasta, cereals, grains, potatoes, legumes, beans, fruits and vegetables. They are God's special nutritional gift to us.

HOW THE BIBLE BAR HELPS YOU LOSE WEIGHT

For most dieters, success or failure in losing weight boils down to a matter of hunger. Too many times, unabated, gnawing hunger pangs are the destroyer of their well-intentioned plans. They think that to lose weight they must drastically starve themselves to the point of suffering. There is nothing worse than that starving, deprived feeling of emptiness tugging at your insides. You can only deprive yourself for so long. Sooner or later such discomfort will lead to a rebound effect and uncontrollable overeating. I have stressed many times in this book that such an approach is always counterproductive.

Therefore, since continuous hunger has the ability to sabotage your weight loss program, what is needed is a healthy and nutritious way to stabilize your hunger while still maximizing calorie burning. This is what the Bible Bar is capable of doing. Because of its high-density nutrition, the Bible Bar works as a great *appetite regulator*. When eaten as a between meal snack, it gives you a satisfied feeling while not overloading you with calories. It actually makes you feel as though you've eaten a full meal. This is because, as numerous studies have shown, eating complex carbohydrates helps trigger the release of *serotonin* and *cholecystokinin*, two brain neurotransmitters that help control food cravings and hunger pangs.

And here's one more excellent suggestion for using the Bible Bar as a weight control aid. Try eating one small Bible Bar approximately a half-hour *before* each meal. This will help normalize your blood sugar and greatly reduce your appetite. As a result, you will eat less at the meal.

With such a good way to control constant, nagging hunger, and also regulate your food intake at meals, the odds of your sticking with a health-building program become much greater. There's no doubt about it. The Bible Bar is a great addition to any diet program.

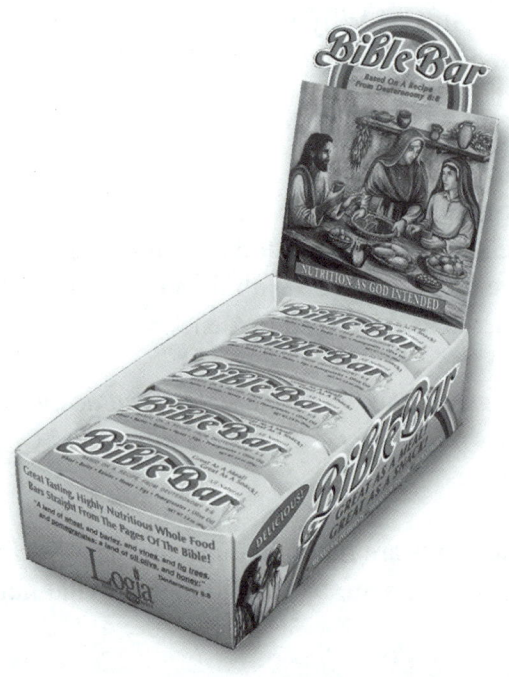

Chapter 16

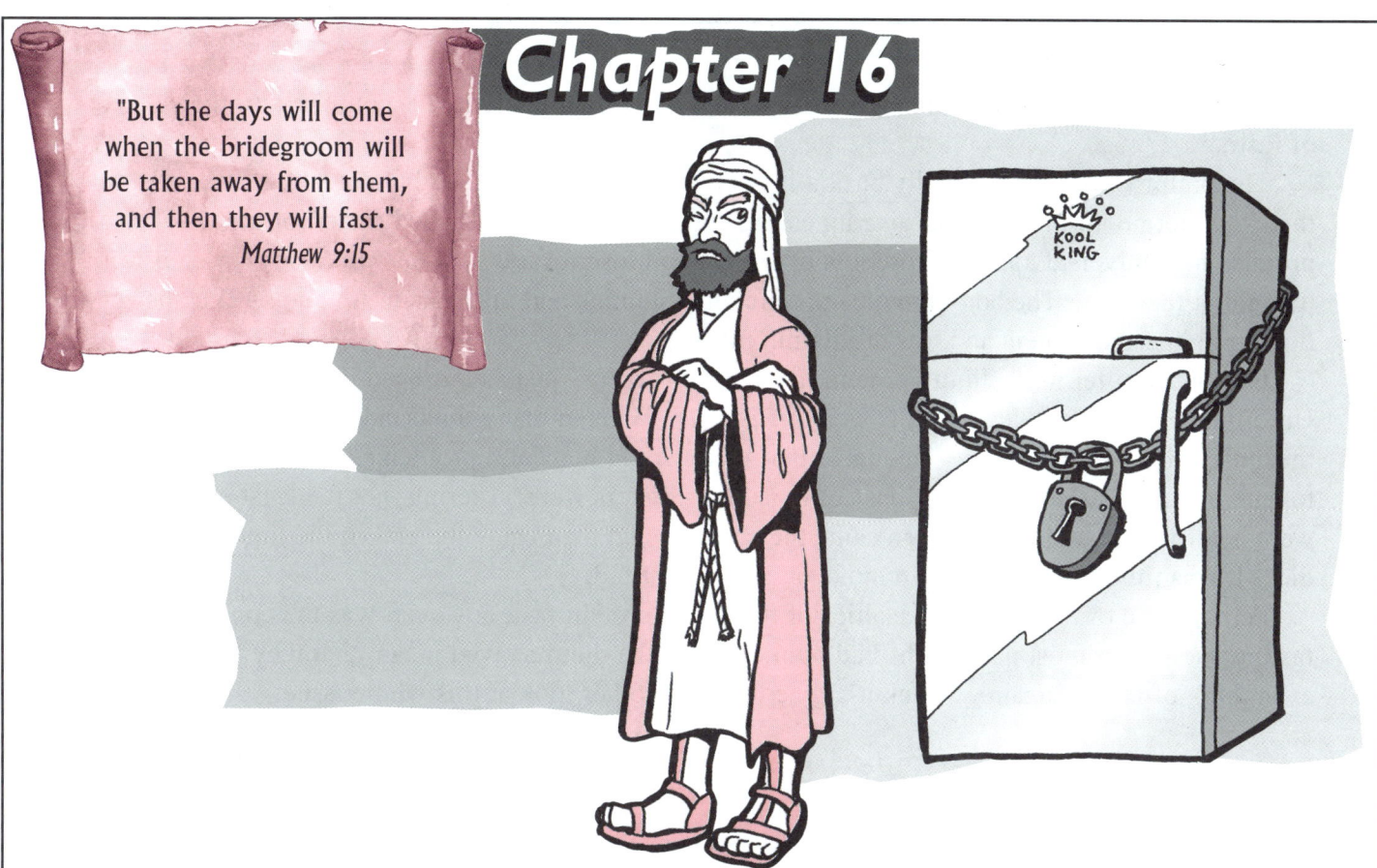

"But the days will come when the bridegroom will be taken away from them, and then they will fast."
Matthew 9:15

Fasting For Physical And Spiritual Blessings.

Discipline Is Doing What Has To Be Done Whether You Want To Do It Or Not.

It was the best of diets and it was the worst of diets. I'll never forget how it swept America like wildfire in the late 1970s. It was one of the biggest weight loss fads to ever hit the country. I had never seen anything like it before nor have I seen anything quite like it since.

I owned a health food store in Utica, New York at the time and my first suspicion that something big was brewing was when I started to receive 20 to 30 calls a day from customers asking if we carried predigested liquid protein. I couldn't help but wonder what was prompting this strange phenomenon. Prior to that time, we were lucky to sell two or three bottles of liquid protein a week. All of a sudden we were selling a case or more a *day*. It didn't take me long to get the answer. I found out that a popular new diet book was making the rounds and propounding the idea of total abstinence from food while recommending predigested protein and a variety of vitamins and minerals. It was called the **liquid protein fast**.

Not only were the usual top Hollywood personalities losing dramatic amounts of weight on this program, but so too were frustrated dieters everywhere. It was just too good to be true. At last, here was a diet program that really worked – and even better than that – it worked *fast*. (Pardon the pun.)

And for many people, this would be their first, and more than likely last encounter with the concept of fasting.

The premise was simplistically basic. If overeating makes us fat, and undereating makes us thin, then why not go all the way and give up eating completely for an extended period of time? The promise had universal appeal. Lose lots of weight and lose it fast. Just one problem – or so it was thought at the time. The body requires protein and vitamins and minerals to function. The answer – liquid predigested protein and lots of vitamin pills.

For the short term, the liquid protein fast really worked – just as most fad diets do. Unfortunately, the long-term results were *disastrous*. With so many thousands of people following this unhealthy program, it was inevitable that there would be health problems. Horror stories started to leak out about some of the serious complications dieters were suffering, not the least of which were heart failure and death. Then came the lawsuits and then came the end of the liquid protein diet. It was time for Americans to move on to the next fad.

Perhaps one of the biggest casualties of the liquid protein fast, however, was the concept of fasting itself. For most people, the bad publicity that the diet received meant that they would never even think of fasting again. I think it's time to take another look at this whole issue.

A TIME FOR EVERY PURPOSE UNDER HEAVEN

Two very important questions need to be asked about fasting. First of all, should it ever be used as a means of losing weight and secondly, is there any biblical justification for still fasting today?

First the issue of weight loss. Let me say right up front and emphatically that you should **never** use fasting as a method of losing weight. Researchers have learned a lot over the last ten years about the effects of radical forms of crash dieting, including extremely low calorie dieting and fasting-starvation. Dieters who tend to go on and off these types of programs repeatedly are setting themselves up for a metabolic catastrophe. Since the body has an intrinsic wisdom placed in it by God, it will automatically slow down its metabolism to preserve existing body fat once it comprehends that dietary calories are being greatly restricted. This creates a vicious cycle whereby the more the dieter restricts calories, the less body fat is burned. The frustrated dieter then reduces calories even more only to be met with even more stubborn resistance from the body. A vicious cycle.

Many dieters tend to overindulge on weekends and then try to compensate for it by abstaining from food on Monday and maybe even Tuesday. Others will overeat at a party or dinner meeting or holiday get together and then force themselves not to eat for one or two days. Not only is this type of eating pattern unhealthy, it will eventually become counterproductive.

Frequent and regular crash dieting such as this also leads to a metabolic reaction similar to that just discussed. After several cycles of such severe calorie restriction, once again the body realizes what's happening. And again as a defensive mechanism against future periods of calorie restrictions, it stores more fat once the dieter resumes normal eating habits. Thus, many dieters actually end up gaining back all of their lost weight and then some, ending up fatter than when they started their diet.

Can you see where all of these crash programs ultimately lead? A dieter's worst nightmare. The harder and more frequently a person diets, the fatter they tend to get. *This is why you must never use fasting as a weight loss technique.*

So if fasting is not recommended for weight control, what is it good for? There are actually two primary reasons for fasting today:

(1) physical purification
(2) spiritual purification

PHYSICAL PURIFICATION

(CAUTION: Diabetics and pregnant and lactating women should not fast.)

Fasting is one of nature's most powerful weapons in the body's fight against illness and disease. There is no better way to purify and strengthen your body Temple than by periodically fasting from all food. Fasting is a natural healing therapy that's as old as the human race. Abstaining from all food intake gives the body a chance to rest and cleanse itself. Just look at some of the great benefits of a fast:

(1) builds energy
(2) restores vigor and vitality
(3) helps regulate the metabolism
(4) helps slow down aging
(5) removes accumulated wastes and toxins
(6) helps with skin problems
(7) helps build discipline

By now, however, you're probably wondering how you can fast effectively and at the same time not harm your metabolism in the ways I discussed above. The answer is *frequency* and *duration*. The ninth commandment of the TEN COMMANDMENTS OF HEALTH listed at the beginning of this book states that you should fast *one full day* each month. This is good advice. A one-day total fast every 30 days will have no adverse affects on your metabolism. I suggest you pick the first day of each month as a total fast day. Furthermore, to keep your fast biblical, you should begin it at sundown of the last day of the month and end it at sundown of the next day.

In addition to these one-day fasts, I also recommend that you go on a 2-3 day total fast once a quarter. (See accompanying story ***Forty-Day Fasts – Not For Everyone!***) Such a fast is also safe and will not contribute to a defensive protective reaction by your body's metabolism. It will, however, require great discipline and motivation. But let me assure you that the rewards will far outweigh any negatives. If you are concerned that a three-day fast may be injurious to your body, you shouldn't be. You have far more health issues to be concerned about from overeating than from an occasional three-day fast.

If a total fast is a bit difficult when you first attempt it, you may modify it slightly by drinking fruit and vegetable juices for a few fasts until you get the hang of it.

HOW TO FAST FOR HALF OF THE REST OF YOUR LIFE

Here's one of the best tips on fasting that I've ever seen. Fasting for half of your life may sound a bit shocking and radical but once you understand the principle, there's hardly anything to it. All you have to do is not eat anything beyond your last meal of the day until 12 hours later into the next morning. For example, if you finish your dinner at 6 p.m., don't eat again until at least 6 a.m. the following day. Thus, you will have successfully fasted for 12 hours or half a day. This tip also works wonders for weight control since eating in the evening and before bedtime is one of the surest ways to gain weight.

SPIRITUAL PURIFICATION

The other question I've set out to answer in this chapter is whether there is biblical justification for us to still fast today. Many Christians believe that with the death and resurrection of Yahshua (Jesus) all need for fasting ended. Are they right? Let's look at what the Bible has to say.

Matthew 6:16 deals with the issue of fasting. In this verse, Yahshua (Jesus) starts out by saying, "Moreover, <u>when</u> you fast, do not be like the hypocrites. . ." Notice that Yahshua's (Jesus') instructions are "when you fast" and not "if you fast." All, well and good you say, but that was before the resurrection while Yahshua (Jesus) was still with His disciples. Then let's keep reading.

In **Matthew 9:14**, the disciples of John the Baptist are quizzing Yahshua (Jesus) as to <u>why His disciples did not fast</u>.

> *"Then the disciples of John came to Him, saying, 'Why do we and the Pharisees fast often, but your disciples do not fast?'"*

Yahshua's (Jesus') answer affirms that we should still be fasting today. Notice what He answered.

> *"Can the friends of the bridegroom mourn as long as the bridegroom is with them? But the days will come when the bridegroom will be taken away from them, <u>and then they will fast</u>."* **(Matthew 9:15)**

The prophetic Book of Joel gives us further evidence that we would still be fasting today. The entire book deals with the end times or what Joel calls "The Day of the Lord." Twice in the book, Joel instructs God's end time people to

> *"Consecrate a <u>fast</u>, call a sacred assembly."* **(Joel 1:14; 2:15)**

The Book of Acts cites several references to members of the early Church fasting *after* Yahshua's (Jesus') ascension into heaven. **(Acts 10:30; 13:2-3; 14:23; 27:9)**

Yes, I think the Bible is quite clear on this point. God still expects us to fast and pray today. And why not? Fasting is a deliberate physical self-denial for spiritual growth. It enables us to have a more focused prayer life while at the same time develop a greater intimacy with God. Fasting also helps deliver us from the bondage of sin and addictions since fasting helps give us power over the flesh.

The Bible instructs us to fast both as a nation (**2 Chronicles 20:3**) and as individuals **(Matthew 6:16-18)**. National fasts were declared as acts of repentance to prevent destruction from coming upon a nation.

> *"Then Jonah cried out and said, 'Yet forty days, and Nineveh shall be overthrown!' So the people of Nineveh believed God, <u>proclaimed a fast</u>, and put on sackcloth. . . Then God saw their works, that they turned from their evil way; and God relented from the disaster that He had said He would bring upon them, and He did not do it."* **(Jonah 3:4-10)**

Our nation of America is in serious moral trouble today and in great need of prayer and fasting. It is highly unlikely that any such decree will be coming forth from Washington any time soon.

Individual fasting was to be done in private and without any public display of discomfort **(Matthew 6:18)**. This is still a good idea today. When you set up your fasting program, keep it to yourself. Don't make a big deal out of it either at home or at work. Friends and family will often try to discourage you and give you all of the reasons why fasting is not good for you. That's why it's best to tell no one when you fast.

Perhaps you should schedule your fast days to fall on non-work or non-school days. This way you will be able to devote as much time as possible to prayer and scripture reading.

There's no doubt about it. Periodic fasting is good medicine for both your body and your soul. That's why it is an essential part of the **Moses Diet & Health Program**. You are going to be a far healthier and holier person as a result of your fasting program. Therefore, please do not underplay its importance or avoid its practice.

Forty Day Fasts – Not For Everyone!

The Bible tells us that Moses, Elijah and Yahshua (Jesus) all fasted for 40 days and 40 nights. Consequently, there are people who try to duplicate this amazing feat – some successfully and some unsuccessfully. Is this the kind of thing we all should be aspiring to or is it something reserved only for a special few?

Fasting is serious business and any fast lasting longer than three days requires special training, monitoring and motivation. Never undertake a lengthy fast – 40 days or otherwise – without the proper training and supervision. To do so could court serious health problems and even death.

However, I would like to give you my interesting variation on the 40-day fast. I call it the *Forty-Hour Fast*. The idea on this program is to divide your fasting time into hours rather than days. Then set out to fast by 40-hour cycles of time. One forty-hour cycle, for example, equals one day and 16 hours. This makes a good target time for beginning fasters to shoot for. And here's a tip. To help you psychologically complete your 40-hour fast, try equating every hour of your fast to one day of your Holy Savior's fasting in the Judean wilderness. Offer it as an act of love and bonding between yourself and Him.

As you get more proficient at fasting, you may want to aim for an 80-hour fast (two 40-hour cycles). This would be a total of three days, eight hours. The 80-hour fast makes a good program to follow for your quarterly fasts.

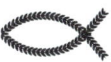

Chapter 17

"Laziness casts one into a deep sleep, and an idle person will suffer hunger."
Proverbs 19:15

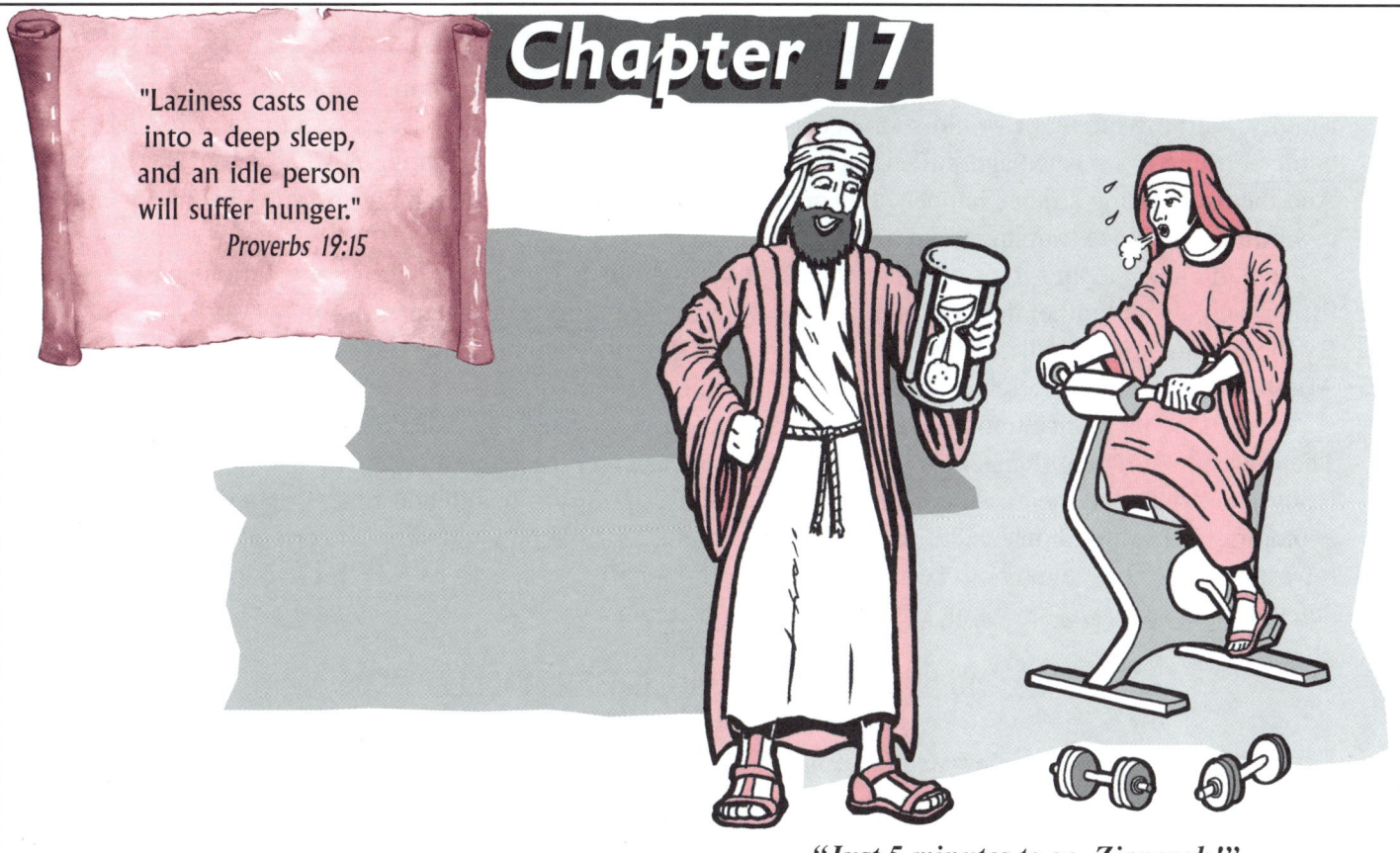

"Just 5 minutes to go, Zipporah!"

To Stay Healthy & Fit, You Have To Exercise.

Your Life Is Like A Field. If You Plant It, Work It And Shape It, It Can Be A Beautiful Garden. But If You Leave It Unattended, It Will Grow Wild And Unkempt.

The year was 1963. I had been away at college for many months and when I returned home, I ran into a high school friend who had been devoting lots of his spare time to what was then a relatively obscure activity called "weight lifting." I couldn't believe my eyes. Since I had last seen him, this formerly lean friend had totally transformed himself into a strapping, muscular marvel. I was shocked by his appearance and couldn't stop talking to him about the remarkable changes he had made in his body. Something clicked deep inside of me and I knew I wanted to do the same thing.

With a college student's income, I could hardly afford the $100 I desperately needed to order my own set of barbells. Thankfully, I had a very supportive and wonderful father who wrote that most important first check for me to the York Barbell Company. About six weeks later, my York **"Big 12 Special"** arrived and my life would never be the same from that day forward.

I couldn't believe the wonderful feeling that exercising with weights was giving me as I pushed myself harder and harder in my crude cellar gym. Working out soon became the most favorite part of my day. My poor mother was nearly losing her mind trying to convince me that I was going to have a

117

heart attack. Friends, family, teachers, coaches – they all tried to dissuade me from this "unnatural" activity, warning me that I would soon become "muscle bound." But the more I was told to quit, the harder I trained. I pushed and pulled and pumped and flexed right through the 60s and into the 70s. And then something strange happened. The rest of the world started to find out just how beneficial and rewarding resistance training could be.

Health clubs began springing up practically overnight in city after city. Professional athletes started lifting weights and rather than become muscle bound, they were actually performing better than ever. By the middle and late 70s, Hollywood rediscovered the muscle man in the likes of icons such as Arnold Schwarzenegger, Sylvester Stallone and Louie Ferrigno.

Next came resistance training for women and a whole new activity called *aerobics*. That was it! There was no stopping things now. At last, exercise was chic. Just about everyone from politicians to Hollywood stars had their own personal trainers. Subscriptions to health and fitness magazines were exploding and selling home exercise equipment became a whole new industry. It certainly was a rewarding time for me too both personally and professionally as an activity which I had loved and defended for years was now quickly becoming mainstream.

BENEFITS OF EXERCISE EXTOLLED

Each year brought us a new exercise and fitness guru who extolled the benefits of exercise as being near miraculous. It was only natural that with all of this exposure, scientists and researchers would start taking a closer look at exercise to see if it really did have any long-term benefits. What they found out was truly amazing! There was no doubt about it. Study after study proved that regular exercise definitely improved overall health and well-being. In fact, the list of exercise benefits proved quite impressive:

(1) builds stronger muscles
(2) strengthens bones
(3) improves flexibility
(4) improves circulation
(5) strengthens heart
(6) helps prevent heart disease
(7) increases endurance and energy
(8) helps regulate metabolism
(9) aids in digestion
(10) helps relieve stress
(11) promotes restful sleep
(12) improves physical appearance
(13) aids in weight control
(14) slows aging process
(15) forestalls onset of degenerative diseases
(16) reduces high blood pressure
(17) helps regulate blood sugar
(18) lessens risk of stroke
(19) helps regulate hormones

Yet with so many health benefits of exercise now conclusively demonstrated, there are still many people who hesitate to include exercise in their health building, weight reduction programs. According to a recent survey by the Center for Advancement of Health, approximately one fourth of Americans do not engage in any physical activity and three-quarters of the population fall far below the recommended 30 minutes a day, five days a week recommendation. If you are one of those people, let me say definitively before going on that **_your health and diet program is doomed to fail if you do not make exercise a regular part of your life!_**

There's just no doubt about it. Exercise is an uplifting experience both physically and spiritually and when done in moderation, it will be a key factor to your success on the **Moses Diet & Health Program**. Therefore, it is not optional – it's *mandatory*! Unfortunately, there are still some diet programs that underplay or even eliminate exercise, stating that it requires too much exercise to burn up significant calories. They base this on the fact that an hour of vigorous exercise burns up between 400 to 600 calories. What they are overlooking is the fact that exercise has an even more profound, long-term effect on the body's metabolism, assisting in weight control in a less obvious manner.

EXERCISE AND METABOLISM

One of the most perplexing things for diet researchers to explain is the fact that many overweight people actually eat as little or less than thinner people do. Consequently, losing weight for these people has meant virtual starvation. And worse yet, once they resume normal eating habits, all of the lost weight is gained back usually with a few additional pounds. Statistics have sadly demonstrated that over ninety percent of the people who lose weight eventually gain it all back again. Isn't this sad that they go through such torture and depravation only to end up back where they started?

The good news is that exercise can help break this pattern. By increasing your physical activity you will increase your metabolism and that will enable you to burn more calories at *rest* than you normally would if you were not exercising. Even moderate exercise will increase your metabolic rate three to eight times. Part of the reason for this is due to the increase in lean tissue (muscle) that often results from following a good resistance exercise program. Muscle tissue requires more calories to maintain than fat. (A pound of muscle burns 20 times more calories than a pound of fat.) Therefore, the more lean muscle you have, the more calories your body burns up.

And as for those critics who say that a 400 to 600 calorie expenditure for an hour's worth of exercise isn't worth it, they are just plain wrong. Evidently, they are unaware that the body's metabolism stays stoked up for hours even after an exercise session is over. One study has shown that the metabolic rate stays elevated for as long as eight hours after an exercise session. This means that your body will continue to burn extra calories for many hours after you've exercised.

And there's still another bonus. Exercise actually helps diminish appetite and relieve hunger pangs. So a trip to the gym may be just the thing you need the next time your stomach starts to rumble.

EXERCISE, APPEARANCE AND LIFESTYLE

In addition to helping you burn up stored fat, a regular exercise program combined with a sensible eating plan can totally change your physical appearance. Dieting will make you thinner but exercise will make you better. While dieting removes fat from the body, exercise actually changes the appearance of the muscle structure to help give you an improved overall look. When you exercise regularly you will soon get pride of ownership of your body. You will carry yourself differently, you will feel more in charge of yourself and you will definitely have more energy and stamina. I can tell you with certainty after more than 30 years in this business that people who keep themselves physically fit have a much higher quality of life. They tend to be healthier, more enthusiastic and more productive. With this kind of track record going for it, I have to wonder why anyone would be reluctant to engage in a regular exercise program.

BUT I'M TOO OLD TO START EXERCISING!

I have one word to say to those of you feel this way. Baloney! Exercise is meant to be a way of life all your life. In fact, people who exercise through their senior years often lead healthier, fuller, more satisfying lives, suffering less from such debilitating diseases as arthritis and Alzheimer's disease. So once you start, never stop; and if you haven't started yet – what are you waiting for? Even something as basic as a one or two-mile walk after dinner is a good place to start. Health clubs have no age limits and you just might be surprised by how many "youngsters" older than yourself are already members. Life by its very definition means activity. So unless you're prepared for the other alternative, then you had better get yourself in motion as soon as possible.

AEROBIC VS. ANAEROBIC EXERCISE

Exercise physiologists describe two different types of physical activity – *aerobic* and *anaerobic*. Here is how they differ.

AEROBIC	ANAEROBIC
• high oxygen requirement	• low oxygen requirement
• steady, non-stop movement	• stop and start movement
• requires at least 12 minutes to achieve training effect	• no time requirements to achieve training effect
• burns fat as principle fuel source	• burns glycogen-glucose as principle fuel source

• examples:
  walking
  jogging
  running
  treadmill
  rowing
  cycling
  jumping rope
  cross country skiing
  swimming
  skating
  aerobics classes
	• examples:
	  sprinting
	  weight training (resistance)
	  golf
	  tennis
	  downhill skiing
	  bowling

AEROBIC EXERCISING:

This type of exercise is also popularly referred to as *cardio training* and the two terms are quickly becoming synonymous. No matter which form of aerobic exercise you choose, there are three basic things you need to keep in mind before you start.

(1) Time. To benefit from the training effect of aerobic exercise, you must perform the exercise for a minimum of 15 to 20 minutes at least three times per week. Thirty to 45 minutes should be your maximum time and be cautioned that over-exercising can actually diminish and even reverse the benefits. The times listed here do not include a one-minute warm up and cool down period which is absolutely required.

(2) Heart Rate. Besides exercising for a measured amount of time, you must also get your heart beating fast enough to achieve the training effect. What's fast enough depends on your age. The maximum heart beat rate decreases with age and no amount of exercise will make it beat faster. For people 20 years old or younger, the maximum heartbeat rate is approximately 200 beats per minute. The average 40-year-old has a maximum heartbeat of around 180 beats per minute. A general rule of thumb for determining your maximum heart rate is to subtract your age from 220.

(3) Intensity. Fortunately, you do not have to exercise at your maximum heart rate to benefit from exercise. As a matter of fact, attempting to do so is very dangerous. Ideally, you should exercise at 75% of your maximum heart rate. This is called your ***target heart rate***. To determine it, subtract your age from 220 and multiply that number by .75. A person 35 years old, for example, would have a target heart rate of 139 beats per minute (220 minus 35 equals 185 times .75 equals 138.75).

ANAEROBIC EXERCISING:

While I have listed several types of anaerobic activities above, the main type of anaerobic exercise that will help you build lean muscle mass is weight training resistance exercise. (There's a complete weight training program for you to use as a guide at the end of this chapter.)

Weight training will strengthen and reshape your muscles while increasing your lean tissue. And remember – it is this increase in lean muscle tissue that helps rev up your metabolism. Most people who don't do any resistance exercise will naturally start to lose muscle mass from around the age of 30 onward. The body is then going to start storing extra fat as the muscle mass decreases making dieting extremely difficult. That's why a lifelong weight training program is so important.

In order to get the best of both worlds, you will need to work out a combination of both aerobic and anaerobic exercise. There are three ways to do this. First of all, you can combine both activities in the same workout, provided you begin with resistance training and finish with aerobics. Secondly, you can do your aerobic exercise at one time of the day (preferably morning when you will burn the most fat), and your resistance exercise at another time of the day. And lastly, you can do your aerobic exercise on one day and your resistance exercise on an alternate day. I suggest that you experiment with the various options to see which one works best for you.

HOW OFTEN AND HOW LONG?

Now that I've hopefully convinced you to start an exercise program, let's address the questions of how often and how long you should exercise. Since most people blame a lack of time as their reason for not exercising, the question of how often to exercise becomes a critical one. So let's start by determining the absolute minimum amount of time you'll need to reap any benefits.

When test subjects were compared on two days of exercise per week verses three days per week, the three-day group showed greater gains in lean muscle tissue along with a greater loss of body fat. However, even those people exercising just two days a week still made noticeable improvements, demonstrating that two days a week is still better than nothing.

Another study demonstrated that three one-hour sessions per week, divided into 30 minutes of resistance training and 30 minutes of cardio-aerobic training is enough to produce a *significant* training effect.

In light of this research, I am going to recommend an absolute minimum of two days of exercise per week. However, three days are even better and four to five days are better yet – provided you do not overtrain at each session.

If you have the luxury of controlling your own daily schedule, here's an interesting suggestion. Exercise for two shorter sessions twice a day rather than one longer one. Not only are briefer workouts easier to psyche up for, studies indicate that they may be even more effective for losing weight quicker. In addition, it's been demonstrated that people who engage in more frequent but briefer workouts, tend to stay with their exercise program longer than those people who train less frequently but for a longer time.

HERE ARE SOME TIPS TO HELP YOU STICK WITH IT

Since exercise is such a fundamental part of the *Moses Diet & Health Program*, I want to give you some suggestions to help you stick with a lifetime exercise program.

1) Try to look upon exercise as a pleasant experience rather than drudgery. Don't just *think* about all of the good it will do for you. Instead, try to also focus on the actual good feelings your body is experiencing while you are performing your exercises. I've been exercising for well over 30 years now and I can honestly say that I've had many enjoyable workout sessions just as an end in themselves.

(2) Never do individual exercises or exercise routines that you don't enjoy. There are just too many options these days for you to have to force yourself through something unpleasant. Keep experimenting until you find things that you like. And never let anyone convince you that you have to do a certain exercise whether you like it or not. That just isn't so.

(3) According to the American College of Sports Medicine, one out of two people who start an exercise program eventually quit. You must beat these odds to be successful on your health program. Therefore, study and learn all you can about exercise. Try to make exercising a passion in your life. Subscribe to health and fitness magazines. Read good exercise books. Exercise physiology is a very dynamic field with lots of good information and exciting new equipment always coming out. Try to stay abreast of all that's going on.

(4) Try to find someone to exercise with. One of the surest ways to stay with an exercise program is to buddy up with someone who shares your interest. You will be able to encourage each other, motivate each other, praise each other, pace each other, spot each other and socialize with each other. I have had some great training partners through the years and there were many times when my commitment to them is what got me into the gym and vice versa.

(5) Vary your exercise routines and your physical activities. If you stick to the same exercise routine day after day, week after week, you're going to quit before you know it. Mix in bicycling, jogging, swimming, cross country skiing, hiking, treadmill, stair climbing, aerobics, kick boxing and so forth and your workouts will always stay interesting and fun.

(6) Never just wing your exercise program. Set up a definite schedule and stick to it. Make fitness a daily priority and don't start missing a workout here and there. Otherwise, before too long you'll be skipping the whole thing.

WALKING YOURSELF TO FITNESS

Before moving on to the weight training program, I want to say a few words about what some authorities consider to be the greatest exercise of all – walking. Here is a form of exercise that, other than a good pair of walking shoes, requires no equipment, no health club membership and no special training. You can literally step out your front door and go. And if the weather's not so great, there's always the local mall.

All things considered, walking is probably the number one fitness option for more people than anything else. In addition to helping control bodyweight, walking at a brisk pace and on a regular basis will also help reduce blood pressure, strengthen the heart and lungs and boost energy levels.

Walking and talking with one or two friends is one of the most therapeutic activities you will ever engage in. You will be able to cover vast distances with hardly being aware of an exertion. No other form of exercise can offer this.

Any time is a good time to walk but a brisk walk after a meal is not only good for weight loss, it's excellent for your digestion too. If you are walking strictly for weight loss, then the faster you walk the greater will be the benefits.

Can You Exercise Too Much?

With so many people needing to be convinced to exercise regularly, it's hard to believe that there are actually people who can become addicted to exercise. Perhaps for some of you, this may sound like a great problem to have but this is not the case. Exercise addiction can cause great physiological damage to the body and, if not corrected, can lead to serious illness.

Listed below are eight signs of exercise addiction:
- Exercising for more than an hour each and every day.
- Feeling guilty when an exercise session is missed.
- Exercising during an illness.
- Exercising with an injury.
- Pushing to exhaustion in every workout.
- Ignoring negative feedback signals while exercising.
- Neglecting other duties and obligations in order to exercise.
- Carrying extremely low levels of body fat.

Setting Up Your Weight Training Program

The rest of this chapter is devoted to showing you some of the basic weight training exercises and how to incorporate them into your *Moses Diet & Health Program*. Here are some basic rules you will need to observe as you begin your training program:
- Never use a weight that makes you strain.
- If an exercise causes pain or aggravates an injury, stop immediately.
- Never exercise the same muscle two days in a row.
- Always exercise larger muscles first working down to the smaller ones.
- Try to rest no longer than a minute between sets.

CHEST

Models: Christine Marton, Gary Birchell

Bench Press
Keep your feet flat on the floor, your back slightly arched and all your body muscles firm. Approximately 30-inch hand space. Lower bar moderately slowly and deliberately to nipple area of chest. Keep elbows out. Do not pause, do not bounce, press bar straight up in a plane (not over your face).

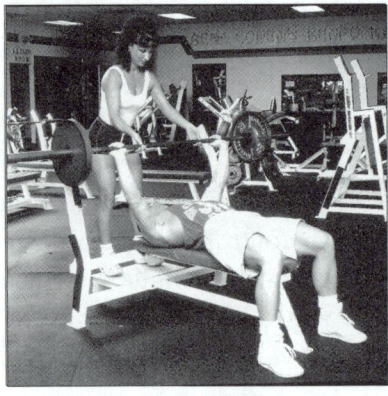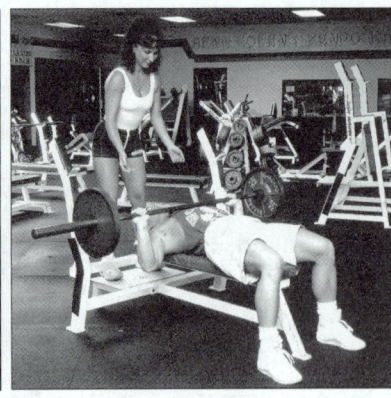

**Try not to wiggle or lag behind with either arm. Do not raise hips off bench.
(3 sets, 8-10 repetitions)**

Dumbbell Flyes
Start with arms locked overhead, dumbbells touching, palms facing each other. Slowly lower dumbbells in an arched movement, keeping elbows slightly bent and back towards shoulders. Lower weights to slightly below parallel to chest and reverse motion back to starting position. Squeeze and flex your chest muscles at the top.

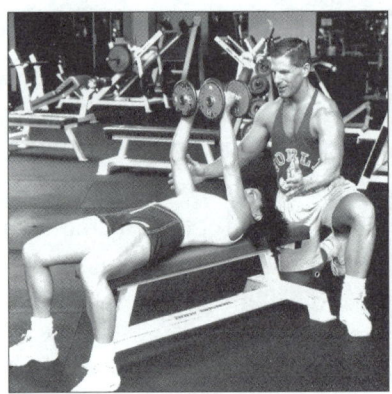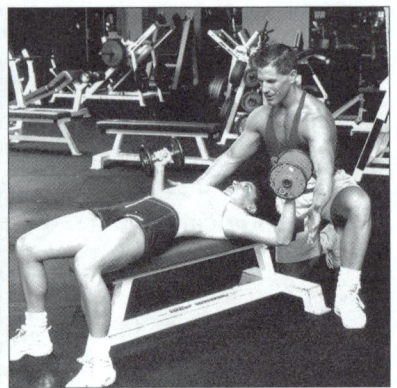

**Always keep elbows slightly unlocked and bent. Lower weights under control of chest muscles and not gravity.
(3 sets, 8-10 repetitions)**

Incline Dumbbell Press
This movement works the tie-in between the upper chest and front shoulders. Set bench angle at about 45 degrees. Start with dumbbells lightly resting on chest palms facing forward. Slowly press weights to an overhead position without changing direction of hands. Weights may lightly touch at top. Lower slowly back to starting position.

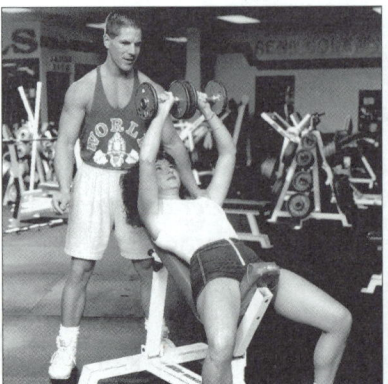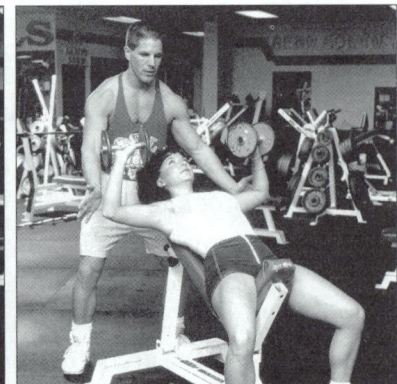

**Keep rib cage uplifted throughout movement. Again try to squeeze chest muscles at top position.
(3 sets, 8-10 repetitions)**

BICEPS

Barbell Curls
Start with barbell resting across front of thighs, shoulder width grip, palms up. Using only the biceps muscles, curl the weight up to under the chin. Try to keep your upper arms fairly stationary. Squeeze the muscles at the top. Lower the bar slowly using muscle control and not gravity.

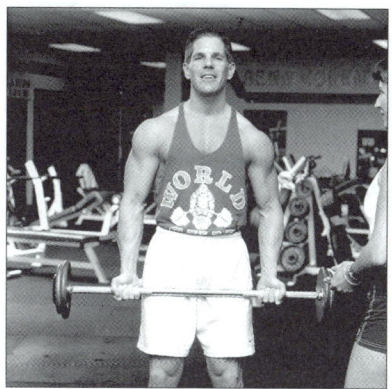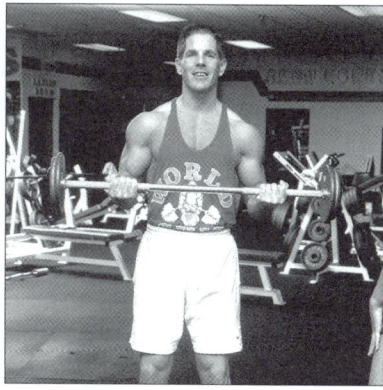

Try not to swing the bar or sway your body. A half-second pause at bottom position between reps is okay.
(3 sets, 8-10 repetitions)

Seated Dumbbell Curls
Sit on the edge of a bench holding dumbbells down at your side, palms facing forward. Using only the power of your biceps, slowly curl the weights up towards your shoulders. Try to keep your upper arms stationary and do not let your elbows drift forward. Squeeze biceps at top. Lower slowly back to starting position.

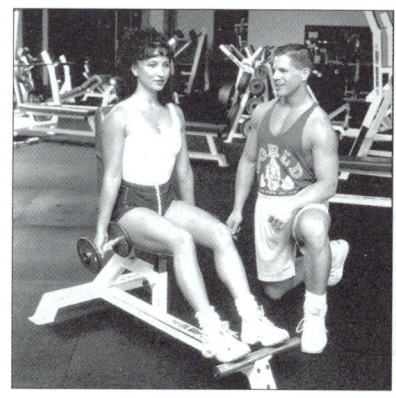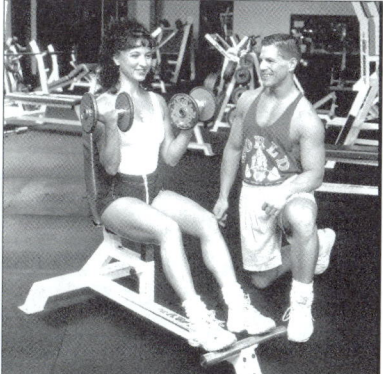

Dumbbells may be raised together or alternately. Keep upper body firm and tight.
(3 sets, 8-10 repetitions)

TRICEPS

Dumbbell Kickbacks
Place one hand and knee on a bench as shown. Start with a 90-degree bend in the elbow and the upper arm almost parallel to the floor. Keeping the upper arm stationary, slowly raise the dumbbell behind you as high as possible and hold and squeeze at the top for a half a second. Lower back to starting position.

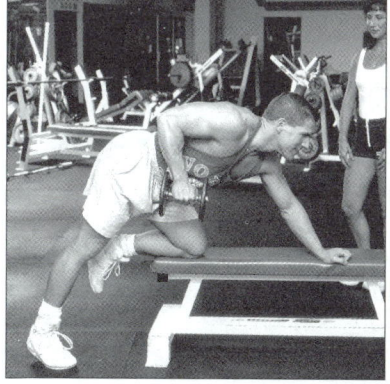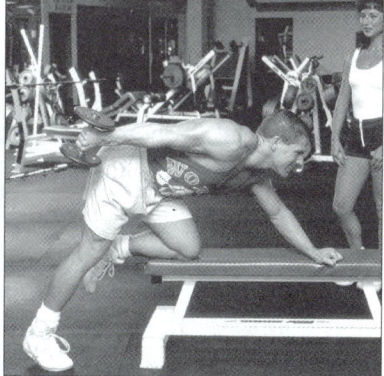

Look forward, keep your upper body still and move only your lower arm.
(3 sets, 8-10 repetitions each side)

TRICEPS

Bench Dips
Place hands on bench at shoulderwidth and heels of feet on opposite bench or chair. Start with elbows locked out. Slowly lower your body towards the floor until fully distended and return to starting position. Try to keep a smooth, steady motion.

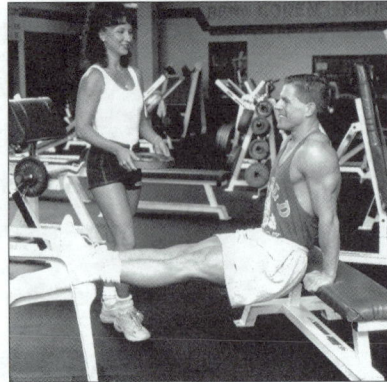 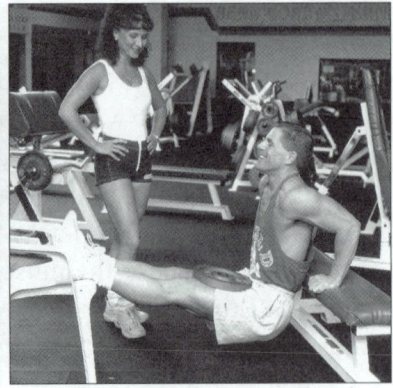

Start with bodyweight only. As strength increases, have partner place weight across thighs.
(3 sets, 8-10 repetitions)

BACK

Chins
Use stool or bench to reach bar. Grab bar a little beyond shoulder width, palms facing away from body. Pull yourself up slowly without body swing until upper chest touches bar. Lower all the way down. Pull up with the strength of the back muscles (latissimus).

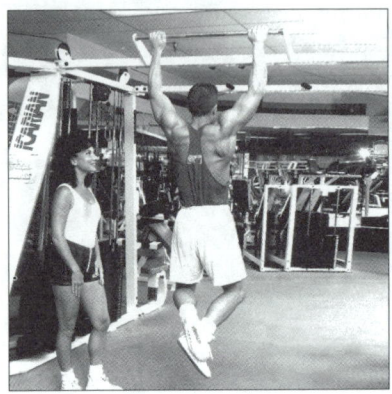 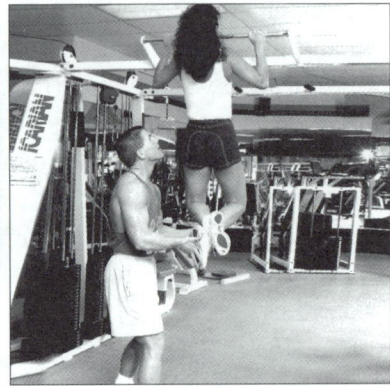

If you are unable to get the required reps, your partner can assist you by pushing up lightly on your feet.
(3 sets, 6-8 repetitions)

Dumbbell Rows
Place hand and knee on bench as shown. Start with dumbbell fully lowered to floor and your body at about 60-degree angle. Slowly pull the weight up towards your chest and point your elbow high to the ceiling. Lower the weight slowly getting an extra long stretch at the bottom.

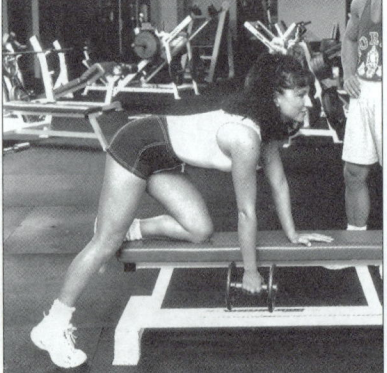 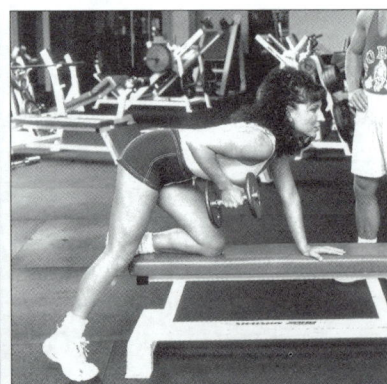

Try not to get too much body swing and pull as much as possible with the back muscles.
(3 sets, 8-10 repetitions each side)

SHOULDERS

Seated Dumbbell Press
Sit on the edge of a bench (preferably a bench with an upright back brace). Start with dumbbells resting on shoulders, palms facing forward, elbows out and back. Slowly press the dumbbells to a lightly touching position overhead, elbows nearly locked. Lower back to starting position.

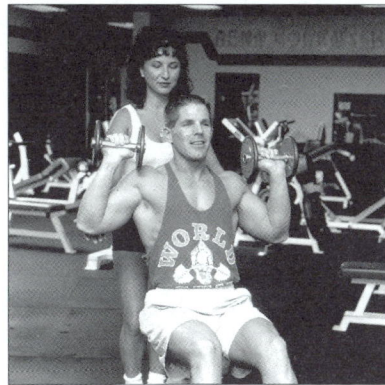 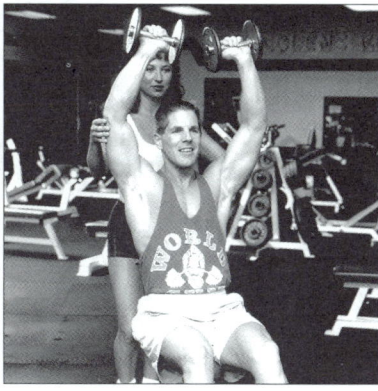

Try not to lean back. Weight lifting belt will help keep your back straight.
(3 sets, 8-10 repetitions)

Dumbbell Laterals
Start with dumbbells held down in front of the body, palms facing each other. Slowly raise out to side, keeping palms facing down as weights are raised. Motion should simulate pouring a cup of coffee. Elbows bent slightly and weights slightly in front of body. Lift only to slightly above shoulder height.

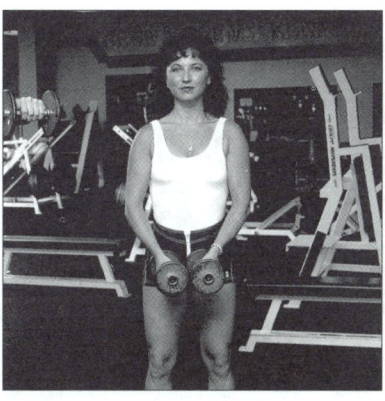 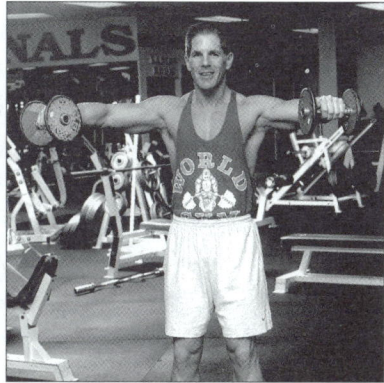

Try not to swing weights up. Instead, lift with the power of the shoulders. Hold briefly at the top and return to starting position.
(3 sets, 8-10 repetitions)

Upright Rows
This exercise is for upper back and shoulders. With bar hanging in front of body, hands about 3 inches apart, pull up on the weight, keeping the bar close to your body. Raise to the chin, hold briefly, flexing shoulders and upper back, then lower.

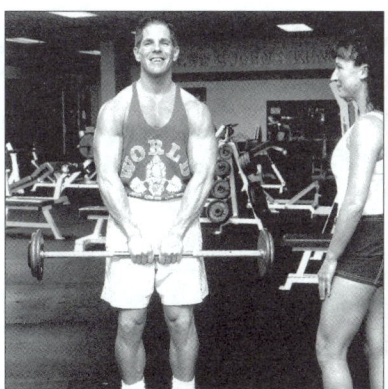 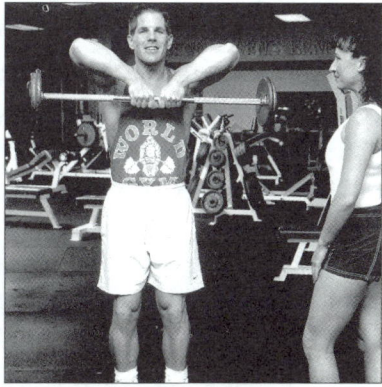

Elbows should flare out to the sides as the weight is raised.. Do not let bar drift away from your body.
(3 sets, 8-10 repetitions)

LEGS

Barbell Squats
Place bar across upper back about 4 inches below the back of the neck. Feet about shoulder width apart and pointing slightly out. Slowly sink down into a deep knee bend and return to upright position. Do not pause at the bottom.

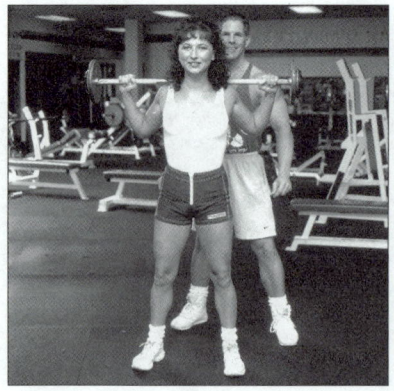
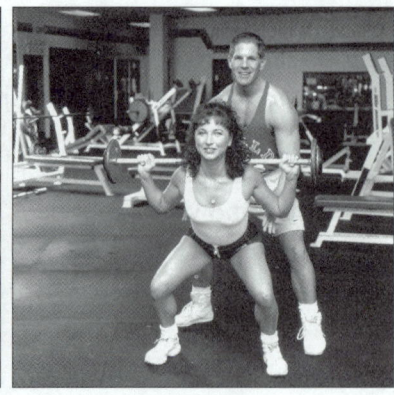

Bouncing down into the low position can damage the knees. Always stay in control.
(3 sets, 8-10 repetitions)

Leg Extensions
Sitting forward on the leg extension machine, place the feet under the front roller. Point the toes slightly outward. Raise the legs slowly forward to the upright position. Hold briefly and flex the thighs hard. Return slowly to starting position.

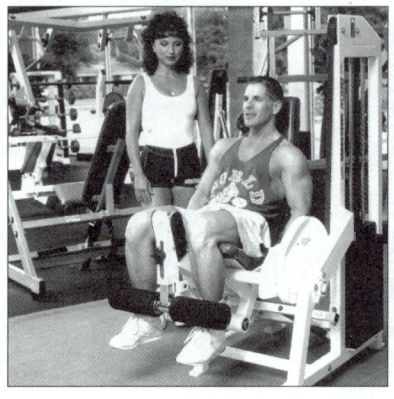
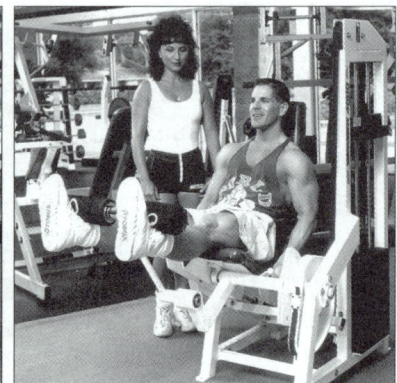

Try not to snap the legs up and down. Stay in control throughout the range of motion.
(3 sets, 10-12 repetitions)

Leg Curls
Lie face down on leg curl machine, legs extended straight out under roller at the ankles. Slowly curl (bend) lower legs back toward buttocks striving for a full contraction. Squeeze the back of the legs (hamstrings) hard at the top of the movement. Gradually lower the legs back to starting position.

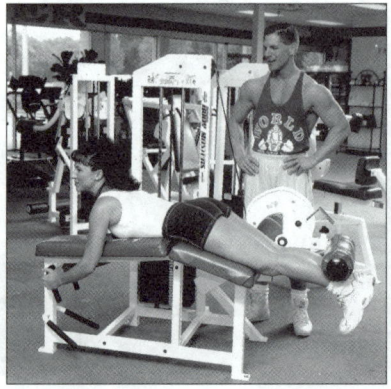
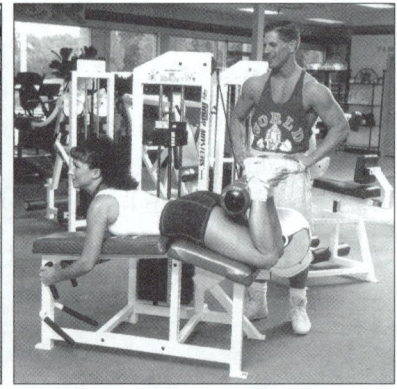

Try not to let momentum swing the machine up and down. Instead, concentrate on pulling with the back of the legs.
(3 sets, 8-10 repetitions)

CALVES

Dumbbell Calf Raise
Stand on a step or a board with one foot and hold the dumbbell in the opposite hand. Brace yourself against a wall or a partner. Just the toes on the edge of the board. Push up off the toes, raising your heel as high as you can and lowering it as low as you can. Squeeze the calf muscles at the top. Calves are tough muscles so push the repetitions on this exercise.

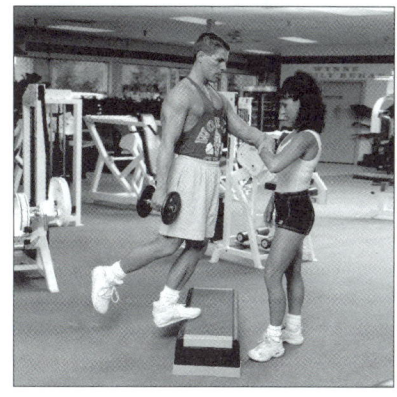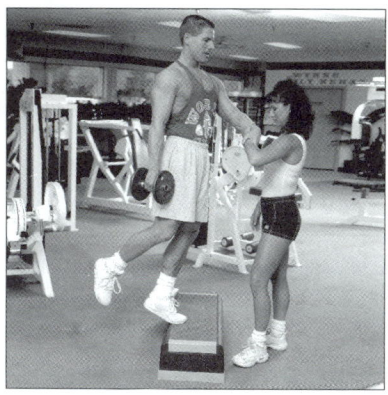

Strive for full extension and full contraction. Experiment with position of toes (pointing straight, out and in).
(3 sets, 15-20 repetitions)

ABDOMINALS

Leg Tuck Ins
Sit with the buttocks on the edge of the bench and grab the sides of the bench with each hand. Lift the body forward to about a 35-degree angle. Keeping feet together, pull them into your chest area, bending your knees as you do. Hold briefly, squeeze the abdominals and extend back out in front of you.

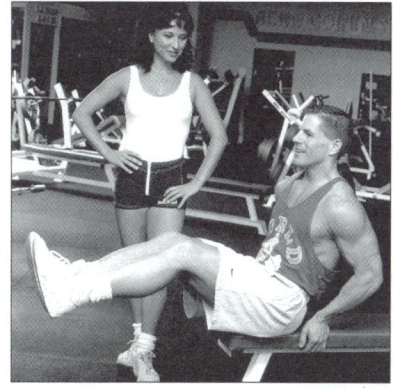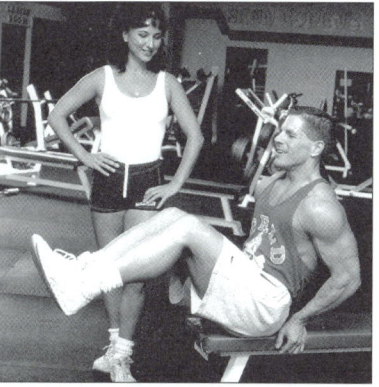

Keep you chin tucked down on your chest. Try to move only your legs, keeping your upper body stationary.
(3 sets, 12-15 repetitions)

Abdominal Rollup
Lie face up on a flat bench, knees bent and hands behind your head. Slowly roll the upper torso off the bench to about 4 or 5 inches. Hold for a full second and squeeze hard on the abdominal muscles. Slowly lower back to starting position, keeping head bent slightly forward.

Twists
Place a broom handle or a bar behind your neck and grip as shown. Slowly twist from side to side bending slightly forward at the full twist position. Try to keep a steady, smooth motion without pausing. Twist with the muscles on the sides of your waist (3 sets, 25 twists) and not with momentum.

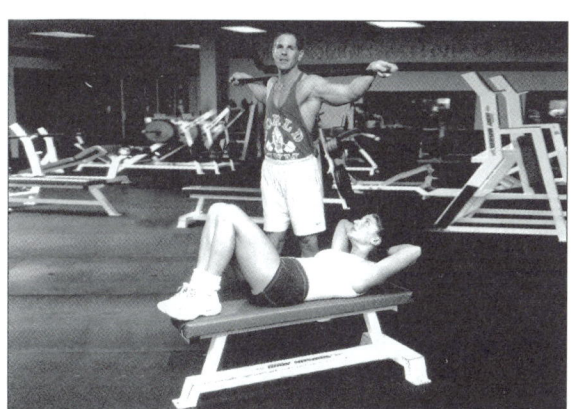

Resist the tendency to lift the lower back off the bench. This is a very effective partial movement.
(3 sets, 15-20 repetitions)

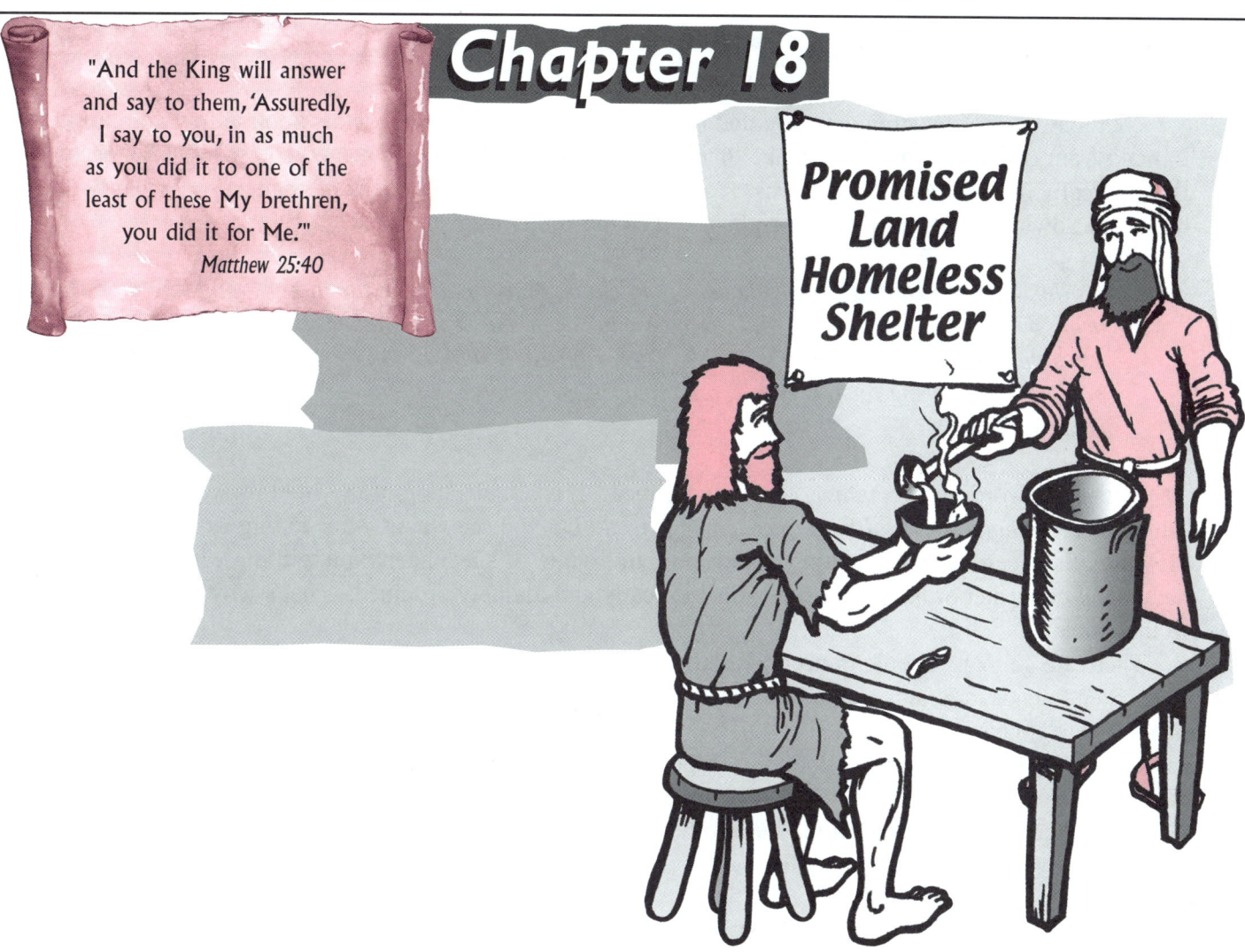

Do Good And Forget It.
Do Bad And Regret it!

The Best Way To Cheer Yourself Up Is To Cheer Up Someone Else.

Important note: Often, when any type of good works program is suggested to Christians, many are quick to retort that we are not saved by our good works.

> "*For by grace you have been saved through faith, and not of yourselves; it is the gift of God, not of works, lest anyone should boast.*" **(Ephesians 2:8-9)**

So before any of you start to write and condemn me for including this chapter, let me state two things. I am not suggesting or implying in this chapter that a good works program is going to earn you your salvation. This chapter is about doing what the LORD expects from us as His loving and caring children and how such good works affect our long-term health. And secondly, isn't it possible to do good works for others and *not* boast about them? Most certainly it is. This is a very important chapter for your health building program. Do not take it lightly.

It may seem a bit strange to you that after spending three-quarters of this book telling you how to make your own life better, I now take time out to tell you how to make someone else's life better. But it's really not so strange as it seems. You see, in making someone else's life better, you actually do make your own life better. It's a principle as old as the Bible itself.

> *"Is this not the fast that I have chosen. . . to share your bread with the hungry, and that you bring to your house the poor who are cast out; when you see the naked, that you cover him, and not hide yourself from your own flesh? Then your light shall break forth like the morning, your <u>healing</u> shall spring forth speedily, and your righteousness shall go before you."*
> **(Isaiah 58:6-8)**

Notice the word *healing* which I have underlined. It is a translation of the Hebrew word **arukah** which means *wholeness, health, perfected, long-lived*. Do you see what God is telling us here? Helping others can make us healthy, whole and long living. It's a concept you will most likely never see in any other diet or health book yet it is biblically and divinely ordained. That's why this chapter is in this book.

There are so many people in need. We all tend to live in our own little worlds, and we don't see that. Step outside, and look around for places or people in need of your help. You'll benefit as much as they will - maybe even more.

Obviously Cain never understood this important point when he answered God as to the whereabouts of his missing brother. *"Am I my brother's keeper?"* **(Genesis 4:9)** His sarcastic answer sealed his fate, for indeed we all *are* our brother's keeper. If the world operated on this principle, we would begin to have heaven on earth.

TO HELP YOURSELF – MAKE TIME TO HELP OTHERS

"When a friend of mine suggested that I help her deliver meals-on-wheels three days a week, I couldn't think of enough excuses to say no. That's why I was surprised when the words 'I guess so' slipped out of my mouth. Now I can tell you that it's the greatest thing I've ever done." So reports Ellen McCabe of Winter Park, Florida. "I have met the nicest group of senior citizens. Some of them would starve to death if it weren't for this wonderful service."

"Volunteering is one of the most satisfying things I've ever done," reports Alan Dougherty, a personal trainer in Lansing, Michigan who spends three nights a week as an exercise instructor to a class of retarded children. "I used to say that nothing felt better than working out in the gym. Now I can honestly say that volunteer work feels every bit as good – maybe better."

Louise Epperson has been the volunteer coordinator for her company Laxion Industries for the last 10 years. According to her, once employees get involved in volunteer work, they get hooked. "So many times a person will come to me more or less out of curiosity or as an afterthought. However once they get a taste of helping others, they become my biggest recruiters."

It's apparent from these comments that doing good and helping others brings untold benefits to the needy while blessing the volunteer with a tremendous feeling of satisfaction. With a track record like this, it's hard to figure out why anyone would hesitate about becoming involved in volunteer programs. The good news is that, according to a recent national survey conducted by Independent Sector of

Washington, D.C., nearly 56 percent of adults in this country do some form of volunteer work every week – averaging about 3.5 hours per week.

There's just no doubt about it. Volunteering is one of the most rewarding things you can ever do both for yourself and others. In fact, a 1999 study performed by the University of Michigan in Ann Arbor found that people live longer when they do volunteer work. According to the study, researchers observed that people who volunteer for as little as one hour a week tend to live longer than those who do no volunteer work. But isn't this exactly what God promised us through the words of his prophet Isaiah quoted above?

HOW TO GET STARTED

Is this all starting to make sense to you? Are you ready to commit yourself to helping others? If so, the Independent Sector (www.indepsec.org) offers 10 tips you should consider before you begin your volunteer work.

(1) Research the causes and issues that are important to you. Look for a group that works with issues about which you feel strongly. If you can't find a group that interests you, perhaps you should start one yourself. Rally your neighbors to clean up a vacant lot, patrol the neighborhood, paint an elderly person's house, take turns helping an ailing neighbor. There is no end to creative ideas just as there is no end to the need for volunteers.

(2) Consider the skills you have to offer. Do you enjoy outdoor work, have a knack for teaching, or just enjoy interacting with people? Look for volunteer work that fits these aptitudes. You may have special skills from your work or a hobby that others can benefit from. By fitting your volunteer work to your abilities and skills, you eliminate training time.

(3) How about trying something new? Perhaps you would like to learn a new skill or be exposed to a new situation. Then volunteering can offer you a change from your daily routine. If you work in an office all day, you may enjoy an outdoor volunteer assignment. Many non-profit groups are willing to teach new skills to their volunteers.

(4) Combine your personal goals with your volunteer work. Perhaps you'd like to combine your volunteer work with your personal goals. If you want to lose weight, pick physical volunteer work such as cleaning a park or working with kids. If you enjoy exercising, teach a senior citizen exercise class at a local nursing home.

(5) Don't over-commit yourself. Make sure the volunteer hours you want to give fit into your lifestyle so that you don't frustrate your family, exhaust yourself and shortchange the organization you are donating your time to. If you are unsure about how much time you can give, see whether the organization can start you out on a limited number of hours as a test. Better to start slowly and stay with it than to jump in gung-ho and end up quitting.

(6) Nonprofits may have some questions too. While most organizations are eager to find help, they do have to be careful when accepting volunteer services. Don't be surprised or upset if an organization you volunteer for asks you to come in for an interview, fill out an application, describe your background and qualifications. It is their job to find qualified volunteers who have the skills they are looking for, are truly committed to helping and whose interests match those of the organization. This is especially true for organizations that deal with children and other at-risk groups.

(7) Consider volunteering as a family. You may want to look for a volunteer opportunity that is suitable for parents and children or a husband and wife to do together. This will help teach biblical values to family members as well as give the entire family a shared volunteer experience.

(8) Virtual Volunteering. If you have computer access and the necessary skills, some organizations now offer the opportunity to do volunteer work over the computer. This could be in the form of free legal advice, typing a college paper for a disabled person, or simply keeping in contact with a shut-in via E-mail. This is a perfect choice for people with limited free time, no transportation or a physical disability.

(9) Bring your heart into your volunteer work. Enter into your volunteer work with cheerfulness, enthusiasm and a good heart. Keep your personal problems to yourself.

(10) Groups looking for help. Here's a list of the various types of groups that are looking for volunteers.

- day care centers
- Neighborhood Watch
- public schools and colleges
- halfway houses
- community theaters
- drug rehabilitation centers
- fraternal and civic organizations
- retirement centers and homes for the elderly
- Meals-on-Wheels
- church and community-sponsored soup kitchens
- prisons
- youth organizations
- after school programs
- Salvation Army
- shelters for battered women and children

For more information on volunteer groups, call **1-800-VOLUNTEER**, or visit www.helping.org or www.pointsoflight.org or go to search engine www.dogpile.com and type in "volunteering" into the search field.

Chapter 19

> "When you lie down, you will not be afraid; yes, you will lie down and your sleep will be sweet."
> Proverbs 3:24

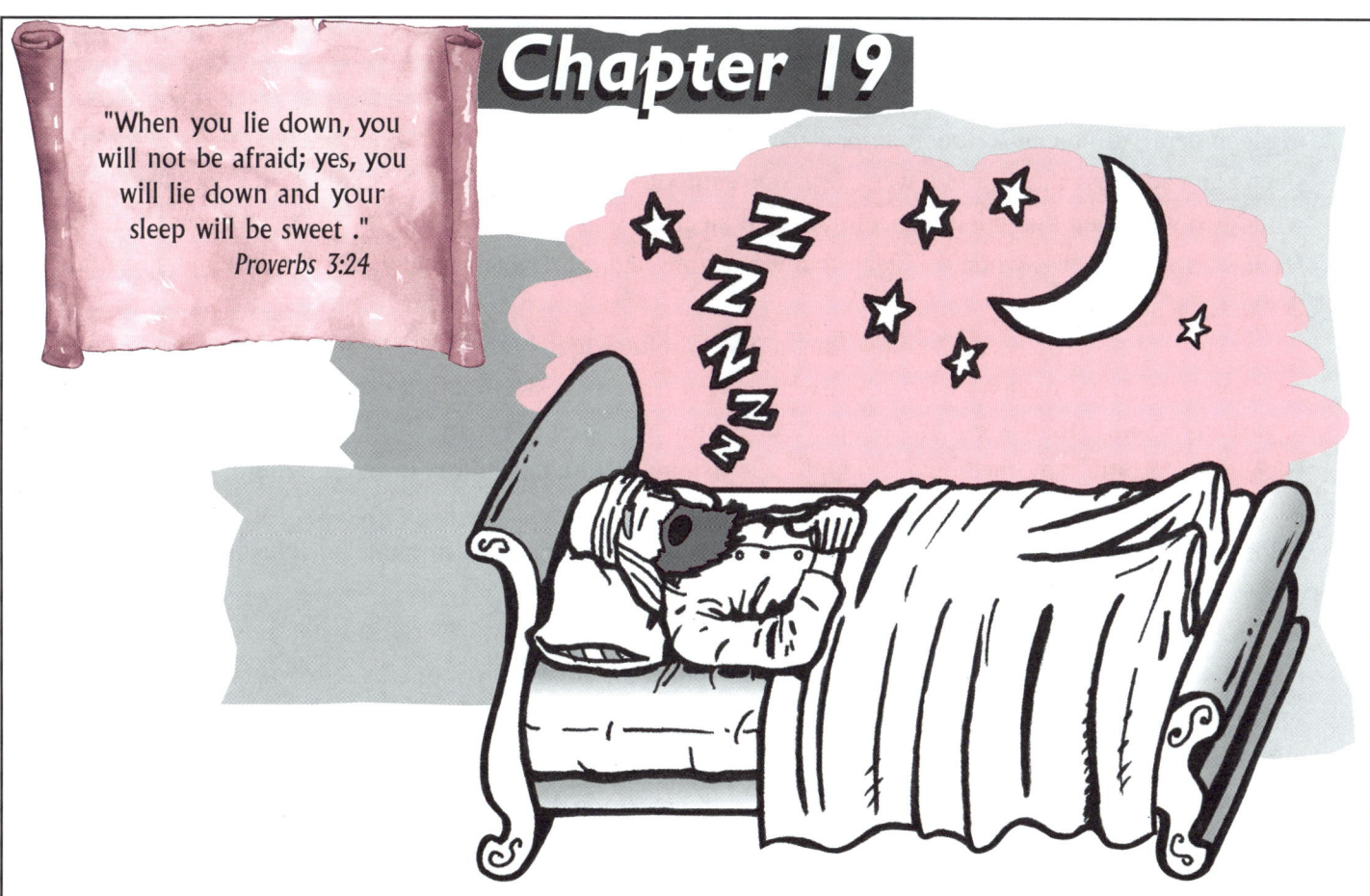

I Pray The Lord My Soul To Keep.

Always Put Off Until Tomorrow What Should Never Be Done At All.

In the very beginning of creation, God established a daily rhythm pattern of night and day.

"God called the light Day, and the darkness He called Night. So the evening and the morning were the first day." **(Genesis 1:5)**

Please note that according to the Bible a new day begins at sundown. Thus the LORD ordained a pattern of sleeping and waking that continues with us to this day. Scientists call this alternating day-night cycle the ***circadian rhythm***. You might recognize it better as your internal biological clock. It has been genetically programmed into all living things on this planet by God. Obviously, something this universal must have a strong reason for being. Indeed – it does.

Sleep is as fundamental to life and health as the air you breathe and the food you eat. In fact, one sleep expert called sleep "the third component of a long and healthy life, right up there with a good diet and exercise." While you can go up to a week without water and a month or more without food, you can go barely a few days without sleep. Sleep is not optional. It's mandatory. Up to three nights of sleep deprivation can seriously impair mental function and judgement. Four to five nights without sleep can cause psychosis and a week or more without sleep can actually be fatal. It almost goes without saying then that good, peaceful, restful sleep is essential for the success of the **Moses Diet & Health Program**. It is while we sleep that we restore and reactivate our physical, mental and spiritual being.

According to sleep researchers, getting a good night's sleep helps make us more alert and productive and puts us in a better mood whereas even a minor sleep deficit can still affect us negatively. Sadly, there are many people today who are trying to get by on reduced amounts of sleep. Busy lives, erratic job schedules, late night television are all contributors to the problem. Research has shown that people who fail to get enough sleep tend to age faster, have increased irritability, suffer mental fatigue and loss of concentration ability, have weakened immune systems and even *experience weight gain*.

Eve Van Cauter, a sleep researcher at the University of Chicago, has investigated the effect that lack of sleep has on weight gain. Van Cutter attributes the link to a decrease in growth hormone brought on by irregular sleeping. She notes that growth hormone plays an important part in controlling the body's proportions of fat and muscle. Men, and to a lesser extent women, secrete much of their growth hormone during the initial hours of deep sleep. Aging reduces the amount of time spent in deep sleep and thus reduces the amount of growth hormone secreted. Young people who scrimp on their sleep could experience a similar growth hormone deficit and thus be contributing to their overweight problems, according to Van Cauter.

Researchers also theorize that long-term sleep debt could be a factor in the high national incidences of diabetes and obesity. There is even some recent speculation that ongoing lack of sleep may contribute to some forms of cancer.

It has become fashionable lately among some high achieving people to push to the limit on awake time. The expectation is that with less sleep, more productive work can be accomplished. However, the research data does not support this. Those people who try to scrimp on sleep may actually be getting less out of their experiment than they bargained for. One study demonstrated that people who stay awake for up to 19 hours scored worse on performance and alertness tests than those with a blood alcohol level of .08 percent – a level high enough to be considered legally drunk in some states.

"Society is being victimized by not getting enough sleep," according to David Dinges, Director of Experimental Psychiatry at the University of Pennsylvania School of Medicine. "Our productivity, our safety, our health are at risk."

Exactly how much sleep do you need a night? Studies have shown that when subjects are allowed to sleep as long as they like without alarm clocks and light, the average night's sleep period is approximately eight hours.

FACTORS THAT CAN DISTURB SLEEP

Unfortunately, one out of three people report that they have trouble sleeping and that percentage goes up with age. The average person requires seven to eight hours of sleep a night and that number also decreases with age. Several factors can interfere with a good night's sleep. These include:

1. Room temperature (best at 60-65 degrees).
2. Caffeine (effects can last for up to seven hours or more).
3. Smoking (nicotine stimulates the central nervous system – you shouldn't be smoking anyway).
4. Exercise (do not exercise too late in the evening).
5. Complete exhaustion (commonly referred to as being over tired).
6. Stress (worry at night makes sleep take flight).
7. Noise (radio, TV, neighbors, dogs, etc.).
8. Arguments (try to avoid them but if you have to, save them for the day time).
9. Medication (some can cause sleep problems).
10. Worrying about not sleeping.

THINGS YOU CAN DO TO HELP YOU SLEEP BETTER

1. Try to stay on the same sleep-wake schedule each day.
2. Eliminate as many distractions as possible (light, sound, etc.).
3. Take a warm-hot shower before retiring.
4. Do not eat a big meal before going to bed.
5. Sleep with a body pillow.
6. Use natural herbs such as chamomile, kava kava, St. John's Wort, valerian, catnip and hops.
   But never resort to sleeping pills.
7. Drink a glass of warm milk.
8. Listen to cassette audio tapes of the Bible.

THE POWER OF POWER NAPPING

Once upon a time it was believed that napping during the day was a bad thing to do – an unproductive time waster and a sign of laziness. Now we know differently. Not only is a brief afternoon *power nap* not bad for you, it actually has some great benefits. Sleep researchers have determined that we actually have *two* regular awake and sleep cycles during the course of a 24-hour day – a greater one in the evening and another lesser one in mid-afternoon. Old world cultures have long acknowledged this phenomenon with a mid-day siesta. Perhaps it's time we in America tapped into this ancient wisdom.

As a matter of fact, some progressive companies have already started to do so by setting up official nap rooms and allowing employees a brief nap time around midday. What they have found out is that after a brief afternoon nap, employees are actually more productive and more energized. It's really like getting two days wrapped up in one.

But there's a catch. To qualify as a power nap, the afternoon siesta cannot be too long or it then becomes counterproductive. This according to Mark Rosekind, a former NASA sleep researcher and currently president of Alertness Solutions, a consultant company that helps businesses reduce fatigue-related errors. Rosekind advises that short power naps up to 45 minutes work best. After that, he cautions, you'll be in deep sleep and will most likely awake groggy and slow.

DON'T FORGET THE SABBATH REST

So important is the seventh day rest that God made it a commandment (the longest):

"Remember the Sabbath day, to keep it holy. Six days you shall labor and do all your work, but the seventh day is the Sabbath of the LORD your God. In it you shall do no work; you, nor your son, nor your daughter, nor your male servant, nor your female servant, nor your cattle, nor your stranger who is within your gates. For in six days the LORD made the heavens and the earth, the sea, and all that is in them, and rested the seventh day. Therefore, the LORD blessed the Sabbath day and hallowed it." **(Genesis 20:8-11)**

The Sabbath day has become quite a contentious issue within Christianity as various denominations debate whether it is Saturday or Sunday, or whether it even needs to be observed at all. Without getting deeply into the theological issues in this book, I do want to say that I believe that God's commandments are eternal and that we should still be observing a seventh day rest as per His orders. What's interesting is that research has demonstrated that a work cycle of six days on and one day off seems to be the most conducive to good health and productivity. And why not? It was set up by the Master Builder Himself. Therefore, if you push yourself through week after week of work without any rest, you are asking for trouble. Your body was designed by God to totally rest every seven days. You better stick to the instruction manual if you want a long, healthy life.

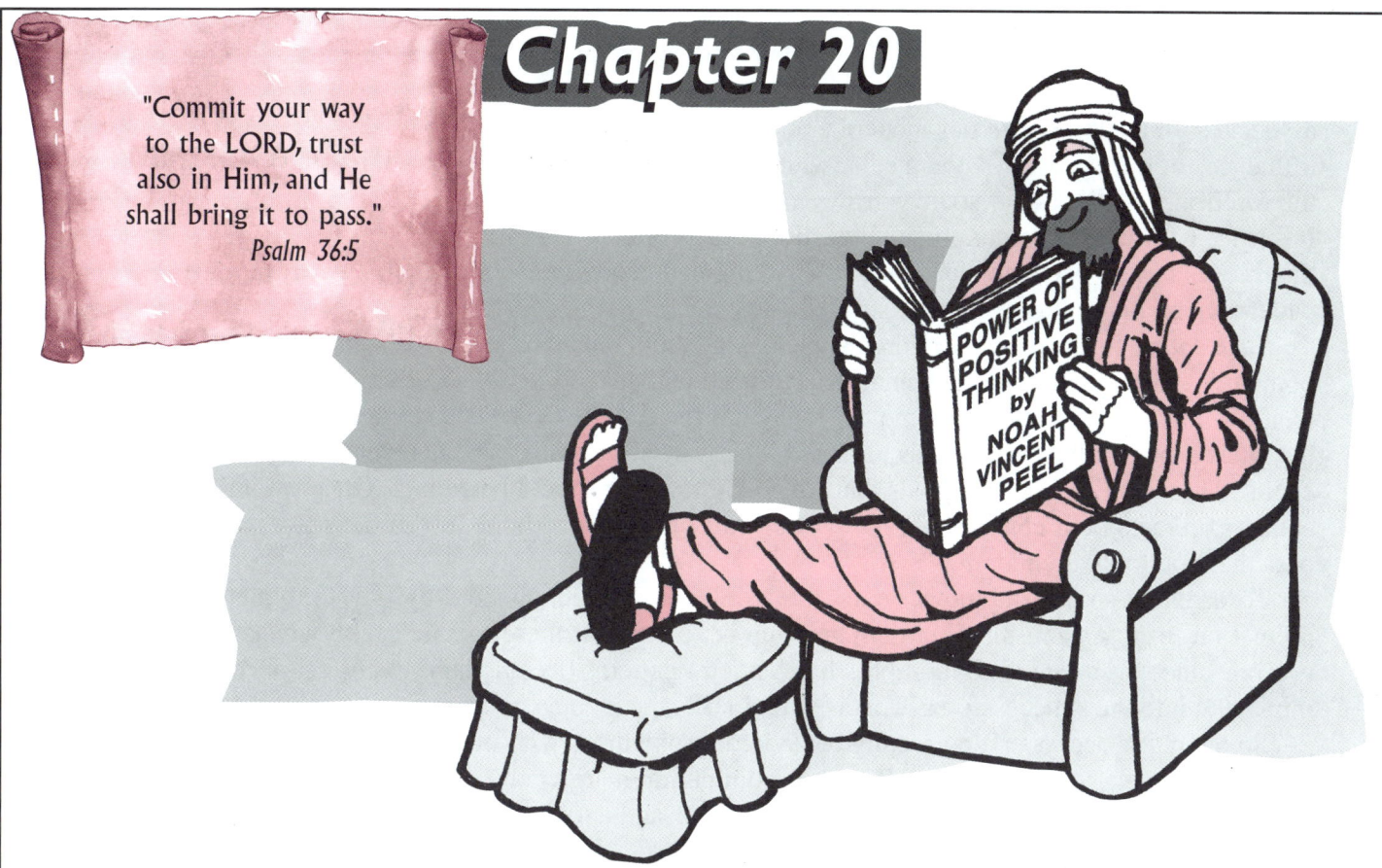

"Commit your way to the LORD, trust also in Him, and He shall bring it to pass."
Psalm 36:5

Chapter 20

Self Control Through Behavior Modification.

If You Truly Want To Move Forward - Then You Must Stop Repeating Yesterday.

For a good many years, diet counselors saw losing weight as simply a matter of calories: *eat less and burn more*. Consequently, many dieters armed themselves with calorie charts and workout clothes as they set out to win the battle of the bulge. While this is undeniably the dynamics behind all sound weight loss programs, we now know that there are many *behavioral* factors that also must be changed in order for a weight loss program to be successful over the long term. In fact, for many people, behavioral modification often means the difference between success and failure in their health building program.

The good news is that behavioral changes can be made rather quickly and once adopted should last a lifetime. In this chapter we will examine some areas of behavior that may be contributing to your weight problems as well as offer some suggestions on how you can change them.

HOW BEHAVIORAL PATTERNS GET STARTED

Every one of us has a template of behavioral patterns that make us exclusively us. We begin learning these patterns as very young children from our parents and other family members. School and teachers continue the imprinting process. So do friends and associates. Interestingly, in our modern era, one of the biggest influences of our behavior is the media, with television of course, at the forefront. Sadly, as our society grows more immoral, this media influence has become predominantly negative. As a result, TV and the movies have played a major role in imprinting bad behavioral patterns upon our culture.

> **What to do when you make a mistake:**
> **(1)** Admit it.
> **(2)** Learn from it.
> **(3)** Try not to repeat it.

Take eating for instance. Children's television continuously bombards our young ones with commercials for all manner of ungodly, processed foods. What mother today has the resolve to withstand the pleas of her children for the latest sugar coated junk cereals, or snacks, or sweets? The message is repeated over and over again. These are the kinds of foods that American families should be eating. Once we inflict these eating patterns on our children, they will often carry them through the rest of their lives and in turn, pass them on to their children.

Teenage TV shows and movies extol the "coolness" of alcohol and drugs – (not to mention premarital sex). As a result, our youth grow up believing that these satanic health wreckers are an okay lifestyle since everyone is doing it. Such behavioral patterns become hard to correct once they are implanted into the subconscious. This is what makes the media so dangerous.

So the real place to start correcting behavioral problems is with our children. As a morally concerned parent, you need to monitor what your children are viewing. You need to explain to them at a young age the importance of eating nutritious foods and avoiding health-wrecking behavioral patterns such as alcohol and drugs.

Furthermore, you need to set an example for them by your own lifestyle and behavioral patterns. Become a disciple of the Moses school of health as presented in this book and then pass it on to your children. Counter the anti-Christian, anti-health philosophy that is being drummed incessantly into the heads of our young people. Make the pursuit of health a family project. Exercise with your children. Study health and nutrition with your children. Let them participate in meal preparation. Teach them respect for their bodies at a young age. Here's some examples of the way Moses put it to the Israelites as they prepared to enter the Promised Land.

> *"Take heed to yourself, and diligently keep yourself, lest you forget the things your eyes have seen, and lest they depart from your heart all the days of your life. <u>And teach them to your children and your grandchildren</u>."* **(Deuteronomy 4:9)**

> *"And (Moses) said to them, 'Set your hearts on all the words which I testify among you today, <u>which you shall command your children to be careful to observe</u> – all the words of this law.'"* **(Deuteronomy 32:46)**

As a matter of fact, Moses warns the Israelites over and over again in the Book of Deuteronomy to follow God's laws and then to teach them to their children and to their grandchildren. This message is so powerful in Deuteronomy that I strongly recommend that you read this book with your whole family.

IDENTIFYING AND CORRECTING COUNTERPRODUCTIVE DIETING BEHAVIORAL PATTERNS

People who are overweight tend to have many counterproductive dieting behavioral patterns. Therefore, it is well worth your while to study these behavioral pattern weaknesses and correct all those that may be holding you back. You must learn all that you can about yourself. What are your behavioral patterns? Why do you do what you do? Who is the real you underneath the person you show to the world? What are your strengths and what are your weaknesses? You will never be able to change behavioral patterns until you become brutally honest with yourself. You must be able to acknowledge both your good qualities and your bad qualities. Only then can you set about the business of strengthening your character.

Now here's the best part. Modern psychologists have discovered a sure-fire technique for correcting a counterproductive behavioral pattern. It has nothing to do with willpower or guilt or rigid restrictions or unrealistic expectations. Instead, you simply replace the bad pattern with a good one. It's that easy! And it works every time.

Below are some of the most common counterproductive dieting behavioral patters along with suggestions on how to overcome them.

(1) SKIPPING BREAKFAST OR EATING SOMETHING QUICK AND NON-NUTRITIOUS FOR BREAKFAST.

Breakfast is arguably the most important meal of the day. You should never skip breakfast or just eat whatever happens to be convenient – like a cup of coffee and a donut. Instead, take the time to plan out a whole week's worth of nutritious breakfasts ahead of time. Make a game out of it. See how many biblically based, delicious variations you can come up with. (See **Appendix F** for healthy breakfast suggestions.) Tell yourself that rather than making breakfast your poorest meal of the day, you are going to make it your best meal. Now go out and do it.

(2) WATCHING HOUR AFTER HOUR OF TV AT NIGHT.

Many people feel that a hard day at work entitles them to an evening of complete passive entertainment in front of the television set. The TV goes on the minute they come home and never goes off until bedtime. This is a very counterproductive behavioral pattern not only for dieters but also for anyone seeking to live a productive life. Television is an absolute time waster and it will chip away your life from right underneath you. You must not fall prey to the night-after-night television addiction.

What a perfect time for you to substitute an exercise program. Why not form a walking club with some friends and take an invigorating walk every evening. Make your walk even better. Pick a biblical topic to discuss each evening. You get two blessings for the price of one.

(3) SLEEPING LATE ON WEEKENDS.

Sleeping too much ranks right up there with television watching as a major time waster. Here again many people feel that they are entitled to sleep in for as long as they like on the weekends. While an extra hour of weekend sleep won't hurt you, you must guard against the temptation to lie in bed until 9, 10 or 11 o'clock. For those people who struggle to find time to exercise, weekends are a great time to pursue your exercise program.

Here's another great way to conquer weekend sleeping. Instead of indulging your self-centered desire to sleep, get up and do a good deed for someone. Remember, it's the 10th commandment of our TEN COMMANDMENTS OF HEALTH. Join a volunteer organization. Visit a nursing home. Go grocery shopping for a shut-in.

(4) ERRATIC EATING HABITS.

Perhaps one of the worst behavioral patterns of overweight people is their tendency to have erratic eating habits. This means eating as much as they like of whatever they like whenever they feel like it. In other words, they have no order or plan or purpose to their dietary habits.

The best way to overcome this counterproductive behavior obviously is to set up a dietary plan for your life such as the **Moses Diet & Health Program**. Set a design to your eating habits. Try to never eat randomly without some forethought of what you are consuming. Write out and follow meal plans such as those contained in **Appendix F**. Strive to eat a variety of Bible foods each and every day. Turn eating properly into a passion. Read and study all you can on health and nutrition. Join clubs of like-minded people.

(5) POOR GROCERY SHOPPING HABITS.

Good eating habits must begin at the grocery store. Never take grocery shopping lightly. Always make a list and become a fervent label reader. Try to avoid junk foods, processed foods and foods with chemical additives. It won't be easy. Buy fresh fruits and vegetables, whole grain breads and cereals, nuts and honey. Avoid impulse shopping. Buy only foods that are life building (vitropic). Think carefully about every purchase. Don't be afraid to try new foods. Visit your local health food store. You will find many more options there that are not available in the supermarket.

(6) ASSOCIATING WITH TOXIC (NEGATIVE) PEOPLE.

They say you are judged by the company you keep and that's probably true. But you can definitely be *influenced* by the company you keep. The Bible stresses this point over and over again as God repeatedly warns the Israelites not to associate with or take on the way of the heathens. (i.e. **Deuteronomy 18:9**) He makes it quite clear that these toxic nations had the ability to totally corrupt His people and pull them away from His law. The only way for Israel to stay holy was through disassociation from these pagan nations.

This is good advice even for us today. Unfortunately, in this current age of physical and moral free fall, there's no shortage of people who can and will sabotage any efforts you make at self-improvement. If your circle of friends is made up of people who are wishy-washy in their faith, out of shape, overweight, and non-goal directed, then you are going to have a difficult time of bettering your life. I am not suggesting here that you become an elitist snob, feeling that you are better than others. But I am suggesting that you need to start cultivating friendships with positive, moral people who are in charge of their lives and who can motivate and inspire you to change your life. Athletes have long known that if they want to get really good at their sport they need to be around other athletes who excel at the sport. Learn from this. Pick your friends and associates carefully. *One motivating, supportive person is worth more than 100 toxic friends*.

(7) USING FOOD FOR PSYCHOLOGICAL THERAPY.

It's no secret that eating offers a temporary therapeutic effect during times of stress and depression. Financial problems, work problems, family problems, marital problems, death of a loved one and so forth can all trigger bouts of uncontrollable eating. For many people, food serves as the perfect "drug" during these low periods. The compulsion to eat is both *physical* and *psychological* making it very difficult to resist. It is physical since the pleasure of eating helps take our minds off of our problems. It is psychological since certain foods increase the levels of the neurotransmitter serotonin in the brain which then produces a calming effect similar to an anti-depressant drug.

This is a very difficult behavioral pattern for many people to break but with a touch of ingenuity it is possible. Exercise makes a perfect replacer for stress related eating. Not only does it give you something positive to do besides eating, it also, like food, releases special calming chemicals to the brain called **endorphins**. These endorphins are naturally produced by the body and will work safer and better than any drug you can take. Thus you get a twofold benefit from exercising. It helps you overcome your urge to eat (and thus gain weight) and it also helps improve the health of your body.

Understand too that Satan knows that you are at a point of weakness and he will move in for an attack. Therefore, another excellent way to overcome the urge to eat during periods of stress is to turn to prayer and scripture reading. Keep a notebook of your favorite prayers (see Appendix D) and always keep your Bible handy. Before reaching for food, reach for your Bible. Tell yourself that you are going to feast on divine food rather than physical food.

"Man shall not live by bread alone, but by every word that proceeds from the mouth of God." **(Matthew 4:4)**

"I am the living bread which came down from heaven. If anyone eats of this bread, he will live forever; and the bread that I shall give is My flesh, which I shall give for the life of the world." **(John 6:51)**

(8) BINGE EATING.

Here is one of the biggest trouble spots for many dieters. Bingeing is one of the most difficult areas for dieters to deal with and it has been the ruination of many well-intentioned health programs. If you are a binge eater you have two clear choices. Either you take steps to control it or you let it wipe you out and become its slave.

There are several causes of binge eating including stress (discussed previously), crash dieting rebound and unrealistic dietary restrictions. Crash dieting by its very nature sets you up for a future binge. Bingeing simply becomes your body's protective mechanism to prevent any future caloric depravation. Virtually every crash diet will lead to a binge. Therefore, to avoid this type of binge, simply avoid crash dieting. It's that simple.

Other people turn to bingeing as a result of severe dietary restrictions. They feel that the best way to make up for years of overindulgence is to totally deny themselves all of the fattening foods they love. Hence, with an all-or-nothing resolve, they vow *never* to eat such-and-such food again. Since it is impossible to abstain completely from foods they have enjoyed for a lifetime, they inevitably crack and eat the forbidden food. This usually gives way to a binge that then leads to another binge that then leads to guilt, low self-esteem and another failed diet.

The best way to break free of this demon is to never say never when trying to change your eating patterns. Total abstinence from your favorite foods will never work. Instead, you must learn to gradually wean yourself off of fattening and mytropic foods. Allow yourself occasional indulgence of your past favorites but be careful not to overdo it. The more you come to understand God's principles of nutrition, the more resolve you will build up to stay away from bad food choices.

Furthermore, if you do give in to a binge, you need to have a game plan to recover from it immediately so as not to derail your health building program. Here is a foolproof binge recovery strategy:

    a. Anticipate that there is always the potential to binge but that you will never be defeated by a binge because you now have a plan to combat it.
    b. If you should give in to a binge desire, you absolutely must take the time to re-read this plan after the binge.
    c. Your initial reaction is always going to be to quit everything in disgust. This is a normal reaction so anticipate it. However, you are now in the critical zone. What action you take immediately after a binge will either make or break your dietary aspirations. Here's the reality of the situation. You have only two choices. You can either let the binge get the

better of you and admit defeat or you can put it behind you as quickly as possible and press forward. Here's a thought that can help. Isn't it highly probable that if you quit your diet after a binge, chances are good that you will go on another diet some time in the future? So why lose all that time? Rather than let weeks or months go by before starting again, simply put the binge behind you immediately and avoid months of lost time.

d. You must never dwell on this or other past failures. Satan would love for you to do this. However, the past is over the instant you cut it loose.

e. Always trust in your ability with God's help to be victorious.

(9) SNACKING ON JUNK FOODS.

One of the most common weaknesses of overweight people is the tendency to snack frequently on junk foods. Soda, chips, candy bars, cookies and other non-nutritious sweets are the snack foods of choice for too many Americans. Such foods provide little or no nutrition while usually packing a high calorie content. This is a guaranteed route to unwanted pounds.

This is an easy pattern to break with just a bit of forethought. Several of the Bible foods discussed in this book, such as fruits, seeds and nuts, make excellent between meal snacks. Just keep a plentiful supply of these nutritious Bible foods around to snack on.

If you just have to have something sweet, I've got some good news for you. There's now a great, whole food nutritional bar called the **Bible Bar**. This delicious bar is made from the seven foods described in Deuteronomy 8:8 and it makes an excellent and nutritious snack and appetite regulator. (To read more on the **Bible Bar** see page 107.)

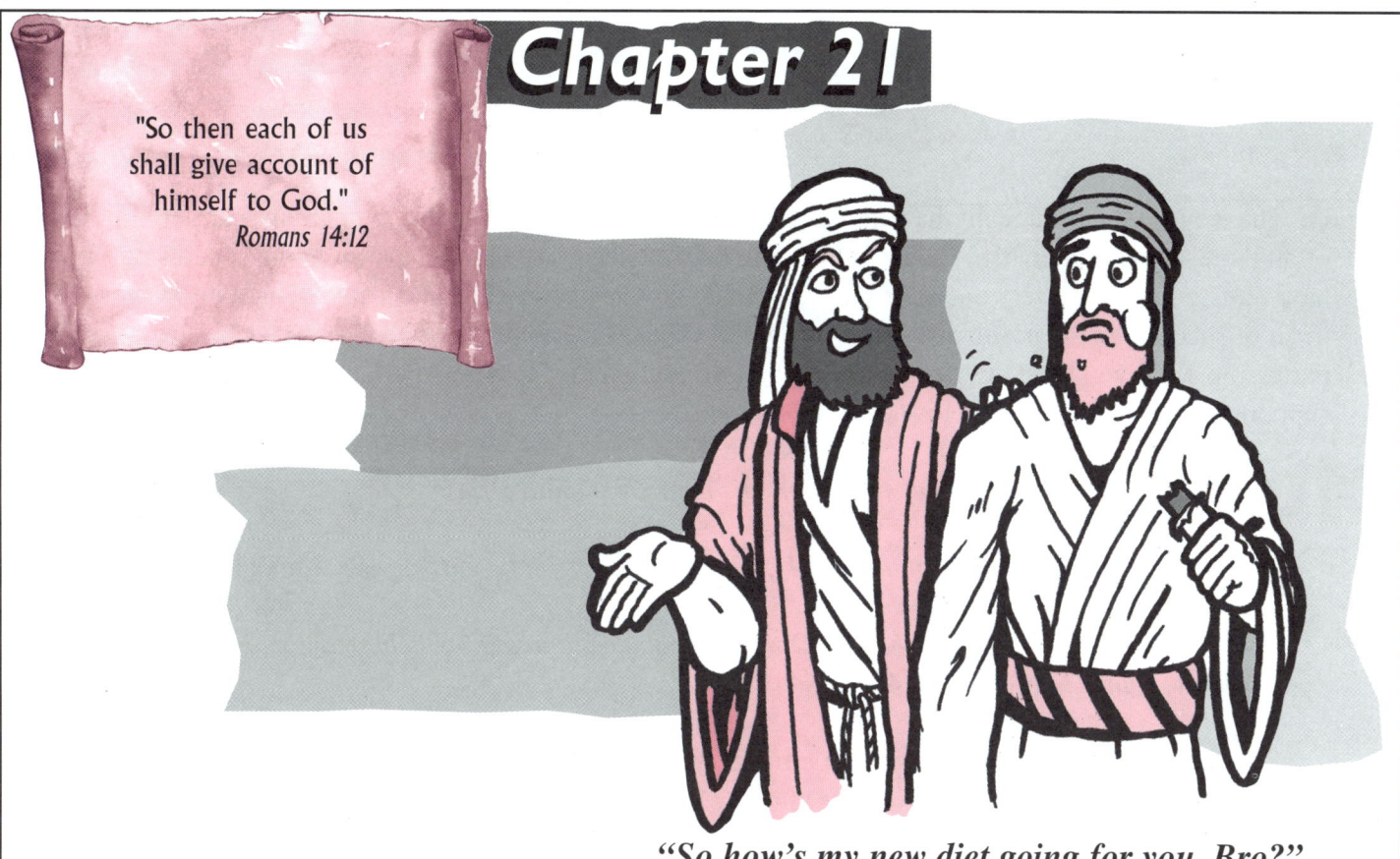

"So how's my new diet going for you, Bro?"

Without Accountability You're Doomed To Fail.

The Main Thing Is To Always Keep The Main Thing The Main Thing!

This is one of the most important chapters in the book for achieving success in your weight loss program. If you do not follow the suggestions offered over the next few pages, there is a good chance you will ultimately fail on the **Moses Diet & Health Program**. I want to talk to you now about the importance of *accountability*.

This book is about changing your life for the better. However, it is never easy to make major changes in our lives. Bad habits are extremely difficult to break even with the grandest intentions. Thankfully, counselors have now learned a few things about behavioral psychology. They now know for instance, that having an accountability partner is one of the greatest tools for successfully making lifestyle changes. For whatever the reason, having to answer to someone for what we do often prompts us to put forth our best efforts. Nowhere is this truer than when following a health building and weight loss program. Just knowing that there is someone else we have to account to for our actions is usually enough to keep us moving forward even through the most difficult times. However, finding the right accountability partner is the hard part.

THREE CHOICES WHEN LOOKING FOR AN ACCOUNTABILITY PARTNER

The way I see it, you really have three choices when looking for your accountability partner. First of all there's God. Of course, He shouldn't even be a choice – He should be a foregone conclusion. I have stressed from the very outset of this book that you must bring God into your life in a big way in order to succeed at any health and fitness program. Therefore, no matter who else you decide to partner up with, you must always make God part of your team. Remember – He is always there to support you and He wants you to succeed.

"Give thanks to the LORD! Call upon His name." **(Psalm 105:1)**

"Our help is in the name of the LORD, who made heaven and earth." **(Psalm 124:8)**

"I am poor and needy; yet the LORD thinks upon me. You are my help and my deliverer; do not delay, O my God." **(Psalm 40:17)**

Yes the LORD truly is your help and deliverer, your strength and your salvation. Do not be afraid to lay your burdens upon Him. Do not be afraid to be honest with Him every single day as you progress through your program. He knows your strengths and your weaknesses better than you do. After all – He made you. He knows when you are sincerely trying to improve and His grace will be sufficient for you. Plan on spending some quiet time every evening with the LORD when you will review your successes and your setbacks. Tell Him you need His help. Ask Him to guide you through each day. There is no other accountability partner on earth who is there the minute you call. But God is always there. Day and night – 24/7/365 – He is there for you. So don't shortchange yourself of such a great resource. Make God your number one accountability partner.

Your second option for an accountability partner is to find a family member or a good friend who shares your hopes and your dreams to improve yourself and is willing to help you through the rough spots. Above all, this person needs to be a good listener. Sometimes just being able to say what's on your mind to someone else is all you'll need for encouragement. It is important that this partner be totally supportive and encouraging rather than judgmental. The last thing you need on a health-changing program is a drill sergeant who's got something negative or condemning to say every time you review your progress. Your accountability partner needs to be someone who knows you well and really loves and cares about you. A newfound friend or a casual acquaintance may not be the best choice.

It is also important that your partner share your belief and faith in God. While they don't necessarily have to be the same denomination as you, they must at least be a moral person who truly loves the LORD.

Now if you can find a friend who also wants to follow this health-building program with you, then that would be the most ideal situation. You would be each other's accountability partners, working together to progress towards your goals. You would also have a built in exercise partner – someone to meet you at the health club or join you for your daily walks. Find that person and you have struck gold.

Unfortunately, as I said earlier, it's not always easy to find the right accountability partner and so that brings us to our third option. Become your own accountability partner. By this I mean that you have to devise a system of accountability procedures whereby you can keep track of your daily progress and effectively answer to yourself. Such a practice is going to be well worth your efforts.

Some recent studies have shown quite impressively that dieters who set up a system of daily accountability tend to be much more successful with their weight loss than those who do not. Fortunately, there are some good ways to set up such a system of checks and balances and I would like to share them with you now. (By the way, even if you find your perfect accountability partner, I strongly recommend that you also set up a personal accountability system similar to what I'm about to recommend.)

Seven Steps To Personal Accountability

(1) Pick The Right Time And The Right Place.

The first and foremost requirement for any personal accountability program to work is for you to set aside a block of time at the end of each day to record and examine your daily efforts. This should only take about 15 or 20 minutes but they will be the most important minutes of your program. Pick a quiet spot where you will not be disturbed and where you can set your notes and charts out in front of you. A kitchen table or an office desk would be ideal. You will soon see that spending this quiet reflective time with yourself is essential for your success. Once you pick your time and place, try to stay consistent with them each day. Remember – your body works best when it is on a set schedule. This is also true for your personal accountability sessions.

Here's a very important point. If for any reason you should miss a day's session, do not at any cost miss the next day. I assure you that once you start skipping days here and there, you will soon give up entirely on these important daily accountability periods.

And one last point before moving on. Personal accountability should be for a lifetime. Don't feel that once you reach your goal weight you can forego this important principle.

(2) Set Up A Three-Ring Binder Accountability Notebook.

As part of your accountability program, you will be recording, tabulating and reviewing several different information charts. In addition, you will need a place to keep your goal sheet, commitment agreement and daily prayers. Therefore, it's a good idea to purchase a three-ring binder notebook at your local office supply store and keep all of your important paperwork in it. You should also purchase colored tabulated page inserts so that you can organize your various materials. Storage pockets on the inside covers of the notebook are also a good idea since they will make a great place for you to keep inspirational stories, photos and miscellaneous materials.

Type or carefully hand write a distinctive title card insert for your notebook. Give it an impressive sounding title like ***Moses Accountability Book***, or ***Mary Smith's Official Daily Progress Journal***. Then, since it will be a very personal record of your life, keep it in a place where only you have access to it. Make this your lifetime partner and no matter whether you move, go on vacation, get married or go off to college, be sure your personal journal always goes with you.

(3) Keep A Personal Progress Journal/Diary.

Keeping a Personal Progress Journal (PPJ) is not quite the same thing as keeping a personal diary of your daily life. I know that some of you are probably already keeping a daily life diary so for you, the PPJ will be an easy thing to do. Your PPJ is a specific diary in which you are going to record each day how you are doing on the **Moses Diet & Health Program**. Write in your entries as if you were writing to a friend but review them as if a friend had sent them to you. Here's an example.

> *Woke up at 6:30, a little bit slow going but once I was up, my motivation came quickly. I rode the exercise bike for twenty minutes and it felt great. Said my morning prayers while riding the bike. Ate a nutritious breakfast according to my menu plan and read three chapters from Book of Matthew while eating. Headed out for work highly driven and motivated. Feeling great and in control of my day.*
>
> *Good day at work. Ate healthy snacks on my breaks. Ate my specially prepared lunch at the office while the rest of the staff went out to a restaurant. I almost gave in and went along but I stopped just long enough to debate my inner voice. I won and felt very much in control of my life. Lunch was good and it gave me a chance to read some more Bible.*
>
> *Felt very tired by mid-afternoon. Recalled the Moses Book commandment about daily sunshine so I took a nice five-minute walk outside the office complex. Tried to concentrate on the feel of the beautiful sunshine on my skin and breathing the fresh, cool air. The walk perked me up.*
>
> *Went to the health club after work and had a good workout. I felt all of the movements working well and I kept picturing in my mind how I want to look by September.*
>
> *Home by six o'clock and had dinner with the rest of the family. So nice to have everyone in the house now willing to eat according to biblical principles.*
>
> *Went grocery shopping for Aunt Marge after dinner. Had a chance to visit with her a few minutes after dropping everything off.*
>
> *All-in-all, a very good day on my program.*

I also suggest that once a week you re-read the previous week's entries. Remember to read them as if you were checking them for a friend. This will help you see the bigger picture of how you are doing. It will tell you where you are strong and where you are weak, where things are just right and where they need more work. Re-kindle your motivation for the next week and vow to do even better.

(4) Read Your Signed Commitment Agreement.

Appendix C contains a sample Commitment Agreement. You may either use the one I give you or write your own. Add the signed Commitment Agreement to your three-ring binder and read it every day. It will rekindle your motivation and keep you focused.

(5) Read Your Goals List.

In Chapter 4 I spoke to you about the importance of writing down your goals. If you haven't done this yet, take a few minutes to do it now. Make a copy of the Goals form in Appendix C and fill it out. Then add it to your three-ring binder. Read this list slowly and deliberately every day. Reflect on each of your goals and whether you are making progress or not in reaching them.

(6) Update Your Daily Review Sheet.

Also in Appendix C you will find the Daily Review Sheet form. Make a copy of this each month and add it to your binder. This will serve as a written reminder and checklist for you to keep track of your daily duties on the ***Moses Diet & Health Program***. I have listed the essentials of the program for you on the form and I have left several columns blank so that you may add whatever else you feel is important for you to keep track of. Appendix C will also show you how to keep a monthly score of your Daily Review Sheet. It is well worth keeping this score since it will show you how you are doing from month to month. Try to compete against yourself by beating your previous month's score.

(7) Read "On Choices" Once A Month.

Appendix E contains an excellent motivational piece called "On Choices" that you should read at the start of each month. Make a copy of "On Choices" and add it to your notebook. And don't forget to read it once a month.

SHOULD YOU KEEP A FOOD DIARY?

Many of the popular diet books recommend that you keep a daily log of the various foods you are consuming. Is this a good idea? Will it help you be more successful on the program? Well there are pros and cons to keeping a daily food diary. On the plus side, a food diary will help you keep track of what you are eating, when you are eating, the amount of calories, fats, protein and carbohydrates you are consuming and where you need to make changes. On the negative side, keeping an accurate food diary requires a lot of work and patience. Either you will need to take the diary with you wherever you go or you will need to record everything in a small notebook and then transfer the data into your diary later. This soon becomes very tedious and boring and most people quit after just a few weeks or less.

Personally, I do not recommend keeping a food diary except perhaps for a very brief time to help you spot problem areas. However, it is totally optional and if you feel that keeping such a diary will help you reach your goals, then by all means go ahead and keep one.

Temple Builders

I know that no matter how hard some of you try to find an acceptable accountability partner, you are going to come up short. That's why there is still one more accountability option I want to bring to your attention. It's a dieter's support group that I have recently founded called ***Temple Builders***. Temple Builders is a weight loss membership club established upon the biblical principles contained in the book ***Moses Wasn't Fat***. My goal is to make Temple Builders your accountability partner in health, prayer and faith.

> *"For where two or three are gathered together in My name, I am there in the midst of them."*
> **(Matthew 18:20)**

And I know further that a good accountability partner as well as a good support group can mean the difference between success and failure in your health building program. As a matter of fact, one study recently showed that dieters who attended weight loss group meetings every week lost nearly twice as much weight as those people who tried to do it on their own. That's why I started Temple Builders. My greatest joy is to help you reach your goals. When you join, you become part of a network of believers who, like yourself, are all working towards physical and spiritual improvement. Just take a look at the great benefits you'll enjoy as a member.

(1) Progress Monitoring. All Temple Builders are eligible for weekly monitoring of their progress by our expert staff of diet counselors. This is done by way of your own private Temple Builder Internet access code. All you have to do is fill in the appropriate weekly dieter's analysis profile on line and then E-mail it to us. Your data will be reviewed by one of our counselors who will return a progress evaluation report to you by E-mail. This great service enables you to have a partner/counselor follow you, advise you, encourage you and give you emotional support throughout your program. This service alone may be all you need to keep going when you otherwise may have given up.

(2) Goal Recognition. There's nothing more encouraging than to receive some form of recognition for your diligent shapeup efforts. That's why all Temple Builders receive certificates of accomplishment as they progress through our three levels of achievement: *Quarrier, Crafter* and *Master Builder*. You'll feel a great sense of pride when you display these beautiful certificates in your home or office.

(3) Monthly Newsletter. Do you try to stay abreast of the latest dieting, nutrition, fitness and health news? If so, then you know what a formidable and overwhelming task that can be. So much research is being done in these areas that it is nearly impossible for the average person to stay current. That's why we publish *The Disciple* every month for all Temple Builder members. You'd have to subscribe to numerous magazines and newsletters and spend hours searching the Internet just to collect the same news you get in each issue of *The Disciple*.

(4) E-mail Updates. In addition to receiving *The Disciple* newsletter every month at your home or office, you'll also receive E-mail updates of all important breaking stories or research that we feel you should know about immediately.

(5) Free Subscription To Temple Magazine. In addition to *The Disciple* newsletter, we also publish **Temple** magazine four times a year. This one-of-a-kind magazine begins where *The Disciple* leaves off. You'll get in depth stories on every aspect of health, dieting, fitness and spirituality that's important to you as a believer. This $19.95 value comes free with your yearly membership to Temple Builders.

(6) 15% Discount On All Logia Products. Here's good news for all of you that use **Logia** nutritional products in your health building program. As a member of Temple Builders, you get an automatic preferred customer discount on all of your Bible foods and supplements that you purchase directly from us. If you use these products regularly, this benefit alone will more than pay for your annual Temple Builder membership dues.

(7) Weekly Drawings For Free Logia Products. Every week five lucky Temple Builder members are each going to win $100 worth of **Logia** nutritional products absolutely free. All club members' names are automatically entered into each weekly drawing. The winner is notified immediately and all winners' names are listed in the subsequent issue of *The Disciple*.

(8) Free Entry In The Moses Transformation Challenge. Every member of Temple Builders is automatically eligible, should they wish, to compete in the Moses Transformation Challenge at no charge. ($20 value) The MTC allows you to compete for some fantastic prizes including an all-expenses-paid trip for two to the Holy Land.

(9) Temple Builder Private Chat Room And Discussion Groups. You never have to struggle through another diet program alone again. Here's a great chance for you to share ideas, tips and success stories with like-minded individuals.

The individual benefits of a Temple Builder membership could easily add up to well over $300 (and perhaps much more depending on the amount of **Logia** products you decide to purchase throughout the year at a 15% savings.) But the annual membership fee to be eligible for all of these great benefits is only $175. However, keep reading because I'm going to do even better than that for all of you who have finished reading *Moses Wasn't Fat*.

When you call or write us to enroll as a member and you say that you read this book, you will be given a special *Moses Wasn't Fat* reader membership price of just $150. But that's not all! We are also going to send you a box of 15 large size **Bible Bars** absolutely free of charge. This is an additional $30 value you're going to get just for reading this book. So be sure to mention it when you apply for your Temple Builder membership.

To enroll in this fantastic program, simply call **1-800-537-7671** with your credit card or send your $150 specially discounted membership fee to **Logia**: *Foods of the Bible*, 731 Kirkman Road, Orlando, FL 32811. Your membership package and free bars will be sent out to you within 48 hours or less.

Set Up Temple Builders Chapter At Your Church Or Organization

There is still one more method of accountability that I would like to recommend. You can start a local chapter of Temple Builders at your church or organization. This would give you and other members of your group a chance to work together locally on your health and fitness program. If you would like more information on how to set up a local chapter of Temple Builders, please call **1-800-537-7671**.

Chapter 22

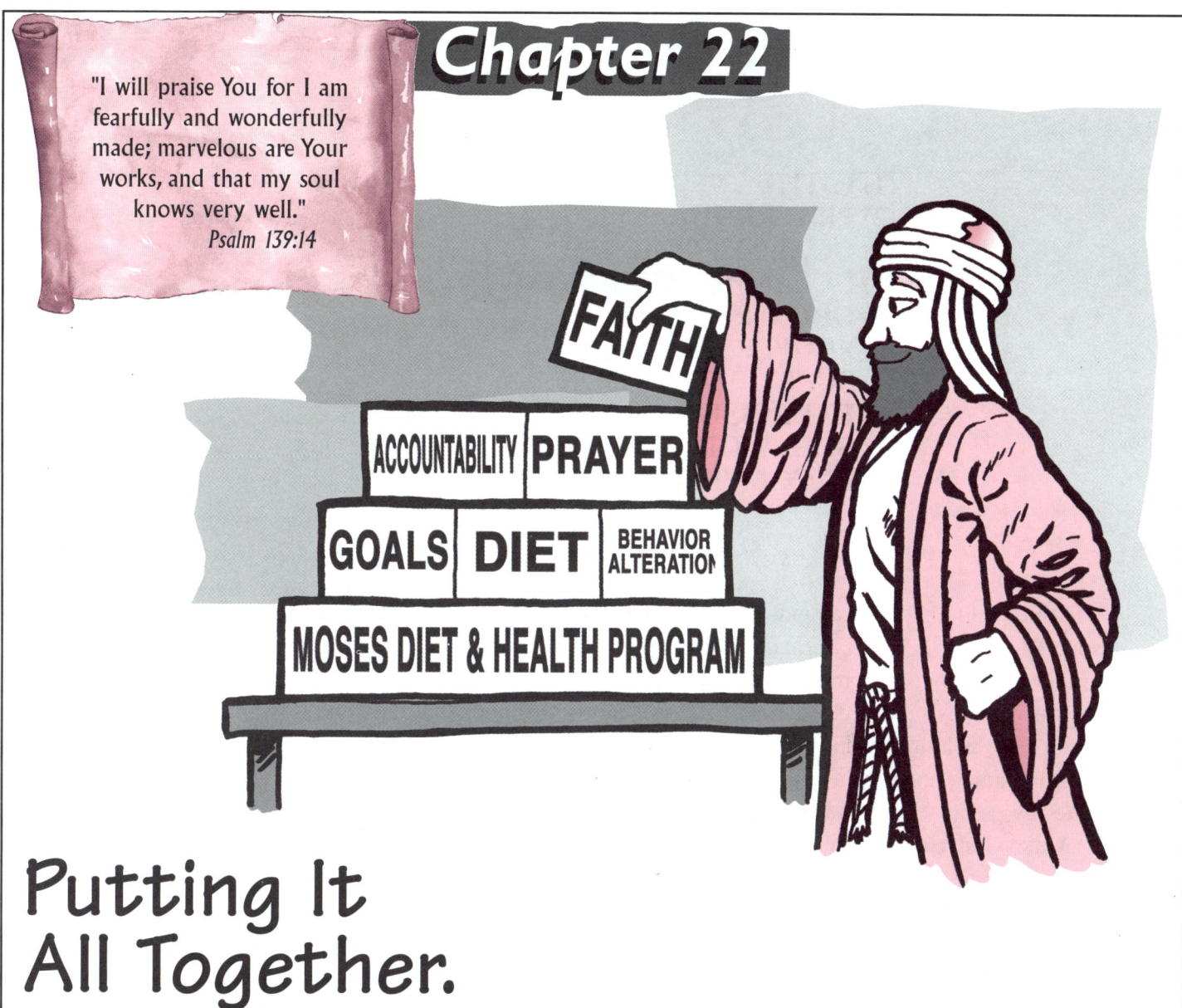

"I will praise You for I am fearfully and wonderfully made; marvelous are Your works, and that my soul knows very well."
Psalm 139:14

Putting It All Together.

Do Things Right Over And Over Again And You Absolutely Must Succeed.

Well here we are at the end of our journey together. Moses and I have taken you to the border of the Promised Land, now it's up to you to cross over the Jordan and begin your new life. I've shared over 30 years of learning with you in this book. I hope it's been helpful to you. I believe that every one of us carries the genetics of God within ourselves. This means that we all have the capability for true greatness. I pray that you will use the guidelines I have given you and begin immediately to build your body into the holy and beautiful Temple that your Heavenly Father designed it to be.

I'd like to take this last chapter to summarize all of the key points of the **Moses Diet & Health Program** putting them together into a handy reference outline form that you can refer to again and again.

153

THE TEN BUILDING BLOCKS OF THE MOSES DIET & HEALTH PROGRAM

    (1) **FAITH**
    (2) **PRAYER**
    (3) **GOAL SETTING**
    (4) **CLEANSING/PURIFYING**
    (5) **ORGANIZATION**
    (6) **PROPER EATING**
    (7) **SUPPLEMENTATION**
    (8) **EXERCISE**
    (9) **BEHAVIOR MODIFICATION**
(10) **ACCOUNTABILITY**

1. FAITH

There are all kinds of diet and weight loss books on the market and many contain good advice. But despite all of their helpful information, something very important has been missing from all of them. This should be obvious from the high failure rate they all have in common.

It has been my main premise right from the start of this book that faith and trust in God must be the anchor of any health, diet and wellness program. Without a burning love and faith and trust in your Heavenly Father, none of the other building blocks of this, or any other program really matter. Here are the key points to always keep in mind as you progress through the program.

- **Make God Your Personal Trainer.** No one wants you to succeed more on your health and wellness program than God Himself. You are made in His image and never forget that. Don't be hesitant to call on him for guidance, consolation and encouragement whenever they are needed. He's the only personal trainer who is at your beck and call 24 hours a day. Use this great resource for success.
- **Never Doubt God Or Yourself.** When you place all of your trust in the Lord, He goes to work instantly changing your heart. But when you have doubts, or try to do it your own way, then you surround yourself with a negative energy field that repels the Holy Spirit making it difficult for God to help you. As you begin this program, cast all of your cares upon the Lord and ask Him to guide you to success. His help is abundant. His help is always free.
- **God Wants You To Be Healthy.** Disease, sickness and eating disorders are not from God. They are from Satan who works both day and night to tear down and destroy our body Temples. God on the other hand, never intended for us to suffer. He granted Moses 120 healthy years of life and He wants to bless us with a healthy, long life. His greatest joy is for us to find peace and for His will to be completed in our lives. However, He will not do all of the work. You must meet Him halfway.

2. PRAYER

Along with your faith in God, you will need to develop a strong prayer life, if you haven't already. Many people take prayer too casually, thinking that an occasional "Lord's Prayer" or a quick formulaic prayer at the end of the day suffices. Prayer is an essential part of the *Moses Diet & Health Program*. It will be through your prayers that you will open up the entry point for God's instruction and guidance in your life. Never neglect to pray!

- **Integrate Prayer Into Your Daily Life.** The Lord loves nothing better than when we acknowledge our love for Him. Therefore, get in the habit of praying to Him morning, noon and night. In addition, try not to let a single hour of the day pass without telling Him at least once that you love Him. If you have a watch with an hour beeper, say a quick prayer every time you hear it. If you work with a computer every day set it to sound on the hour, and once again, use that as a reminder to say a quick prayer. I have given you several prayers in this book. **(See Appendix D)**
- **Write Your Own Prayers.** God loves nothing better than when you speak to Him honestly and directly from your heart. I suggest you take time occasionally to sit and write some of your own prayers. This is one of the greatest gifts you can ever give to the Lord. David composed many beautiful Psalms and the Lord called him His beloved.
- **Pray Diligently In Your Moments Of Weakness.** No matter how motivated and dedicated you are on this program, there are going to come times of weakness and temptation. Perhaps to miss a workout, or to eat something unhealthy, or even to quit all together. These are the times you need to pray with all your heart for God to give you strength.
- **Pray After A Setback.** I talked at length in this book about setbacks. They are inevitable and they are part of all success journeys. I am warning you ahead of time. Satan is going to try and tempt you to give up after a setback. This is his time of strength and your time of weakness. You may be so upset after a setback that the last thing you want to do is pray. You may feel like you let God down and that now it's too late to pray. This is totally wrong and it is Satan reasoning with your subconscious mind to try and pull you completely away from God. As a matter of fact, it is after a setback that you need prayer the most. So whatever you do, don't break the link with God just because you're an imperfect human being.

3. GOAL SETTING

Without definite written goals and a plan of action, you are dooming yourself to failure. No great accomplishments in life just happen by accident. The one thing all successful people have in common is a written goals sheet and a plan of action for achieving them.

- **Always Know The Reason Why.** Before beginning any difficult undertaking, it is imperative that you have a clear vision of what you want to accomplish and more importantly, the reasons why. Never begin a health and wellness program to make someone else happy. This will not work. I'd like to think that this book has given you plenty of reasons why you should begin the *Moses Diet & Health Program*.
- **Set Realistic Goals.** Your subconscious mind plays a big part in reaching your goals. It doesn't matter how thorough you are in writing out your goals, if they are unrealistic, your subconscious mind will automatically know that they are unachievable and fight you every step of the way. Consistent achievement of realistic, beneficial goals will be one of the greatest motivators you will ever have.
- **Goals Must Have Deadlines.** Goals without deadlines are simply dreams. A goal doesn't become real until you put a target completion date to it. Deadlines create urgency and urgency gets things done.
- **Goals Must Be Measurable.** How will you know if you are making headway if you have no way to keep track of your progress? By breaking a big goal down into smaller bite size pieces, and then progressing from one piece to the next, you will eventually reach your goal. Football teams love the dramatic 90 yard score play, but it's the smaller, consistent yardage plays that score the

most touchdowns. Learn to keep moving your goal ball forward yard by yard and before you know it, you will be in the end zone.
- **Plan Your Strategy.** Once you've listed your goals, don't just sit around waiting for things to happen. Set down a realistic game plan on how you will achieve your goals. I have given you many suggestions in this book on how to put together your winning strategy for a lifetime of health and happiness. Never try to just wing it.
- **Evaluate Your Progress.** You must constantly evaluate and reevaluate your progress or lack thereof. If you are moving forward, you need to be able to see it. If you are stuck or regressing, you need to know why. Don't become a slave to a rigid strategy. Plans and strategies are simply guidelines. Wisely adapt them and change them as necessary.
- **Take One Day At A Time.** Constantly looking at a big goal that's hard to achieve can be very daunting. Break big goals down into a series of smaller goals and then simply take one day at a time. Patience and the calendar will eventually get you to where you want to be.
- **Make It Fun.** Our bodies are programmed by God to seek pleasure and avoid pain. While we have the ability to forge ahead through unpleasant and painful experiences, it is highly unlikely that anyone can stick to a health and wellness program that is unpleasant or downright painful. Therefore, do all in your power to make your program fun.

4. CLEANSING/PURIFYING

God originally designed the human body for life and not death. It was only as a result of sin that entropy or breakdown entered our genetics. Fortunately, God left us with a powerful immune system to fight off disease. In addition, He also equipped our bodies with an amazing ability to cleanse and purify themselves from the various toxins and environmental poisons that are all around us. Nevertheless, long periods of indiscriminate living and/or subjection to external pollutants takes a toll on the body. Therefore, it is a good idea to observe a periodic cleansing and detoxification program.
- **Fast And Pray.** One of the best ways to cleanse and purify the body is through regular fasting and prayer. Fasting for three or four days every quarter is an excellent way to keep your body functioning at optimal levels. Abstinence from eating also gives your prayer life a chance to be more intense.
- **One Day Fasting.** Fasting should never become burdensome. Instead, you should learn to welcome a fast as a pleasant respite from a busy life. Some people enjoy following a one-day fast every week. This can either be a day of total abstinence from food, or a day when only juices are consumed. CAUTION: Never fast as a means of dieting or weight control.
- **Use Natural Herbal Detoxifiers.** God has given us many natural herbs that are highly beneficial as internal body cleansers. They should be used just before or during a fast to assist the body in removing the various toxins. **Logia** has developed an excellent Bible-based herbal cleansing product called *Thoroughly Cleansed* (see page 96). I recommend the use of this product for 14 days at the beginning of the **Moses Diet & Health Program**.
- **Go On A TV Fast.** You may never have thought of it this way, but a steady diet of television is also toxic to the mind. Therefore, to purify yourself from the media pollution of immorality and time wasting, go on regular fasts from TV. This will be rather difficult for some people in the beginning (harder in some cases than giving up eating), but with steady practice you should be able to go weeks at a time. Some might even want to follow a lifetime television fast.

5. ORGANIZATION

To succeed at this or any life-changing program, you need to get organized and stay on a schedule. Remember that God brought order out of chaos when He created the earth which was without form and void. God's system of order then is for everything to become progressively more organized. After all, isn't that what the six days of creation are all about? Therefore, the more organized your life is, the more Godlike you become.

• **Set Up A Daily Schedule.** It's amazing how many people have no order to their lives, simply living from hour-to-hour, day-to-day, week-to-week with no underlying structure to their lives. This is a guaranteed recipe for boredom and failure. What you need to do therefore, is to set up a fairly rigid daily schedule and do your best to stick to it. Our bodies function best when they are on a routine schedule.

• **Eat On A Schedule.** You will be much more successful on your diet program if you eat your meals on a regularly scheduled basis. Write the schedule down and try not to vary from it by more than a few minutes. Meals scheduled approximately three hours apart throughout the day will do wonders for your metabolism and weight loss program.

• **Schedule In Snack Time.** You must never let yourself get hungry since this is a sure way to sabotage your weight loss program. Therefore, when you set up your daily eating schedule make sure to include between-meal time for snacking.

• **Never Skip A Meal.** Anyone can lose weight by not eating. And skipping meals will definitely lead to *temporary* weight loss. But such deprivation comes with a sharp rebound effect. Excessive hunger usually leads to excessive eating. Far better is it for you to take action to control your hunger pangs with sensible snacking than to willpower your way into a crisis.

• **Try Overnight Fasting.** If you don't eat anything from six o'clock at night to six o'clock the next morning, you will effectively have fasted for a half day (12 hours). Do this henceforth and you will have fasted for half of your remaining life. Perhaps there's some ancient wisdom behind this idea which is why our first meal of the day is called *break-fast* (breakfast). Many successful dieters attribute this technique alone to their success. If this sounds a bit too severe, you may want to adapt it to no food after 7 PM. This technique really works and you should give it a try.

• **Don't Overlook The Importance Of Rest.** As you set up your schedule, be sure to schedule in a set time for sleep and rising. Once again, your body will operate at peak performance when you sleep and rise at the same times each day. And don't forget the Sabbath Day. It's so important to rest on the seventh day that God made it a commandment rather than a suggestion.

6. PROPER EATING

One of my main goals in writing this book has been to get you to change your eating habits. It is my contention that the more you eat according to the wisdom of the Bible, the healthier and holier you are going to be.

• **Eat Bible Foods.** The Book of Genesis is explicit when it tells us that every herb that bears seed and every tree that bears seed shall be for our food. According to this instruction then, all of the following food categories qualify as original Eden Bible food. Fruits, vegetables, legumes, beans, grains, nuts, seeds, sprouts, herbs, spices. Choose wholesome, natural unprocessed foods from these food categories as the main part of your diet.

• **Eat Meat Sparingly.** Even though God gave permission to man after the flood to eat meat, His original diet for us was 100 percent vegetarian. Therefore, to get as close to the original *perfect* human diet, you should eat little or no meat. In addition, the meat raising and meat packing industry is now engaging in practices that can cause serious illness. Once again then, the best way to avoid these health problems is to reduce, or even eliminate the use of meat. And besides, a diet composed of Bible foods is much more nutritious anyway.

• **Keep An Eye On Fiber Intake**. Be sure to keep your daily intake of dietary fiber high. Fortunately, this happens automatically when you eat lots of Bible foods. Caution: meat, dairy foods, refined cereals and breads, sugar, vegetable oils and eggs contain little or no fiber. You may want to insure that you are getting enough fiber by using a good natural fiber supplement.

• **It's Not A Diet. It's A Lifestyle.** This book is not about going on a diet. It is about creating a whole new lifestyle. Dieting is something you do temporarily – and usually unsuccessfully. This program is about changes you make for a lifetime – not to lose weight, but to live according to God's law. Regulation of bodyweight is simply a by-product of this biblically sound lifestyle.

• **Never Eliminate Or Drastically Reduce Any Food Category.** Beware of those popular diet programs that encourage you to reduce or eliminate carbohydrates, fats or proteins. Bible eating by its very nature will give you a balance of these nutrients. That should be a clue to us that God's diet for man was not exclusionary. A rule of thumb guideline for dietary balances of these foods is protein 25%, fat 25 % and carbohydrates 50%. But I caution you not to become a slave to ratios. Eat a variety of Bible foods and the ratios will basically take care of themselves.

• **Use Complex Carbohydrates.** Complex carbohydrates are God's perfect energy food. He designed our energy system to function optimally by burning complex carbohydrates. Eliminating or reducing carbohydrates forces the body to convert to fat and/or protein for energy, neither of which are the body's first choice. Wise selection of carbohydrates will actually facilitate weight loss. Include generous amounts of the following whole grains in your diet: wheat, barley, oats, rye, millet and buckwheat.

• **Use Olive Oil Regularly.** Olive oil seems to be God's number one choice of fatty acid for our bodies. Olive oil is the only mono-unsaturated oil and its health benefits are legend. It is particularly effective in combating and preventing cardiovascular disease. Be sure to use 100 percent extra virgin olive oil regularly, if not daily. In fact, a bit of olive oil at each meal may be the very best thing you could ever do for your health.

• **Don't Count Calories.** Develop calorie *awareness* rather than calorie *slavery*. For years, most dieters have put their primary emphasis on counting calories. Could this be the reason why 95 percent of diets fail? Counting calories is a burdensome, unnecessary chore. It's a far better idea to count portion size rather than calories. Studies have shown that people can actually *lose* weight on a higher calorie diet just by changing the types of food eaten, the amounts eaten at one time and the spacing time between meals.

• **Taper Your Food Intake As Your Day Progresses.** Get the majority of your calories earlier in the day, preferably at breakfast and lunch. This is when your body demands the most energy. Avoid large dinners late in the evening. Overeating at any meal is a guaranteed prescription for weight problems.

• **Never Allow Yourself To Get Hungry.** Hunger is the bane of dieters. It is difficult to concentrate on anything else when hunger pangs are gnawing at your stomach. And while you may have the willpower to fight them off for awhile, they always have the potential to lead to uncontrollable overeating. Better that you regulate your hunger by sensible snacking with things like **Bible Bars** and fruits and raw vegetables, than to prolong it into a diet-wrecking event.

- **Drink Copious Amounts Of Water.** Water is the very essence of God who is the Living Waters that comes down from Heaven. Every cell in your body is bathed in an ocean of water. And it is water that helps remove many toxins from the body. Therefore, drink generous amounts of water throughout the day. Just make sure it's not from the tap. Bottled spring water or purified water is best.
- **Foods To Avoid.** Here is a list of foods you should try to avoid, not only for weight control, but also for a healthy life and clean temple. White sugar, white flour, white rice, fried foods, tap water, sodas and colas, candy, foods with chemical additives, pork, processed luncheon meats, hot dogs. Here is a list of foods you should eat sparingly. Eggs, red meat, chicken, chips, ice cream, cake, cookies.
- **Leave Room For Occasional "Junk" Foods.** It would be ideal if you could just walk away from all of the foods you know are bad for you, but realistically this is difficult, if not impossible. So rather than say you will never eat a certain food again (and risk psychological meltdown when you inevitably do), schedule an occasional break day or break meal where you allow yourself a brief indiscretion. This will sure make life a whole lot easier. And you may be surprised some day that your cravings for those no-no foods actually disappear.

7. SUPPLEMENTATION

God certainly did not mention nutritional supplements in the Bible and in an ideal world there would never be a need for them. However, because of our farming indiscretions, overprocessing, long-term storage and bad cooking habits, our food is not as nutritious as God intended. Supplementation technology when practiced properly can do a lot to fill in the missing pieces. That's why I strongly urge you to consider using high quality supplements as part of the *Moses Diet & Health Program*.

- **Enzymes.** Very few people are aware of just how important digestive enzymes are to a health and nutrition program. Quite simply, without digestive enzymes there is no life. Even if your diet contains all of the nutrients you need but you are lacking enzymes, you are going to have problems. Therefore, I would like to recommend that you take one or two *Eden's Enzyme* capsules with each meal.
- **Meal Enhancers.** Eating a balanced meal is like putting together a picture puzzle. Each piece must fit properly in its place to make the whole picture. It's the same way with eating. Your body takes the various proteins (amino acids), fatty acids, carbohydrates, vitamins, minerals, co-factors and still undiscovered nutrients and puts them all together into a complete picture. If the foods you eat at a meal are lacking in certain nutrients, your body will have to work harder to finish the puzzle or worse yet, leave the puzzle unfinished. This is where a good meal enhancer comes in. A meal enhancer is a high nutrient liquid or powder that is consumed with a meal that makes sure your body has all the pieces of the puzzle – a nutrient insurer if you will. In addition, a good meal enhancer may actually be used as a meal replacer. There are several good meal enhancer supplements on the market but I would like to suggest *Back To The Garden* since I personally designed this product based on the foods of the Bible. It is all-natural with no artificial flavors or sweeteners.
- **Detoxifiers.** These food supplements have become extremely popular over the last 10 years. They are meant to assist the body in removing stored toxins and waste material. They are meant to be taken only for a short time (up to 14 days) rather than indefinitely. **Logia** has developed an excellent detoxifying formula using several Bible-based herbs and cleansers. It's called *Thoroughly Cleansed*.

• **Vitamins And Minerals.** While I prefer that you get your vitamins and minerals from your diet and from meal enhancer powders like **Back To The Garden**, there are some good multiple vitamin and mineral pill formulas on the market. Let me caution you, however, that it is very difficult to get sufficient quantities of *both* vitamins and minerals in one pill. Therefore, look for those products that put several individual pills in one packet. This should enable you to get the sufficient quantities you need, especially of the all-important minerals like calcium and magnesium.

I rarely, if ever, recommend that you take *individual* vitamins or minerals. This can throw off the balances in the body. Instead, strive to get your vitamins and minerals as part of the complete spectrum. And another thing, always take your vitamin/mineral supplement with a meal and never on an empty stomach. Your absorption rate will greatly increase and your chances of stomach distress greatly decrease.

8. EXERCISE

No weight control program or health building program will ever be successful without including regular exercise. Numerous studies have shown that exercise is one of the main factors in contributing to sustained weight loss.

• **Set Up An Exercise Schedule.** For exercise to work, it must become a regular part of your life. You must never be hit-or-miss about something so important. Therefore, you need to set up a specific exercise schedule that you commit yourself to following.

• **Never Miss A Workout.** Once you have established your routine, never miss a workout (other than for illness). The benefits of exercise are cumulative and this can only happen if you are consistent. Starting and stopping exercise programs is hardly better than not exercising at all. So once you begin, make it a lifetime commitment.

• **Blend Aerobic Training With Resistance Training.** Your body has two key areas that need and benefit from regular exercise: (1) cardiovascular-respiratory (CVR) system and (2) skeleto-muscular (SM) system. The CVR system benefits from rather long, non-stop training sessions (20-30 minutes) that elevate the pulse and breathing rate. This is called *aerobic* exercise and it has the ability to burn stored fat.

The SM system on the other hand, benefits from brief, full range movements with a weight resistance (barbell, dumbbell, machine). This type of training strengthens muscles and bones and does not elevate the pulse or breathing rate substantially. It contributes to weight loss indirectly by increasing the body's lean muscle mass. Lean muscle mass burns more calories than stored fat. Therefore, the more lean tissue, the more calories burned.

Both forms of exercise are beneficial for regulating the body's metabolic rate. Aim for a program of 3-5 days a week of both types of training. They can either be done together at the same workout or at different times of day.

• **Morning Aerobics Burns Fat.** The very best time to do your aerobic exercise for losing weight is first thing in the morning on an empty stomach. If you can arrange your schedule to do this regularly, your fat loss will be dramatic.

• **Keep An Exercise Log.** It's a good idea to keep a log of your various exercises, dates, length of workout, amount of weight used, amount of time on treadmill, or bike, and so forth. Consult your log weekly and set up small steady goals for yourself.

• **Vary The Exercises And The Routines.** There is no law that says you must perform the same exercises and exercise routine over and over again for the rest of your life. In fact, research has proven that people who put variety into their training tend to last longer on an exercise program. So don't be afraid to mix things up. And be sure to include walking as a regular part of your program. It's one of the best exercises in the world.

• **Flex Every Hour.** This may sound crazy but it's a fantastic way to firm up all of the muscles of the body. Just give every muscle in your body a tight flex for about five seconds and then relax. When you get good at this, you can do it anywhere without anyone ever knowing.

And as long as you are going to flex every hour, it's a great time to also say a prayer. Remember – our program is about both *physical* and *spiritual* improvement.

9. BEHAVIOR MODIFICATION

No health or weight loss program is going to be successful over the long haul without changes in behavior. There will be a direct correlation between your success on this health and wellness program and your ability to change behavior patterns. Thankfully, behavioral changes can be made rather quickly and once adopted, they should stay with you for life.

• **Make It A Family Affair.** It does little good for one member of a family to work at bettering his or her health while the rest of the family overindulges and under-exercises. Therefore, try to share your interest in health and fitness with the rest of the family. Perhaps you should start by letting them read this book. Things go much easier when health becomes a family affair. Don't nag or force anyone, just use patience, knowledge and example. A little prayer won't hurt either.

• **Avoid Negative People.** As much as you want family support, that's how firm you should be about staying away from negative people. For some strange reason, there are some people who, once they know you are trying to better yourself, will do all in their power to discourage you or sabotage your efforts. The best way to answer the skeptics is with *results*. Nothing you say or do is going to stop them so the best thing to do is simply avoid them. This is not snobbery – it's survival! Try to foster relationships with like-minded people who will motivate you and encourage you to press forward.

• **Break Free From Television.** I spoke about this above but it bears repeating here. Television for the most part today has become a purveyor of satanic immoral filth. We let characters on the TV get away with things in our home that we would never allow from friends or visitors. What's the difference? Television has become a corrupter of the mind. Give it up for exercise, prayer, charitable work, reading or visiting. You may be surprised how little you miss it once you make the break.

• **Don't Sleep Late On Weekends.** Try to stick to a good schedule even through the weekends. Sure, it's okay to grab an extra half-hour of sleep, but don't lie there until nine, ten or eleven o'clock. Besides, weekends make a great time for uninterrupted, focused exercise. Head to the gym instead.

• **Don't Use Food For Therapy.** It's easy to get into the habit of eating every time you feel depressed, nervous, worried or tired. Food makes great therapy for a whole bunch of reasons. But you must learn to control this urge since eating under stress usually means excessive amounts of poor food choices. Exercise and prayer make good substitutes for food therapy.

• **Learn To Eat Slowly.** Here's a good gimmick used by many successful dieters. By eating slowly, you give your blood sugars a chance to normalize which makes you feel satisfied which makes you want to eat less. Besides that, food tastes a whole lot better when you take the time to eat it slowly and enjoy it.

• **Never Overeat.** This isn't as hard as it sounds. If you are following a timed eating schedule of nutritious Bible-based foods, there's a good chance you will no longer have the need to overstuff yourself at a single meal. Always stop when you feel pleasantly full. Eating to excess puts a terrible strain on the digestive system as well as your other internal organs.

• **Try To Walk After Every Meal.** This is a great tip if you can manage the time. A brief 5 to 10 minute walk after a meal is very therapeutic for body and soul. Not only that, a post-meal walk is one of the best ways to improve digestion and help prevent the storage of excess fat. It's a winner. Give it a try!

10. ACCOUNTABILITY

If you can set up a good system of accountability, you are almost guaranteed success on the **Moses Diet & Health Program**. Accountability is a system of checks and balances. It is a way to answer for your progress or lack thereof.

• **Find An Accountability Partner.** You must always be accountable to God first and then to yourself, but it will be a great help for you to also find an accountability partner. Do you want to see your level of success go right through the roof? Then find someone you love and respect and report to them regularly on your health and fitness progress. Be honest with them. If you can find someone who also starts the program with you, that's even better. You can be each other's accountability partner.

• **Account To Yourself.** Regardless of whom you pick for an accountability partner, you still need to also be accountable to yourself. The way to do this is by keeping an accountability notebook of schedules and progress charts and updating it and reviewing it every single day. (See **Appendix C**)

• **Write An Official Commitment Agreement To Yourself.** This idea may sound a bit silly to you but it has great merit. Type out a formal letter of commitment just as though it were a legal document. List all of the things you are committing yourself to accomplishing. Sign the form and add it to your accountability notebook. Read it every day.

• **Read Your Goals Every Day.** Make a written list of all your goals and add it to your accountability notebook. Read it at least once every day. Be sure to amend your goals as the need arises.

• **Weigh Yourself Regularly.** There is an on-going debate among diet counselors as to how often you should weigh yourself. Some say once a week while others say every day. I believe that every day weighing has great merit. It keeps you closely attuned to where you are. Now, of course you are not going to register a weight loss every day, and in fact there will be days when your weight is actually up a bit. But by weighing yourself every day, you will never have any surprises. And if you are up more than you think you should be, you can take corrective action much quicker.

By the way, if you purchase a doctor's balance scale, you will actually be able to weigh yourself to within fractions of a pound and thus see a weight loss that may not show on a regular floor bathroom scale. And beware of those cheap bathroom scales. You can "gain or lose" a pound or two just by stepping on and off a few times.

• **Join A Club.** If you'd like the support of like-minded people to help get you through the rough spots, why not join a walking club or a dieter's club. Most areas have them and they can be very helpful to keeping you on track. If you'd like more help from me, I've set up a dieter's support group called **Temple Builders**. Your yearly membership dues get you all kind of benefits besides just accountability. (See page 149 for complete details.)

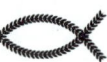

162

Epilogue

Some Parting Thoughts

Well now our time together has come to an end. It has been a real joy for me to write this book. I hope it has been as equally enjoyable for you to read it. I feel that even if only one person improves his or her life as a result of reading **Moses Wasn't Fat**, then it has been well worth all of the time and effort.

Perhaps you are that one person whose heart I have touched. Perhaps I have convinced you to start making some positive changes in your life. If so, I pray that the Holy Spirit moves you to start *immediately* and not put off for another day such an important matter.

Oh. . . and by the way. . . would you do me a small favor? If you do follow this program, would you write to me and let me know how you are doing? I would love to hear from you.

Meanwhile, I wish you all of the best blessings from God, both now and forever.

Shalom-Shalom

Tom Ciola

Tom Ciola

P.S. I do have one last request. If you found this book to be beneficial, would you share it with a friend?

APPENDIX

Appendix A

Answering Your Questions

The Moses Diet & Health Program appears to be very high in carbohydrates. Yet I have read several magazine articles that urge dieters to restrict carbohydrates since carbohydrates boost insulin in the body which then encourages fat depositing. Who's right?

This is far and away the most frequently asked question about this program. While I did discuss this whole issue of carbohydrates several times in this book (see Chapter 8 & Chapter 15), let me briefly recap here.

Carbohydrates are God's primary energy nutrient and they are found in abundance in nearly every type of Bible food. This should be an indication to us that God not only doesn't want them restricted in the diet, but in fact desires that we eat lots of them.

The average person requires at least 1,400 to 1,800 energy calories a day just to maintain all bodily functions. Carbohydrates are the body's first choice for fuel to satisfy this energy requirement which is why they burn more efficiently than protein or fat for this purpose. The low carbohydrate diets that are now in vogue force the body to convert to either protein or fat for its energy requirements. While the body is capable of making this conversion, it does so hesitantly and somewhat less efficiently since it much rather prefers carbohydrates.

Furthermore, high carbohydrate Bible foods also tend to be high in vitamins, minerals, enzymes and fiber – all important nutrients for good health. To reduce or exclude such an important food group in the diet makes no sense at all and usually leads to deficiencies in these important nutrients. Prolonged carbohydrate restriction may also lead to health complications.

The *glycemic index* (see page 53) which measures how quickly individual foods convert to blood glucose, may have some merit for diabetics and hypoglycemics, but it is questionable as a diet aid tool. The reason for this is that a food's glycemic index may change considerably when it is combined with other foods in the stomach.

Let me conclude then by saying that carbohydrate foods are among the most nutritious, delicious and satisfying foods known to man. God gave them to us as a wonderful gift. To drastically restrict them in the diet is a travesty and an insult to God.

Do I have to use your food concentrates in order for the Moses diet program to work?

Absolutely not! This is a lifestyle program that is designed to teach you how to build good health using God's Bible-type foods. Everything you need to follow this program effectively is available at your local grocery store and health food store.

The **Logia** Bible food concentrates recommended in this book are simply convenient tools or aids that you can use to help you achieve your health and fitness goals. They have been carefully formulated from natural food sources in order to maintain the integrity of the biblical nutrition principles espoused in this book.

Can children follow this program?

The Bible rules of good health apply equally as much to children as they do adults. In fact, the Bible admonishes us in several places to teach our children God's Law (e.g. **Deuteronomy 4:9**).

Therefore, it makes excellent sense for children to learn respect for their bodies as young as possible. In fact, the sooner you start your children out on the principles explained in this book, the better chance they have of leading a healthy, disease-free, holy life.

I absolutely hate to exercise. Do I have to follow an exercise program in order for this diet to work?

Exercise is an essential part of this program and without it your diet and health building plan will suffer. More than likely, the reason you hate to exercise is because you have been involved with exercise programs that are not enjoyable. The key then, is to find a form of exercise that is fun. There are so many options these days that this should not be a difficult assignment. Check out Chapter 17 for a choice of exercise plans.

I'm really not a person for details. Just how necessary is it to keep the daily accountability charts?

Studies have shown that people who have to account to someone for their actions tend to have greater discipline and stick-to-it power. While it would be ideal to find someone you respect as an accountability partner in order to help keep you on your health building program, this is not always easy. Therefore, I have found out through personal experience that you can be your own accountability partner. But the only way for this to work is for you to keep accurate daily charts of your actions and review them daily. Prepare them with the diligence due as if you were to present them to God each day as an accounting of your life. In fact, that is exactly what you are doing. So in answer to your question, the daily accountability charts are absolutely an essential part of the *Moses Diet & Health Program*.

What exactly is the Bible Bar?

The *Bible Bar* is a highly nutritious, all natural food bar made from the seven foods listed in the Book of **Deuteronomy 8:8**: *whole grain wheat, whole grain barley, organic raisins (vines), organic figs, pomegranates, extra virgin olive oil* and *raw honey*. It is unbaked and contains no added synthetic vitamins, no additives, no refined or artificial sweeteners, no high fructose corn syrup, no artificial flavoring or coloring. It has a delicious and wholesome fruit and grain flavor with just the right amount of sweetness from raw honey, brown rice syrup and the natural dried fruits. Each bar is bursting with God-given nutrients: protein, mono-unsaturated fats, complex carbohydrates, vitamins, minerals, enzymes, and fiber. But yet, it is more than just a health bar. It is a *spiritual* bar too since its seven main ingredients have been singled out by God Himself as being good. When you eat a *Bible Bar*, you are getting maximum nutrition as God intended and in a form that is easy and convenient to eat.

What makes the Bible Bar good for weight control?

Weight loss actually has more to do with what you eat than what you don't eat. Because of the powerful nutritional array achieved by combining the seven healthy foods of **Deuteronomy 8:8**, the *Bible Bar* is a nutritious and healthful snack and yet contains only 270 calories. Thus, it can be eaten along with a meal or as a between meal snack. Its strong nutritional profile assures you of getting complete biblical nutrition in every bar.

Additionally, when consumed between meals, the *Bible Bar* makes the perfect appetite regulator while helping to control and normalize the body's metabolic processes. When used as a diet aid between meals, the *Bible Bar* helps to relieve hunger pangs and that starving feeling that so many dieters hate. Thus, the *Bible Bar* helps people to lose weight while feeling satisfied.

I noticed on the Bible Bar label that it contains 6 grams of fat and 53 grams of carbohydrates. This seems way too high for a weight control aid. What's the story?

Unfortunately, there are some currently popular diet programs that recommend cutting fats or carbohydrates to very low levels, and in some cases, almost zero. This is not only wrong – it is *dangerous!* We need to let the wisdom of the Bible speak to us on this point. God gave us a variety of foods to consume: seeds, grains, nuts, fruits, vegetables, oils, honey, milk. A healthy, well-balanced diet of biblical foods will automatically contain higher levels of fats and carbohydrates than some of today's diet experts are recommending. Fats and carbohydrates play a very important role in our health and well being. The key then, is not so much the *amount* of fats and carbohydrates in the diet, but the sources and balance of the fats and carbohydrates. Nutritional studies continue to show, for instance, that olive oil helps protect the arteries against heart attack and has a very positive effect on the overall health of the body. Not surprisingly, olive oil is one of the foods of Deuteronomy and hence, an ingredient in the **Bible Bar**. This is the primary source of the 6 grams of fat.

Additionally, complex carbohydrates as found in grains are excellent for the body's health. They regulate blood sugars and provide a sustained source of energy to both the brain and the muscles. Two grains – wheat and barley – are used in the **Bible Bar** and account for much of the 53 grams of carbohydrates. The remainder of carbohydrate comes from the raw honey and dried fruits.

It is the very sources and balance of the protein, fat, and carbohydrate in the **Bible Bar** which makes it so effective for weight control, whereas other diets that are super low in fats or carbohydrates are ultimately doomed to failure.

Can diabetics eat the Bible Bar?

While we have gotten several reports back from diabetics who are using the **Bible Bar** quite successfully, I strongly recommend that you consult with your doctor before using this product.

Where can I purchase the Logia Bible food concentrates?

These products are now being sold in many health food stores, Bible bookstores, as well as select pharmacies, specialty stores and grocery stores. If they are unavailable in your area, you may purchase them directly from us (see order form in back of book) or ordering directly from our web site at www.logia.net.

How quickly can I expect to lose weight on this program?

Please remember first and foremost that the **Moses Diet & Health Program** is about lifestyle changes and not necessarily rapid weight loss. The goal of the program is to get you to permanently normalize your bodyweight by following biblical principles of health and nutrition.

Some people with a lot of weight to lose experience very quick weight loss, while others who are closer to their ideal weight, will take longer to normalize. Your goal on this program should not be *quick* weight loss but rather *lasting* lifelong weight loss and health.

Can pregnant or nursing mothers follow this program?

It is never a good idea for pregnant or nursing mothers to be on any *calorie-restricted diet*. Nevertheless, the biblical food recommendations in this book are very valid for pregnant and nursing mothers since these are the very high nutrition foods needed for both the mother's and the child's health. Therefore, other than restricting calories, everything else in this book will be most beneficial to pregnant and nursing mothers.

You seem to come down very hard on prescription medicines in this book. I am currently on three different medications. Does this mean I shouldn't follow the program?

As you have guessed, I am not a fan of the pharmaceutical industry and I do believe we have become an overmedicated society. Nevertheless, discontinuance of prescription medicines, especially after prolonged usage, is a very serious matter and should only be done with the input and approval of a doctor.

People on medication can successfully follow this program and hopefully, as the health benefits accrue, they will be able to drastically reduce if not eliminate completely their drugs. Once again, however, any changes in prescription drug use should never be done without a doctor's consent.

A friend of mine told me that I needed to reduce my daily fat intake to less than 10 percent of total calories in order to lose weight. Is this true?

This gets us back to the same issue I discussed earlier regarding carbohydrates. Should the intake of any macro-nutrient food (protein, fat, carbohydrate) be greatly restricted in order to lose weight? Once again the answer is no. Fats, like carbohydrates, play an important role in overall health and well being and should account for 25 to 30 percent of total daily calories. What should be restricted, however, are the saturated animal fats that can lead to many health complications. Replace them with naturally extracted vegetable oils, including the greatest oil on earth – *olive oil*.

I have been hearing a lot lately about something called GMO's. What exactly are they?

GMO stands for *genetically modified organisms* and refers to a relatively new procedure whereby scientists are able to take a gene from one organism and splice it to the genes of another organism in hopes of producing a better plant or animal. For example, genetic engineers have injected tomatoes with the antifreezing gene of a flounder in an effort to give the tomato a longer growing season. Some crops are being genetically altered to resist certain forms of insects. Foods that have been so altered are also referred to as GMs, bioengineered foods and "Frankenfoods."

GM foods were introduced into the world's food supply in 1996 without any great fanfare or media attention. According to a report by Barbara Keeler and Shirley Watson, today there are three GM varieties of soybeans, ten varieties of corn, as well as GM papaya, squash, canola, potatoes, tomatoes and even dairy products and meat.

As this book goes to print, great debates are raging as to the safety and wisdom of such genetic modification. The big agri-business companies argue that GMOs will lead to lower food costs, help feed the world's poor, save the environment and require fewer pesticides. Opponents argue that genetic engineering is a risky venture that can have both serious environmental and bodily health consequences.

Where do I stand on this issue? I am totally against it. The extra-biblical book of Jasher says that before the flood of Noah, human beings were heavily involved in cross species experimentation and that this was one of the main offenses that angered God. It's a very powerful incrimination. Here it is in its entirety.

> *"And the sons of men in those days took from the cattle of the earth, the beasts of the field and the fowls of the air, and taught the mixture of animals of one species with the other, in order therewith to provoke the Lord; and God saw the whole earth and it was corrupt, for all flesh had corrupted its ways upon the earth, all men and all animals."* **(Jasher 4:18)**

Don't you find it somewhat interesting that Yahshua (Jesus) warned us that the world would be like the time of Noah before His Second Coming **(Luke 17:26)**. Furthermore, the Bible tells us in Genesis Chapter 1 that God made everything according to its kind (species). Obviously then, God made each species to be self-contained and any attempt by man to cross-splice genes from one species to another is immoral. Genetic engineering bodes very ominously for the future of the human race.

Aren't you just using the Bible as a gimmick for making money?

Absolutely not! As I've said both in this book and at our web site (www.logia.net), I have dedicated my life and my various business enterprises to bringing the knowledge of biblical nutrition and health to as many people as possible. I see the human body as the temple of the Holy Spirit and therefore, I believe with my whole heart that people should be working to keep their bodies healthy and fit. My goals then, are never about making lots of money, or using the Bible as a gimmick to line my own pockets. Instead, my goals are to reach as many people as possible with this important message and secondly to bring them quality food products and information on this topic.

Until the time that Godly love replaces economics, we must all, unfortunately, function within this world's monetary system. To compensate for this, here at **Logia**, we tithe both corporately and individually to a charity called **"Over The Rainbow"** (www.overrainbow.org).

Appendix B

Dieter's Profile

REASONS FOR DIETING

Before you begin the *Moses Diet & Health Program*, it would be a good idea to determine your reasons for dieting. There are a variety of reasons why people start diets. Some are good and some are not so good.

Listed below are some of the main reasons people give for losing weight. Check as many reasons as apply to you. If you are dieting for the right reasons, you will have a better chance of losing weight and keeping it off. If you begin this or any other program for the wrong reasons, you are ultimately doomed to fail.

RIGHT REASONS FOR DIETING

- ❑ **Because my body is the Temple of the Holy Spirit.**
- ❑ To improve my overall health.
- ❑ **Because of an illness or medical problem.**
- ❑ To improve my overall appearance.
- ❑ To have more energy and vitality.
- ❑ To demonstrate self control.
- ❑ To participate in sports.

   Other positive reasons:
- ❑ _____
- ❑ _____

WRONG REASONS FOR DIETING

- ❑ To look good for an upcoming event.
- ❑ To please another person.
- ❑ At the insistence of another person.
- ❑ To find a mate.
- ❑ To get a new job or promotion.
- ❑ To win a bet.

   Other negative reasons:
- ❑ _____
- ❑ _____

EXCUSES FOR NOT DIETING

There are lots of reasons why people put off dieting. Perhaps you too have been stalling for one or more of the reasons listed below. If so, you should know that none of these excuses is valid. Each is precisely that – an excuse. Hopefully, this book has given you the motivation you need to put these excuses to rest once and for all. Check all the excuses you are currently using to prevent you from improving your life. Be brutally honest with yourself. Now see them for the stalling tactics that they really are and get going on your self improvement program immediately.

- ❑ I'm really not that fat.
- ❑ I've tried too many times and failed.
- ❑ I like to eat too much.
- ❑ I don't know how to get started.
- ❑ My mate likes me just the way I am.
- ❑ I don't have any willpower.
- ❑ My family won't support me.
- ❑ I don't have time to prepare good meals.
- ❑ I like to cook too much.
- ❑ I eat out too often.
- ❑ I'll start next (week, month, year).
- ❑ My weight problem is genetic.
- ❑ I don't have time to exercise.
- ❑ I use food to control stress.

Appendix C

Good Record Keeping Will Keep You On Track

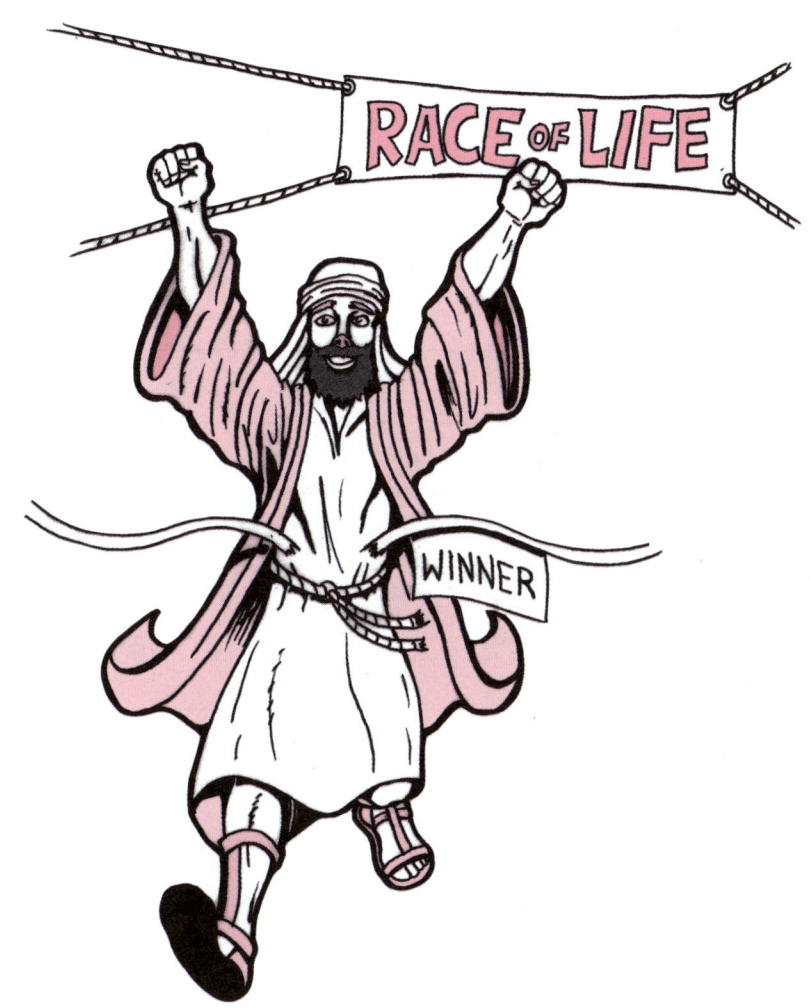

As I discussed in Chapter 21, it is extremely important that you maintain accurate accountability charts of your progress. As you begin the *Moses Diet & Health Program*, feel free to photocopy and use the various forms and charts in this Appendix.

GOALS

Be it declared on this _____ day of _____, that I_____, do hereby resolve to the best of my abilities, and with the help of the eternal God of heaven and earth, to meet the following goals:

(1) _____

(2) _____

(3) _____

(4) _____

(5) _____

(6) _____

(7) _____

(8) _____

(9) _____

(10) _____

Signature: _____

Witnesses: God the Father and His Son Yahshua (Jesus Christ)

COMMITMENT AGREEMENT

I _____ , after careful consideration of all that is required of me and under my own free will, do hereby commit all of my resources, talents and energy to the goal of losing weight and keeping it off for the rest of my life. In undertaking this endeavor, I realize that I must make a total commitment both to myself and to God. I also acknowledge that there will be setbacks, but I will never let them deter me from reaching my goal. I know that with God's grace and the power of the Holy Spirit, I will be successful.

I further acknowledge that I will utilize all of the knowledge that I have gained from reading the book ***Moses Wasn't Fat*** knowing that it contains biblical wisdom for health and well being. I refuse to let myself get discouraged since I am now on a program I can follow for life. I am confident that I will succeed since I have finally taken charge of my life. I know that by reaching all of my goals, I will look better, feel better, and draw closer to God the Father and to His Son Yahshua the Messiah (Jesus Christ).

Furthermore, I agree to exercise regularly even on those days when I would rather not. I will strive to avoid all foods which are not good for me and attempt to eat only the most nutritious, biblically based foods.

I realize that the sought after changes will not happen overnight but instead, I do know that every day in ever so slight a way, I am getting better and better. I know also that if God is for me, nothing can be against me. Therefore, I will let nothing stop me from reaching my goals. I can do all things through Christ who strengthens me.

Signed _____

Dated _____

Witnesses: God the Father and His Son
               Yahshua (Jesus Christ)

12 POINT PLAN FOR DEALING WITH SETBACKS

1. When you suffer a setback or a make a mistake, let it go as quickly as possible. Just say to yourself: "<u>It's OVER!</u>" and then move on.

2. Setbacks dwelled upon quickly become failures. Therefore, never dwell on your past mistakes or setbacks. The past is over the second that you cut it loose.

3. See conquered setbacks as something that actually makes you stronger.

4. See a setback as a chance to start again with a fresh new resolve and renewed vigor.

5. Your chance of success is going to be in direct proportion to the number of times you have a setback and keep on trying.

6. If you dwell on your previous setbacks, you are destined to repeat them. Instead, dwell on God's grace, your plan, and your goal.

7. Strive to re-ignite your original desire as quickly as possible after a setback.

8. Remember that regardless of how many setbacks you encounter, the future is always a clean slate.

9. Never have enough "common sense" to stop.

10. Accept God as your partner and "personal trainer" and then place your trust in Him during periods of setback.

11. Write down your goals and read them daily, and let nothing ever deter you from reaching them.

12. Always remember how the Success Shuffle works. "Three steps forward and one step back." You're never going to change it. That's just the way things work. So you might as well learn to live with it.

DAILY MENU PLANNER

Breakfast

_____
_____
_____
_____

Mid-morning Snack

_____

Lunch

_____
_____
_____
_____

Mid-afternoon Snack

_____

Dinner

_____
_____
_____

DAILY MENU PLANNER

Breakfast

_____
_____
_____
_____

Mid-morning Snack

_____

Lunch

_____
_____
_____
_____

Mid-afternoon Snack

_____

Dinner

_____
_____
_____

DAILY MENU PLANNER

Breakfast

_____
_____
_____
_____

Mid-morning Snack

_____

Lunch

_____
_____
_____
_____

Mid-afternoon Snack

_____

Dinner

_____
_____
_____

How To Fill Out The Daily Review Sheet

It is important that you keep daily accountability records. The **DAILY REVIEW SHEET** in this Appendix will enable you to do so. Be sure to make plenty of photo copies of this sheet and keep them in your three-ring binder.

On the next page is a filled out sample of a **DAILY REVIEW SHEET**. Let's review the sample so that you can get an idea on how to keep your daily records.

First of all, be sure and fill in the month and year at the upper right. (You should keep all of your monthly review sheets in your binder as an ongoing record of how you are doing.

The numbers in the first column are the days of the month. In the next column, you will record your weight regularly. It is for you to decide how frequently you wish to weigh in. But please weigh in at a minimum once a week. Our sample person chose to weigh in quite frequently (20 days) out of the 31. This column will give you an overview of how you are progressing on your weight loss if that is your goal.

The **Prayer** column is to record whether you remembered to say your prayers. You must decide how often during the day you wish to pray and then keep track of it here. If you fail to say all of your prayers, you must leave this column blank. Our sample person missed only one day of prayer during the month. The score is determined by dividing the total prayer days (30) by the total days in the month (30 ÷ 31 = .967 or .97)

Thus, you will proceed across the sheet each day, giving yourself a check mark or a blank. Once again, you will determine your score at the end of each month by dividing the total check marks by the number of days in the month. Under **Read Goals**, for example, our sample person missed three days. Therefore, their score is 28 ÷ 31 = .90

Notice under **Exercise** that **NA** is entered on those days when you are *not* scheduled for exercise. Also note, then, that this changes the total days of the month in this column. Rather than 31 days, for instance, this column total is 23 days (31 days less 8 **NA** days).

Finally, under **Diet**, you are going to assign yourself a number up to 10 depending on how well you did on your diet. This will be a subjective number so try to be honest with yourself. If you had a perfect day of dieting, you will assign yourself a 10. If you were near, but not quite perfect, give yourself a 9. And so forth. Six or lower would mean you really blew it for the day. At the end of the month, add up all of the numbers in this column and divide that number by the total potentially perfect days in a month. In the sample case, for instance, a perfect score would be 310 (31 days x 10). Our sample person totaled 253. This number is divided by 310 giving a score of .816 rounded up to .82.

Daily Review Sheet

SAMPLE

MONTH: __February__

DAY	WEIGHT	PRAYERS	READ GOALS	READ COMMITMENT AGREEMENT	READ BIBLE	EXERCISE	GOOD DEEDS	DIET	SUPPLEMENTS
1	162	✔	✔	✔	✔	✔	✔	9	✔
2	162	✔	✔	✔	✔	✔	✔	9	✔
3	---	✔	✔	✔	✔	✔	✔	9	✔
4	161	✔	✔	✔	✔	NA	✔	9	✔
5	160	✔	✔	✔	✔	✔	✔	10	✔
6	---	✔	✔	✔	✔	✔	✔	8	✔
7	159	✔	✔	—	✔	✔	✔	8	—
8	158	✔	✔	✔	✔	NA	✔	8	✔
9	---	✔	✔	✔	✔	✔	✔	9	✔
10	156	✔	—	—	✔	✔	✔	9	✔
11	156	✔	✔	✔	✔	✔	✔	7	✔
12	154	✔	✔	✔	✔	NA	✔	10	✔
13	153	✔	✔	✔	✔	✔	✔	8	✔
14	---	✔	✔	✔	✔	✔	✔	8	✔
15	153	✔	✔	✔	✔	✔	✔	9	✔
16	153	✔	✔	✔	✔	NA	✔	8	✔
17	---	✔	✔	✔	✔	NA	✔	9	✔
18	---	✔	✔	✔	✔	✔	✔	10	✔
19	152	✔	—	—	—	✔	—	6	✔
20	153	✔	✔	✔	✔	✔	✔	8	✔
21	151	✔	✔	✔	✔	NA	✔	8	✔
22	150	✔	✔	✔	✔	✔	✔	9	✔
23	---	✔	✔	✔	✔	✔	✔	6	✔
24	---	✔	✔	✔	✔	✔	✔	8	✔
25	149	—	—	—	✔	NA	✔	6	✔
26	149	✔	✔	✔	✔	✔	✔	10	✔
27	---	✔	✔	✔	✔	✔	✔	8	✔
28	148	✔	✔	✔	✔	✔	✔	9	✔
29	---	✔	✔	✔	✔	NA	✔	8	✔
30	---	✔	✔	✔	✔	✔	✔	8	✔
31	148	✔	✔	✔	✔	✔	✔	8	✔
SCORE:		.97	.90	.87	.97	1.00	.97	.82	.97

Daily Review Sheet

MONTH: _____

DAY	WEIGHT	PRAYERS	READ GOALS	READ COMMITMENT AGREEMENT	READ BIBLE	EXERCISE	GOOD DEEDS	DIET	SUPPLEMENTS
1									
2									
3									
4									
5									
6									
7									
8									
9									
10									
11									
12									
13									
14									
15									
16									
17									
18									
19									
20									
21									
22									
23									
24									
25									
26									
27									
28									
29									
30									
31									

Daily Review Sheet

MONTH: _____

DAY	WEIGHT	PRAYERS	READ GOALS	READ COMMITMENT AGREEMENT	READ BIBLE	EXERCISE	GOOD DEEDS	DIET	SUPPLEMENTS
1									
2									
3									
4									
5									
6									
7									
8									
9									
10									
11									
12									
13									
14									
15									
16									
17									
18									
19									
20									
21									
22									
23									
24									
25									
26									
27									
28									
29									
30									
31									

Daily Review Sheet

MONTH: _____

DAY	WEIGHT	PRAYERS	READ GOALS	READ COMMITMENT AGREEMENT	READ BIBLE	EXERCISE	GOOD DEEDS	DIET	SUPPLEMENTS
1									
2									
3									
4									
5									
6									
7									
8									
9									
10									
11									
12									
13									
14									
15									
16									
17									
18									
19									
20									
21									
22									
23									
24									
25									
26									
27									
28									
29									
30									
31									

Measurements

DATE: _____

WEIGHT: _____

UPPER ARM: _____

CHEST: _____

WAIST: _____

HIPS: _____

THIGH: _____

CALF: _____

UPPER ARM
CHEST
WAIST
HIPS
THIGH
CALF

DATE: _____

WEIGHT: _____

UPPER ARM: _____

CHEST: _____

WAIST: _____

HIPS: _____

_____

CALF: _____

DATE: _____

WEIGHT: _____

UPPER ARM: _____

CHEST: _____

WAIST: _____

HIPS: _____

THIGH: _____

CALF: _____

DATE: _____

WEIGHT: _____

UPPER ARM: _____

CHEST: _____

WAIST: _____

HIPS: _____

THIGH: _____

CALF: _____

DATE: _____

WEIGHT: _____

UPPER ARM: _____

CHEST: _____

WAIST: _____

HIPS: _____

THIGH: _____

CALF: _____

Appendix D

Additional Prayers

Here are some additional prayers that may help give you strength, motivation and comfort as you progress through the *Moses Diet & Health Program*.

COMMUNION TO THE HEAVENLY FATHER

All creation and life spring forth from You – Heavenly Father, for it is Your Wisdom and Love, which begot all that, is. As the Creator, You are worthy of all my love and respect. There is only one way – Your Way! And Your Way is perfection. As Your Child, it is my destiny to be perfect just as You, Heavenly Father, are perfect. When I am in harmony with Your Wisdom and Your Health Laws, I become a perfect replica of Your Holy Essence and thus, worthy to be called a Child of Light. Light from Light – Truth from Truth – Spirit from Spirit. To be one with You, Heavenly Father is to be one with all of Your creation and this makes for a perfect Shalom. I become light when I know I am of the Light. I become spirit when I know I am of the Spirit. I become peace when I know I am of the Eternal Peace.

PRAYER BEFORE MEALS

Heavenly Father, I praise Your Holy Name and acknowledge You as the Creator and Giver of Life. Father, You in Your infinite wisdom, set up the cycle of life whereby this food which I am about to eat nourishes my physical body, just as the Word, Your Son, Yahshua (Jesus Christ), the Bread of Life nourishes my spirit.

Most loving Father, I thank You with my whole heart for this life-sustaining food that You now provide for me and I look forward to the day when I can be in Your everlasting Kingdom and eat freely from the Tree of Life.

AN HOURLY PRAYER

My Father, sometimes I get so wrapped up in the activities of the day that I forget to give You praise. Nevertheless, I will make every effort to honor You my Lord at least once every hour. If I could, I would spend every minute of every day praising, honoring and worshipping You. The next best thing I can do is to let all of my actions reflect the kind of person You want me to be. Father, I love You.

PRAYER WHEN READING SCRIPTURES

My Lord Yahshua (Jesus Christ), as I now set out to read the sacred words of the Holy Scriptures, I ask that You guide me in my studies just as You guided Your disciples to a deeper understanding of Eternal Truth two millennia ago. O Great Teacher, I beseech You to send forth the Holy Spirit into my heart so that what I read now may become alive for me just as You are the Living Word which came down from heaven.

But most importantly, my Savior, let the wisdom of this Blessed Book inspire me to lead a holy and pure life so that I may be worthy to share everlasting life with You in the Kingdom of Heaven.

MY DEEPEST LOVE

My Lord and my God – You are my love and You are all around me. You live deep inside of me and I can feel our spirits uniting. Your Wisdom is ancient and eternal and it is soothing as the sea breeze. It is the core of energy that keeps my heart beating. What would I be without You and where would I go? Where would I stand tall and free and safe? Who would nurture me and watch over me.

Dear God – the love I feel for You is overwhelming. Sometimes I sit in solitude and simply ponder Your majesty. I picture my spirit just floating gently in the living waters of Your tranquility. When I first came to know You, my soul felt a peace as never before and I knew I wanted to be with You forever – to share Your Love and to bring You joy. I have loved You for many years now and yet our relationship is still growing and unfolding. Each evening, as the moon and stars make their way across the heavens, I feel a certain closeness to You. Each day in Your Love is better than the day before.

You have taken me to heights beyond the mundane. With You, I skip across the mountains, over the hills and valleys. You are my firmament, my light, my shining star, my reason for being. You are my strength, my hope, my dreams, my love. Some day we will laugh and sing together. But until that longed for time comes, I send out my prayer to You morning, noon and evening. O Great and Eternal One, I love You.

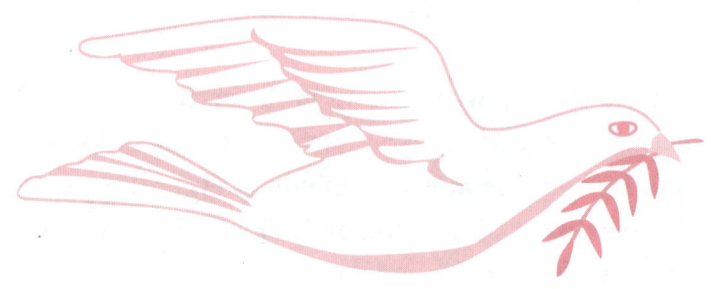

Appendix E

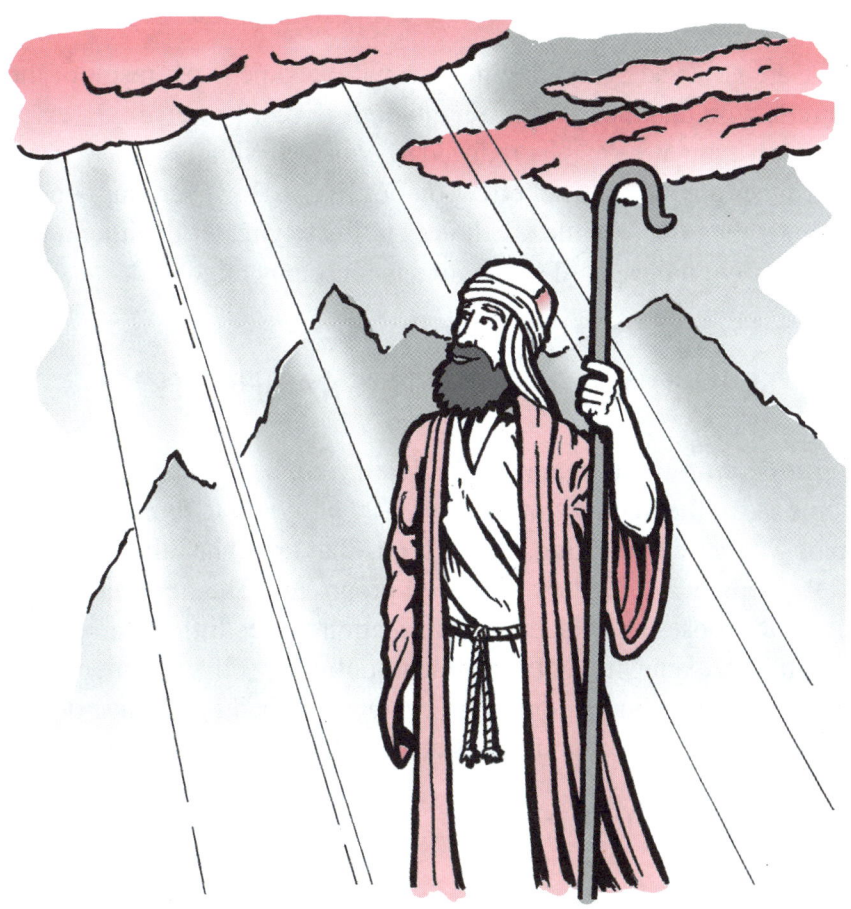

Sometimes, just knowing that something is true is not enough. In order to live a truth, we need to periodically remind ourselves of its importance. The following Truth Message is so valuable, so important to your health program success, that I am requesting that you read it on the first day of each month for the rest of your life.

On Choices

Everything that we are now and everything that we will become is the result of the *choices* that we make. Just stop and reflect on that thought for a minute. It is very powerful. Everything that we do throughout each day that we are alive can be reduced to *choices*. Simply speaking, we can refer to each choice as having either a good or a bad effect on our lives. However, our decision-making process goes much deeper than that. While all choices ultimately result in either a positive or negative effect, we must be constantly on our guard since our subconscious mind seeks to interpret every choice as good.

BEWARE OF IMMEDIATE GRATIFICATION

The concept of *gratification* (both immediate and delayed) is closely linked to the process of choosing. Most people make the majority of their choices based upon *immediate gratification* (pleasure). Some examples would be overeating, eating foods that are unhealthy, wasting time, sleeping late, talking on the telephone, watching bad television programs. The important thing to remember is that nearly everything we choose for immediate gratification serves little or no purpose in the bigger picture of our lives (self improvement, goal fulfillment, holiness, self-fulfillment, job skills). The truth is that immediate self-denial builds long-term character. Therefore, since our natural instincts want us to opt for immediate gratification, it takes a special person to choose long-term results over short-term pleasure.

IT BEGAN IN THE GARDEN OF EDEN

Here is a MYSTERY. This all began in the Garden of Eden with the bad choice made by Adam and Eve. Satan presented the *Tree of the Knowledge of Good and Evil* to Eve as a source of immediate gratification-satisfaction.

> *"She saw that it was good for food and pleasant to the eyes and a tree to make one wise, so she took from it and ate."* **(Genesis 3:16)**

Yet, it was God's plan that the man and woman would delay their immediate gratification, grow in wisdom and understanding by eating from the *Tree of Life*, and then share eternity with Him in everlasting bliss. But it was not to be. Adam and Eve chose immediate gratification and as a result, they passed this weakness on to all of us. This is why we have the tendency to always make hasty and bad choices.

WE WIN DURING SELF TALK

Since everything we do or don't do in life is based on this principle of choices, it is imperative that we stop long enough before each decision to go through a rational thought process. This process of choice analysis is known as *self-talk*. It is a form of internal debate whereby we decide whether or not to do something. Most of the time, self-talk is so brief that we are hardly aware that it has happened. And at other times, there is no doubt that a debate is taking place. <u>It is important to realize that it is during self-talk that we will rise or fall, succeed or fail.</u>

TWO OPPOSING FORCES

As a result of the fall in the Garden of Eden, we now are composed of two opposing entities – the natural (material) man and the spiritual (heavenly) man. We must be aware that in all self-talk, it is the natural man that will always push for dominance. This voice will always give us all of the apparently rational reasons for choosing immediate gratification. Since the natural man ultimately dies, this voice and this logic are anchored in the here and now. This voice cares nothing for things eternal and it will always push for immediate, sensual gratification. This is why we must always be suspicious of this voice. **CAUTION**: It will *always* be the first to speak. *(The first shall be last.)*

The voice and logic of the spiritual man on the other hand, since it is eternally directed, will always strive to preserve the long-term well being of the individual. Once we are aware that the natural voice will shout the loudest and push the hardest, we can anticipate this and learn to restrain it. The ability to do this is called *discipline*. When we comprehend that the spiritual voice is the one that actually leads to long-term well being, then we will be more inclined to listen to it. *(The last shall be first.)*

THINK BEFORE ACTING

Armed with this knowledge of how the mind works, we are now prepared and equipped to make correct and positive choices. Every day will be filled with hundreds of choices – from the time we rise until the time we retire. Therefore, we must learn to think carefully about every choice we make during the course of each day. Our choices are cumulative and will ultimately determine our success or failure in life.

Choose wisely! Choose life!

Appendix F

Using Bible Foods To Plan Your Meals

Would you like some meal planning guidelines to follow as you begin your **Moses Diet & Health Program**? Here are some Bible-based daily meal plans that you can either follow as given, or adapt to suit your personal preferences. Please note that all meal plans in the first column are vegetarian.

SAMPLE BREAKFASTS

whole wheat cereal (mixed with soy or rice milk)	*Bible Granola**	4 scrambled egg whites
1 orange	10 ozs. orange juice	1 slice whole grain toast
1 tbs. flaxseed oil*	1/2 cup plain yogurt	1 banana
5-6 raw almonds	1 tbs. flaxseed oil*	1 tbs. flaxseed oil*
1 *Eden's Enzyme**	3 dried figs	sm. handful walnuts
	1 *Eden's Enzyme**	1 *Eden's Enzyme**

3 Bible pancakes*	barley or oat cereal	large *Bible Bar**
1/2 grapefruit	handful of grapes	10 ozs. grape juice
1/2 cup plain yogurt	1/2 cup cottage cheese (low fat)	1/2 cup plain yogurt
1 tbs. flaxseed oil*	1 tbs. flaxseed oil*	1 tbs. flaxseed oil
sm. handful raw peanuts	sm. handful unsalted mixed nuts	sm. handful *Caravan Mix**
1 *Eden's Enzyme**	1 *Eden's Enzyme**	1 *Eden's Enzyme**

SAMPLE LUNCHES

tossed vegetable salad (olive oil-vinegar dressing)	broiled fish	tuna sandwich-grain bread (empty water from tuna and mix with olive oil)
2 slices whole grain bread	1 slice whole grain bread	1/2 cup beans of choice
lentil soup	10 ozs. pomegranate juice*	cup low fat milk
10 ozs. apple juice	small *Bible Bar**	sm. handful pitted dates
1 *Eden's Enzyme**	1 tbs. olive oil or 4 olive oil capsules*	1 *Eden's Enzyme**
	1 *Eden's Enzyme**	

1 cup beans of choice
mixed with olive oil
tossed vegetable salad
   (olive oil-vinegar dressing)
10 ozs. tomato juice
1 *Eden's Enzyme**

grilled chicken breast
1 slice whole grain bread
1 cup vegetables of choice
   (corn, peas, carrots)
sm. handful *Caravan Mix**
1 tbs. olive oil or
   4 olive oil capsules*
1 *Eden's Enzyme**

low fat turkey sandwich on
whole grain bread
4-5 olives
1 apple
10 ozs. low fat milk
1 tbs. olive oil or
   4 olive oil capsules*
1 *Eden's Enzyme**

SAMPLE DINNERS

bowl of lentils and rice
tossed vegetable salad
   (olive oil-vinegar dressing)
10 ozs. *Pomegranate Juice**
1 cup grapes
small *Bible Bar**
1 *Eden's Enzyme**

broiled fish
1 cup broccoli
1 cup stewed tomatoes
1 slice whole wheat pita
1/2 fresh melon
1 tbs. olive oil or
   4 olive oil capsules*
1 *Eden's Enzyme**

baked skinless turkey breast
3 bean salad mixed
   with olive oil
scoop low fat cottage cheese
sm. handful *Caravan Mix**
1 *Eden's Enzyme**

vegetarian burger on
   whole wheat bread
tossed vegetable salad
   (olive oil-vinegar dressing)
10 ozs. grape juice
4-5 dried apricots
1 *Eden's Enzymes**

bowl of pasta (whole wheat)
   or Jerusalem artichoke)
1 slice whole grain bread
1 cup mixed fruit salad
sm. handful mixed nuts
1 *Eden's Enzymes**

3 egg omelet
1 whole grain muffin
10 ozs. orange juice
1/2 cup plain yogurt
small *Bible Bar**
1 tbs. olive oil or
   4 olive oil capsules*
1 *Eden's Enzyme**

*Available from **Logia**: *Foods of the Bible*, **1-800-537-7671**.
See order form in back of book.

FOOD GUIDE PYRAMID
A Guide to Daily Food Choices

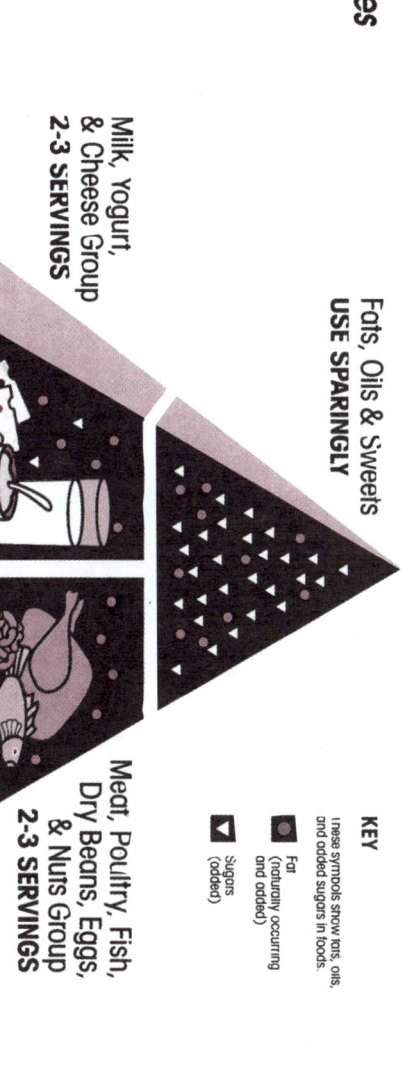

Fats, Oils & Sweets
USE SPARINGLY

KEY
- ● Fat (naturally occurring and added)
- ▼ Sugars (added)

These symbols show fats, oils, and added sugars in foods.

Milk, Yogurt, & Cheese Group
2-3 SERVINGS

Meat, Poultry, Fish, Dry Beans, Eggs, & Nuts Group
2-3 SERVINGS

Vegetable Group
3-5 SERVINGS

Fruit Group
2-4 SERVINGS

Bread, Cereal, Rice, & Pasta Group
6-11 SERVINGS

Source: U.S. Department of Agriculture and the U.S. Department of Health and Human Services

Provided by: the Education Department of the National Cattlemen's Beef Association

Appendix G

Blends, Recipes, Shakes

If you'd like some suggestions on how to put various Bible foods together, this chapter's for you. Here are some great suggestions on how to combine the foods of Eden into delicious and nutritious blends, recipes and shakes. Let's start with a list of some of the various foods that qualify as Bible foods according to **Genesis 1:29**.

FRUITS
Apple, Apricot, Avocado, Banana, Blackberry, Blueberry, Boysenberry, Cantaloupe, Carob, Casaba, Cherry, Coconut, Cranberry, Currant, Date, Elderberry, Fig, Gooseberry, Grape, Grapefruit, Guava, Honeydew Melon, Huckleberry, Kumquat, Lemon, Lime, Loganberry, Mango, Muskmelon, Nectarine, Nutmeg Melon, Olive, Orange, Papaya, Peach, Pear, Persian Melon, Persimmon, Pineapple, Plum, Pomegranate, Quince, Raspberry, Sapodilla, Sapota, Tamarind, Tangerine, Tomato, Watermelon

DRIED FRUIT
Dates, Figs, Prunes, Raisins

GRAIN (CEREAL)
Amaranth, Barley, Buckwheat, Corn, Flax, Millet, Oat, Rice, Rye, Wheat

LEGUMES & BEANS
Black-eyed Pea, Chick Pea (Garbanzo), Green Bean, Kidney Bean, Lentil, Lima Bean, Mung Bean, Navy Bean, Pea, Peanut, Pinto Bean, Pole Bean, Soy Bean, String Bean, Wax Bean, Yam Bean

NUTS
Almond, Brazil Nut, Cashew, Chestnut, Filbert (Hazel Nut), Macadamia Nut, Pecan, Pine Nut, Pistachio Nut, Walnut

SEEDS
Pumpkin Seed, Sesame Seed, Sunflower Seed

VEGETABLES
Artichoke, Bamboo Shoot, Beet, Broccoli, Brussels Sprouts, Cabbage, Carrot, Cauliflower, Celery, Chicory, Collard Greens, Cucumber, Dandelion, Eggplant, Endive, Jerusalem Artichoke, Kale, Kohlrabi, Leek, Lettuce, Okra, Parsnips, Peppers, Potato, Radish, Rutabaga, Spinach, Squash, Sweet Potato, Turnip, Watercress, Yam

MISCELLANEOUS (Not in Genesis 1:29 but in Bible)
Coriander, Cow's Milk & Cheese, Garlic, Goat Milk & Cheese, Honey, Olive Oil, Onion, Vinegar, Yogurt

Recipes

UNLEAVENED BREAD
1 cup whole wheat flour
1/4 teaspoon coriander
1/4 teaspoon sea salt
1/2 cup spring water

Mix flour, coriander, salt in a bowl. Add water slowly, kneading with other ingredients for about 5 to 10 minutes (until dough is elastic). Cover with damp cloth and let stand for 1/2 hour. Knead again lightly and form into small round balls. Flatten balls with palm of hand and lightly flour each side and place on breadboard. Roll out thinly. Heat ungreased griddle or frying pan on medium heat. Cook one or two flat breads at a time, turning as bread browns and rises. Rotate gently and press lightly on edges. Turn and lightly brown on the other side. Serve hot.

FRUIT & NUT BIBLE BITES
1 cup mixed dried fruit (raisins, dates, figs)
1/2 cup raw honey
1/4 cup oat flour
1/2 cup raw wheat germ
1/4 cup wheat bran
2 cups chopped nuts (per preference)
2 tablespoons olive oil
purple grape juice

Mix all ingredients well. Add just enough grape juice to make thick batter. Spread into greased 8 inch square baking pan. Bake at 300° for 30 to 40 minutes or until firm. Cut into squares immediately but allow to cool before removing from pan.

GETHSEMANE LOAF
15 pitted black olives sliced
15 green olives, sliced
2 tablespoons olive oil
2 tablespoons softened butter
1/4 cup Parmesan cheese
4 garlic cloves, minced
1/2 cup shredded cheese (cheddar or Mont. Jack)
1 teaspoon dried parsley
1 loaf French bread, sliced in half horizontally

Mix all ingredients together in medium bowl. Heat oven to 400°. Spread olive mixture over each half of French bread. Place on a cookie sheet or pizza pan and bake until bread is brown and crispy around the edges (5-10 minutes). Slice and serve.

HOLY LAND RAISIN HONEY CAKE

2 cups raw honey
3/4 cup olive oil
1 1/4 cups pineapple juice
1 cup raisins
1 teaspoon each (cinnamon, nutmeg, cloves, allspice, baking powder)
2 3/4 cups whole wheat flour
1/4 cup soy flour
2 teaspoons baking powder
1 teaspoon sea salt
3 cups chopped nuts (per preference)

Mix honey, oil, juice, raisins, cinnamon, nutmeg, cloves, allspice and baking powder together in saucepan. Stir and cook over low heat for 5 minutes. Combine flours, baking powder and salt. Pour honey mixture into flour mixture and mix well. Stir in nuts. Pour into oiled, floured 9 inch tube pan. Bake at 350° for one hour and 15 minutes. Cool and refrigerate.

JOHN THE BAPTIST COOKIES

1/2 cup warm water
2 tablespoons butter
1/3 cup powdered milk
1/2 cup carob powder
2 tablespoons lecithin granules
1 cup raw peanuts
1 cup raisins

Place water, butter, powdered milk, carob and lecithin in blender and blend until smooth. Combine peanuts and raisins in mixing bowl and pour carob mixture over combination. Stir well. Spoon clumps of batter onto lightly oiled baking pan. Start in cold oven middle rack and bake at 300° for 10 to 15 minutes. Remove and allow to dry for several hours.

GALILEAN CAROB DELIGHT

1 cup almonds
2 1/2 cups carob chips
3 tablespoons powdered milk
3 tablespoons olive oil
3 tablespoons lecithin
1 1/2 cups shredded coconut
1 cup chopped cashews
1 teaspoon sea salt
2 teaspoons pure vanilla

Coarsely chop almonds and spread in baking pan and roast at 300° for 15 minutes or until lightly browned. In top of double boiler, mix chips, powdered milk, oil and lecithin. Stir over hot but not boiling water until the chips are melted and the mixture is smooth. Combine all other ingredients in a bowl and pour melted mixture over them. Spoon clumps of batter onto waxed paper. Refrigerate to set.

ISAIAH'S FALAFEL FAVORITES

1 can chick peas, drained and rinsed
1 can pinto beans, drained and rinsed
1/2 cup green onions, sliced
1 celery stalk sliced thin
2 garlic cloves, minced
1 tablespoon olive oil
2 tablespoons lemon juice
1/2 cup whole wheat bread crumbs
1/2 teaspoon cumin
1/2 teaspoon sea salt
1/4 teaspoon pepper

Place drained chick peas and pinto beans in a blender or food processor and pulse until smooth. Heat oil in a small skillet over medium heat and add onion, celery and garlic. Cook until soft (about 5 minutes). Set aside. In a large bowl, combine mashed beans, lemon juice, cumin, salt, pepper and bread crumbs. Add the cooked vegetables and mix well. Form into patties and cook in a large skillet over medium heat until lightly browned on both sides.

JACOB'S LENTILS AND RICE

1 small onion, chopped
1 celery stalk, finely chopped
2 carrots, shredded
2-3 garlic cloves, minced
1 tablespoon olive oil
1/3 cup sherry
1 cup uncooked brown rice
1/3 cup lentils
1/2 teaspoon basil
1/4 teaspoon cumin
1/2 teaspoon salt
3 dashes hot pepper
2 cups vegetable broth

Heat oil in a large skillet. Add onion, celery, carrots and garlic. Cook 2-3 minutes. Add rice, lentils, broth and spices. Bring to a boil. Cover and reduce heat to low. Cook until all liquid is absorbed (15-20 minutes). Serve hot.

HONEY FRUIT BALLS

2 large bananas
1 cup ground nuts (per preference)
2 tablespoons raw honey
shredded coconut

Mash bananas in a bowl. Mix in honey and nuts. Form into small balls and roll in shredded coconut.

Blender Drinks

JEREMIAH JUICE COOLER

1 cup frozen blueberries
1 medium banana
2 tablespoons frozen orange juice concentrate
1 cup plain yogurt
1/2 cup pineapple juice

Mix all ingredients in blender until smooth. If too thick, add more pineapple juice.

SINAI STRAWBERRY SPLASH

12 ounces orange juice
1 cup frozen strawberries
1/2 cup crushed pineapple
ice cubes

Mix all ingredients in blender until thick and smooth. May be eaten by the spoon.

SAMSON'S ULTIMATE POWER SHAKE

12 ounces apple juice
1 cup plain yogurt
1 medium banana
4 ounces orange juice
2 tablespoons lecithin granules
1 tablespoon pollen granules
1-2 tablespoons raw honey
ice cubes

Mix all ingredients in blender. Drink immediately and look for nearest jaw bone of an ass.

Appendix H

Web Sites

There is now a wealth of health, fitness and spiritual information available to you over the Internet. Here are some web sites that you may find helpful as you pursue the *Moses Diet & Health Program*.

HEALTH & FITNESS

- http://www.naturalproductsinsider.com
- http://www.100hot.com/directory/sports/health.html
- http://www.healthandfitness.com
- http://www.healthshop.com/healthcenter
- http://www.healthwell.com
- http://www.nutrition.com
- http://www.onhealth.webmd.com
- http://www.phys.com
- http://www.thehealthnetwork.com
- http://www.fitnessonline.com
- http://www.cooperinstitute.org
- http://www.myvites.com
- http://www.herbnet.com
- http://www.dietsite.com
- http://www.cyberdiet.com
- http://www.drkoop.com
- http://www.dsqi.org
- http://www.healthcentral.com
- http://www.clickwell.com
- http://www.consumerlab.com
- http://www.supplementwatch.com
- http://www.nutrasolutions.com
- http://www.pandamedicine.com
- http://www.altmedicine.com
- http://www.ificinfo.health.org

- http://www.fatfree.com
- http://www.earthmed.com
- http://www.healthtalk.net
- http://www.sciencekomm.at/journals/medicine/med-bio.html
- http://www.gsu.edu/~wwwfit
- http://www.fitnessatlast.com
- http://www.getjorge.com/html/onlinetv.html
- http://www.global-fitness.com
- http://www.worldfitness.org
- http://www.fitnesslink.com
- http://www.fitnesslink.com

VEGETARIAN

- http://www.planetveggie.com
- http://www.vegetarianbaby.com
- http://www.jesusveg.com
- http://www.vegetarianrecipe.com
- http://www.members.gotnet.net/walter
- http://www.ivu.org
- http://www.veganet.com
- http://www.vegetariantrader.com
- http://www.becomevegetarian.com

SPIRITUAL

- http://www.liveprayer.com
- http://www.christianityonline.com
- http://www2.oneplace.com
- http://www.cptryon.org/prayer/day.html
- http://www.gbgm-umc.org/lhumc/prayer/prayer.htm
- http://www.Christ.com

The Hand Behind The Artwork

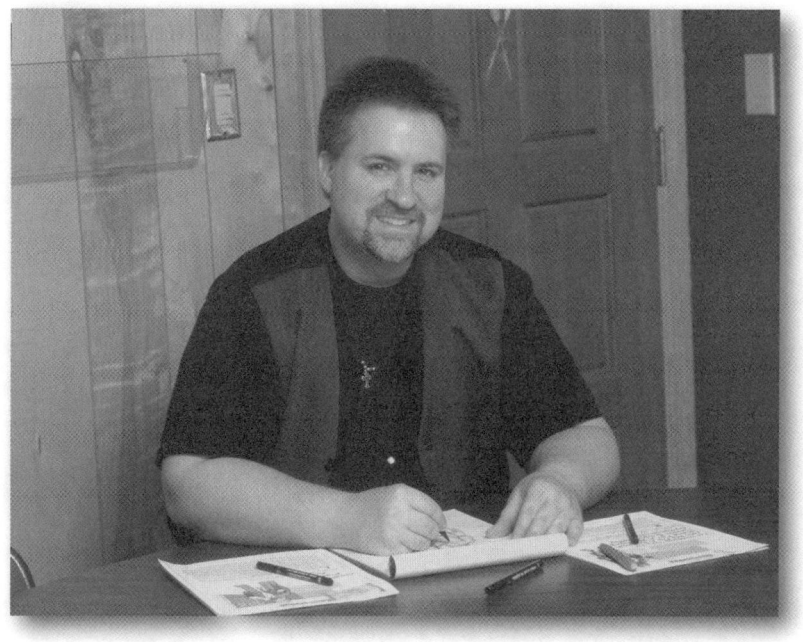

Special thanks to artist Tracy Lesch whose wonderful and amusing renditions of Moses et al. have helped bring this book to life.

Special Thanks To

William Gallagher, without whose diligence, patience and skill, this book would never have been published.

I'm Inviting You To Join Me On A Tropical Island For A Week-Long Health & Spirituality Symposium!

Come With Me To A Beautiful Christian Resort/Retreat Center For An Experience That Is Going To Change Your Life Forever!!

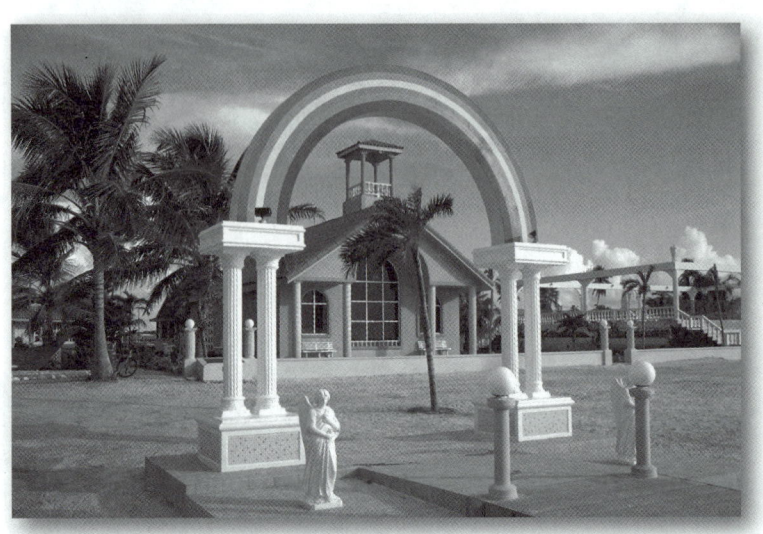

Remember those defining moments I spoke to you about back in the Dedication of this book? Those singular events that happen to us that can change our lives forever? Well I'd like to suggest such a possible defining moment to you right now.

How would you like to join me and a small group of other like-minded Christians for a Week-long **Health & Spirituality Symposium** at a gorgeous tropical retreat center in the beautiful Caribbean? An event-filled week of study, fellowship, exercise, prayer and recreation. A time to learn more about God and the Bible, health, nutrition, fitness, herbs, natural healing, weight loss and so much more.

I'm so certain that this Symposium will change your life for the better that I want to make you this most unusual guarantee. *If this week doesn't prove to be a life transforming experience for you, then I'll see to it that your entire enrollment fee is refunded*. That's how anxious I am to have you participate in this fantastic, one-of-a-kind event.

How This Great Idea Got Started.

After I finished writing *Moses Wasn't Fat*, I received lots of calls, letters and e-mails from readers who wanted to know if I ever did any personal counseling or if I knew of any health centers that they could visit to learn more about the Bible and health. While there indeed are many good health centers and many good spiritual retreats, I was hard pressed to recommend one that I thought did a good job of combining both concepts. That's when I decided it was time for me to sponsor my own health and spirituality symposium vacations. And I knew immediately where the perfect place would be.

In the middle 90s, I was instrumental in raising funds for the building of a Christian resort and retreat on a tropical island off the coast of Belize in Central America. It's called *The Essene Way* and it is truly a magnificent place. Twenty acres of lush, tropical island paradise located directly on 1,200 feet of sandy Caribbean beachfront. Check it out for yourself at www.esseneway.com. It has absolutely everything I needed for a symposium of this kind. Eighteen beautiful seaside cottages all with a spectacular ocean view, fully equipped health club, quaint chapel at the water's edge, meticulously landscaped grounds and gardens, conference rooms, natural foods restaurant, outdoor tennis and basketball courts, game hall, Grecian above ground swimming pool and so much more. I can honestly say that everything about this special complex has been designed to reflect the awe-inspiring beauty of God's limitless creative power. I can think of no better place for you to begin your program of physical and spiritual renewal than this Eden-like paradise.

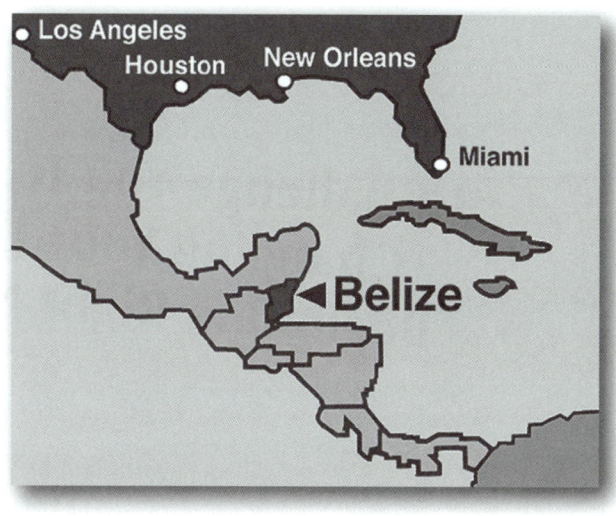

I've Assembled A Panel Of Expert Teachers To Guide You In Your Studies.

To assure you that you'll be getting the very best and latest health and biblical information, I've assembled a top-notch Christian team of nutritionists, naturopathic doctors, Bible scholars, and exercise and fitness experts to share the teaching responsibilities with me. Each one is an expert in his and her field and each shares a view similar to mine on the importance of biblical wisdom and the physical-spiritual connection.

In addition, I also deliberately limit the number of symposium participants to no more than 30 people per week so that you will have plenty of one-on-one time with the instructors while also getting to know the other attendees. Be prepared to return home with several newfound friends.

Your week will be filled with lots of activities from workshops and seminars, to exercise classes and chapel worship services. We'll even take a great one-day side trip to an ancient Maya ruin. Oh yes, and by the way, you'll also have plenty of free time for snorkeling, fishing, boating, diving and sight seeing. But there will also be quiet and reflective time for you to talk with God.

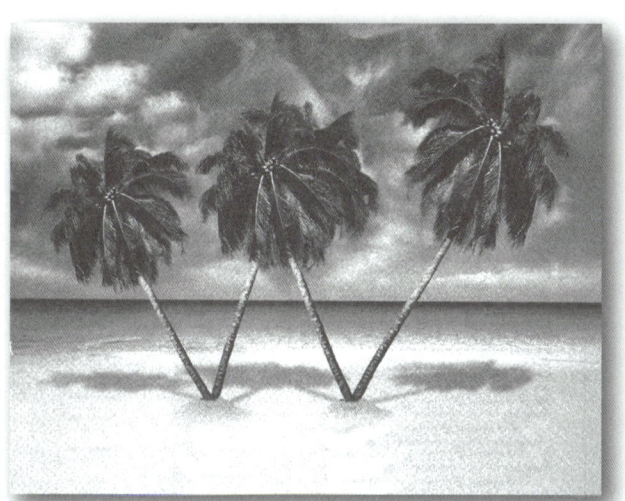

This unforgettable and unique **Health & Spirituality Symposium** will alter your whole attitude on life and health. All of the teaching is straightforward and practical so that you will be able to incorporate it into your life immediately. I promise that you will not leave the Symposium or *The Essene Way* the same person you were when you arrived. You will leave healed, renewed, focused and motivated.

If you enjoyed *Moses Wasn't Fat* and you're ready to take another big step in your health building program, then I strongly recommend that you join me at the Symposium in Belize. For a complete package of information on teachers, curriculum, upcoming dates, travel arrangements and pricing call **1-800-537-7671**. But a word of caution. Each Symposium books up quickly so make your plans so that you won't be disappointed.

Come alone or come with a companion but please do yourself a great big favor and come.

"I Challenge You To Start Changing Your Life – Beginning Right Now!"

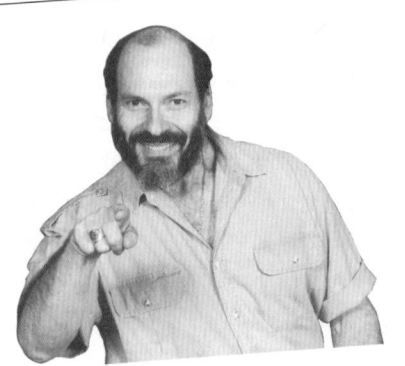

Dear Reader,

Congratulations on finishing *MOSES WASN'T FAT*. I hope you enjoyed it and benefited from it. <u>Now the big question is whether this book gets tucked away on a shelf somewhere or will you take the necessary steps to begin your own life-changing program?</u> I'd like to think that by now I've convinced you to start taking action to improve your health. <u>The decision you make over the next few days can impact your life radically</u>. I'm hoping and praying that you decide to move forward.

I want so much for you to better your life that I've come up with a wee bit of an incentive that might help you make up your mind. I've inaugurated <u>a fantastic new self-improvement contest like none you've ever seen before</u>. In keeping with the theme of this book, the contest is based on both *physical* and *spiritual* improvement. I call it the **Moses Transformation Challenge (MTC)** and this exciting and fun event may very well be just the impetus you've been waiting for to change your life forever.

And the best part of the **MTC** is that you don't win this contest by beating anyone else or losing the most weight. (In fact losing weight is only one part of the Challenge). <u>You win by making the most improvement within yourself – physically and spiritually</u>. So it really doesn't matter if your 18 or 88. What matters is how effectively you transform yourself into a better person.

Sure I'm going to ask you to send in some before and after photos. But in addition to that I'm also going to ask you to make an effort to improve your physical fitness, spirituality and charitable works. (Like I said, it's like no other contest you've ever seen.)

I learned a long time ago, and I stressed it in this book, that <u>working towards definite goals really helps keep us motivated</u>. That's why I felt that the **MTC** might be just that extra incentive you needed to begin your program. <u>I've set it up to award as many prizes as possible (100 winners per award period) so that you all would have a chance of getting something for your efforts</u>.

But even if you don't win a single thing, <u>you're still truly a winner</u>! You will have dramatically improved your body Temple – and that, in the long run, is even better than any prize.

So what do you think? Are you up for this Challenge or will you continue to live your life as you always have? <u>Can you think of any better time to get started changing your life than RIGHT NOW?</u> Send for your entry form and make that commitment. It's "D-Day."

Shalom,

Tom Ciola

Tom Ciola

P.S. Seven happy first place winners are each going to win an all-expenses-paid trip for two to the Holy Land. There's no reason why it can't be you.

"ARE YOU READY TO COME OUT OF BONDAGE AND GET BACK IN SHAPE? THEN CHECK THIS OUT!"

Moses Transformation Challenge!

Do You Have What It Takes To Transform Yourself Physically And Spiritually?

YOU CAN WIN
★ **TRIPS**   ★ **GREAT PRIZES**

Have you read the popular new diet and health book ***Moses Wasn't Fat?*** Well that's how this whole transformation idea got started. If you've been looking for motivation to get yourself back in shape, here's a self-improvement contest like nothing you've seen before! You don't win this contest by beating anyone else or even by losing the most weight. Instead, winners are selected by the amount of physical and spiritual improvement they make from their original starting condition. So in a way, you're really competing against yourself. And the best part is that just improving your health and well being is a form of winning.

100 WINNERS PER AWARD PERIOD

This is an ongoing contest with two award periods per year and we've got lots of prizes to award, including all-expenses-paid trips for two to the Holy Land for seven lucky transformers. As a matter of fact, we're selecting 100 total winners per award period. You could be one of them! Give us a call today for an entry package and then get ready to change your life.

LOOK WHAT YOU CAN WIN!

1st PLACE

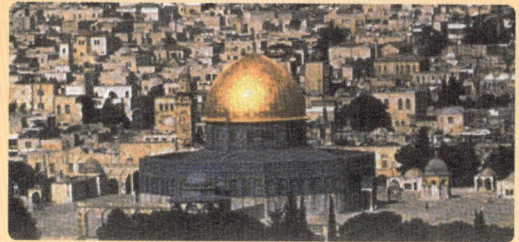

ALL-EXPENSES-PAID TRIP FOR TWO TO THE HOLY LAND

$4000 VALUE   SEVEN WINNERS

2nd PLACE

ALL-EXPENSES-PAID LUXURY CARIBBEAN VACATION.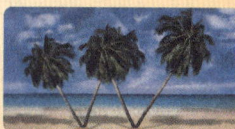

$1500 VALUE   SEVEN WINNERS

PLUS
MANY OTHER GREAT PRIZES

Your Body Is God's Temple. Are You Ready To Start Construction?

THIS CONTEST SPONSORED BY
Logia: Foods Of The Bible

FOR ENTRY FORM OR MORE INFORMATION 1-800-537-7671

If You Enjoyed This Book –

WHAT IT'S ALL ABOUT

What is TEMPLE magazine?

TEMPLE is a brand new and uniquely different body-mind-spirit magazine that combines health, fitness, exercise, religion and spirituality all into one publication. TEMPLE seeks to forge a solid link between our physical being and our spiritual being. Each issue is jam-packed with great articles on nutrition, dieting advice, exercise programs, self-improvement articles, book reviews, motivational stories, and so much more, all from a biblical and religious perspective.

Why is it called TEMPLE?

The Bible refers to the body as the *temple* of God's Holy Spirit (**1 Corinthians 3:16 and 2 Corinthians 6:16**) and as such, it should be kept as pure and holy and healthy and fit as possible. The staff of TEMPLE magazine agrees totally with this belief and thus the word *temple* perfectly embraces the goals and philosophy of this magazine.

How often is it published?

TEMPLE is published four times a year.

What does it cost and where can it be purchased?

TEMPLE's cover price is $5.95 per issue and a one-year subscription is $19.95. It is sold at many newsstands, health food stores, religious book stores and magazine shops. In addition, the magazine is mailed directly to subscribers.

What types of articles can someone expect to read in TEMPLE?

TEMPLE magazine covers a broad spectrum of topics dealing with health, fitness, exercise, nutrition, the Bible and spirituality. Our unique emphasis of course, is on how all of these topics work together for the complete development of the body, mind, and spirit.

Each issue also features in-depth stories on individuals whose personal lives reflect this holistic spiritual philosophy and who can thus serve as an inspiration and role model for our readers.

TEMPLE also places a heavy emphasis on drug-free living, whether street drugs, athletic enhancement drugs (steroids, etc.), or prescription pharmaceuticals.

Is this magazine affiliated with any particular religion or denomination?

TEMPLE magazine is definitely a Christian-oriented publication but it is also non-denominational. We try to show respect and editorial fairness to all denominations and we hold firmly to the belief we are all children of God and that Jesus died for all men's sins.

Who publishes this magazine?

TEMPLE is published and distributed by **Axion Publishers** of Orlando, Florida. The Editor/Publisher is Tom Ciola, author of *Moses Wasn't Fat* and the President of **Logia**: Foods of the Bible. The magazine has put together an expert staff of writers on fitness, health, nutrition and spirituality and we are pleased to note that all contributors to this magazine are themselves believers and practitioners of the Temple philosophy. This staff includes: doctors, nutritionists, exercise physiologists, personal trainers, athletes, theologians, pastors, and spiritual counselors. Such an eclectic staff assures TEMPLE readers that they are always getting the very best information possible.

SUBSCRIBE TODAY!

> "Do you know that you are the temple of God and that the Spirit of God dwells in you? If anyone defiles the temple of God, God will destroy him. For the temple of God is holy which temple you are.
> 1 Corinthians 3:16

HERE ARE THE KINDS OF STORIES YOU'LL READ ABOUT IN TEMPLE

Each issue of TEMPLE covers great topics like this:

- WEIGHT CONTROL ADVICE
- HERBS & FOOD SUPPLEMENTS
- EXERCISE TIPS
- ALTERNATIVE HEALTH NEWS
- VEGETARIANISM
- HEALTH PRODUCTS REVIEWS
- CHRISTIAN ATHLETES
- FAITH & HEALTH
- BIBLE FOOD RECIPES
- LATEST HEALTH RESEARCH
- MOTIVATIONAL ADVICE
- LATEST BOOK REVIEWS
- ADVICE FROM HEALTH PROS
- BIBLICAL NUTRITION
- HEALTH & FITNESS PRAYERS
- PERSONALITY INTERVIEWS

Some of the tough issues we're not afraid to cover:

- ASPARTAME CAN KILL YOU
- ORGANIC FOODS DEBATE
- SOY PRODUCTS YES OR NO?
- ABORTIONS & BREAST CANCER
- EATING DISORDERS
- GMO CONTROVERSY
- DANGERS OF BOTTLED WATER
- MAKING KIDS RITALIN ADDICTS
- FOOD SUPPLEMENT DECEPTION
- PHARMACEUTICAL MADNESS

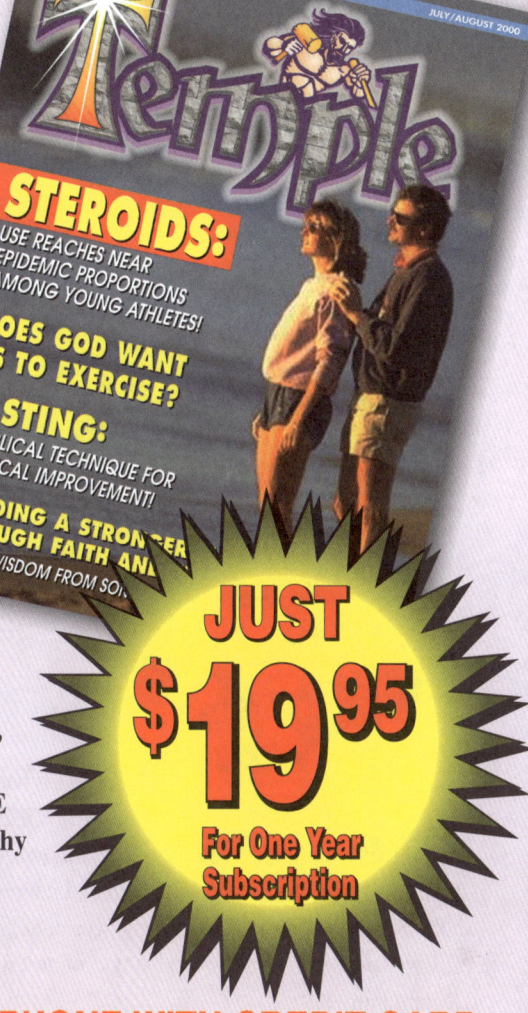

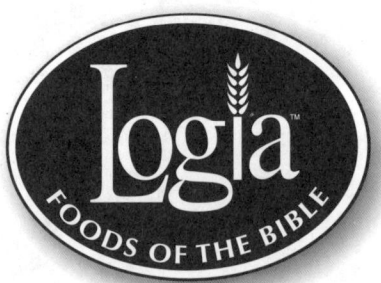

LOGIA: FOODS OF THE BIBLE
BIBLE BASED PRODUCTS

Let The Bible Be Your Guide To Health

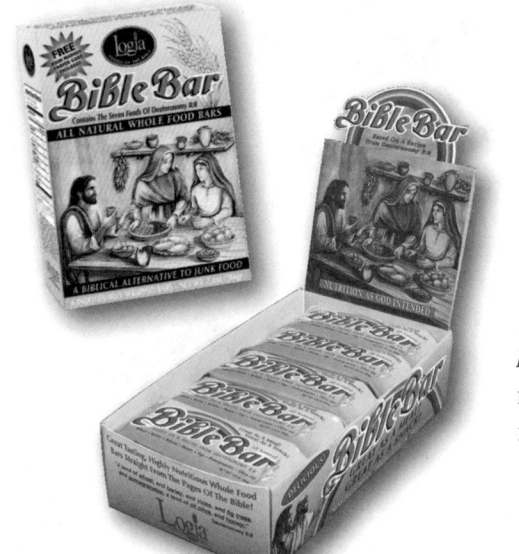

The *Bible Bar* is a fantastic-tasting, all natural whole food bar that contains the seven foods which the Lord calls good in Deuteronomy 8:8: Wheat, Barley, Honey, Figs, Olive Oil, Grapes, and Pomegranates. The *Bible Bar* is a complete, wholesome food packed with nutritional and spiritual goodness. When consumed between meals, *Bible Bars* make the perfect appetite regulator while helping to control and normalize the body's metabolic processes. When used as a diet aid between meals, the *Bible Bar* helps to relieve hunger pangs and that starving feeling that so many dieters hate. You will love this unique, first-of-its-kind nutritional bar with its refreshing, natural fruit flavor.

At long last here it is — another great food of the Bible! It's a high potency **Royal Jelly, Pollen** and **Honey** combination that's unequaled by anything else on the market. It's called **Sacred Nectar** and this unique honey product is now available for shipment. Honey truly is a Bible food and both honey and honeycomb are mentioned more than 60 times in the Scriptures. In fact, on several occasions God refers to the Promised Land as *"a land flowing with milk and honey."* Honey is also one of the seven principle foods of the Holy Land singled out in Deuteronomy 8:8

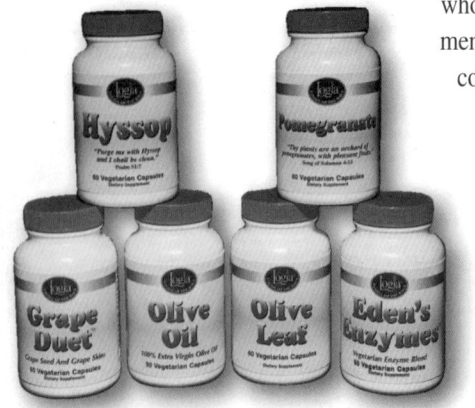

Here at **Logia**, we truly believe that our bodies are meant to be God's Temple and we have a moral obligation to keep them as healthy as possible. Therefore, we now offer several new **Logia** foods of the Bible. *Back to The Garden* is a perfect food supplement for those people who have a difficult time trying to consume five servings of fruits and vegetables every day as recommended by nutritionists. *Da' Udder Milk,* an organic, non-fat, wholesome and unique milk powder, comes exclusively from cows that are not treated with antibiotics or hormones, never receive any form of animal by-products in their diet, and no pesticides, herbicides or chemical fertilizers are ever used on their feed. For those people looking to cut down on their meat consumption, organic *Lentils*, with their high protein content, will make the perfect meat replacement. *Thoroughly Cleansed* is a carefully selected blend of several Bible-based herbs noted for their cleansing and purifying qualities. *Eden's Enzymes* contain all three of the essential digestive enzymes produced by the body (protease, amylase and lipase). For those people who would like to use a Bible-based herbal product to protect themselves from harmful microscopic invaders, *Olive Leaf* capsules make the perfect answer. *Grape Duet* contains *Resveratrol,* a bioflavonoid found in the grape skin which scientists now believe may be helpful in the prevention and treatment of cancer. *Pomegranate Juice* is a powerful anti-oxidant capable of both reducing the amount of harmful cholesterol in the arteries while neutralizing its bad effects, and additionally, our all-vegetarian *Pomegranate Capsules* contain 150 milligrams of pomegranate fruit extract in each capsule.